Reducing the Odds

PREVENTING PERINATAL TRANSMISSION OF HIV IN THE UNITED STATES

Michael A. Stoto, Donna A. Almario, and
Marie C. McCormick, *Editors*

Committee on Perinatal Transmission of HIV
Division of Health Promotion and Disease Prevention,
Institute of Medicine, and
Board on Children, Youth, and Families,
Commission on Behavioral and Social Sciences and Education,
National Research Council and Institute of Medicine

NATIONAL ACADEMY PRESS
Washington, D.C.   1999

NATIONAL ACADEMY PRESS • 2101 Constitution Avenue, N.W. • Washington, DC 20418

NOTICE: The project that is the subject of this report was approved by the Governing Board of the National Research Council, whose members are drawn from the councils of the National Academy of Sciences, the National Academy of Engineering, and the Institute of Medicine. The members of the committee responsible for the report were chosen for their special competences and with regard for appropriate balance.

The Institute of Medicine was chartered in 1970 by the National Academy of Sciences to enlist distinguished members of the appropriate professions in the examination of policy matters pertaining to the health of the public. In this, the Institute acts under the Academy's 1863 congressional charter responsibility to be an adviser to the federal government and its own initiative in identifying issues of medical care, research, and education. Dr. Kenneth I. Shine is president of the Institute of Medicine.

Support for this study was provided by the Department of Health and Human Services and the Centers for Disease Control and Prevention (Contract No. 200-97-0651).

Library of Congress Cataloging-in-Publication Data

Reducing the odds : preventing perinatal transmission of HIV in the
United States / Michael A. Stoto, Donna A. Almario, and Marie C.
McCormick, editors ; Committee on Perinatal Transmission of HIV,
Division of Health Promotion and Disease Prevention, Institute of
Medicine [and] Board on Children, Youth, and Families, Commission
on Behavioral and Social Sciences and Education, National Research
Council, Institute of Medicine.
    p. cm.
  Includes bibliographical references and index.
  ISBN 0-309-06286-1
  1. AIDS (Disease) in pregnancy—United States. 2. AIDS
(Disease)in infants—United States—Prevention. 3. HIV
infections—United States—Prevention. 4. AIDS (Disease) in
women—Treatment—United States. I. Stoto, Michael A. II. Almario,
Donna A. III. McCormick, Marie C. IV. Institute of Medicine (U.S.).
Committee on Perinatal Transmission of HIV. V. Board on Children,
Youth, and Families (U.S.)
  RG580.A44 R43 1998
  618.3—dc21

                                98-40214

Additional copies of this report are available for sale from the National Academy Press, 2101 Constitution Avenue, N.W., Lock Box 285, Washington, DC 20055. Call (800) 624-6242 or (202) 334-3313 (in the Washington metropolitan area). This report is also available online at **www.nap.edu.**

For more information about the Institute of Medicine, visit the IOM home page at: **www2.nas.edu/ iom.**

The serpent has been a symbol of long life, healing, and knowledge among almost all cultures and religions since the beginning of recorded history. The image adopted as a logotype by the Institute of Medicine is based on a relief carving from ancient Greece, now held by the Staatliche Museen in Berlin.

COMMITTEE ON PERINATAL TRANSMISSION OF HIV

Marie McCormick, M.D., Sc.D. (*Chair*),[*] Professor and Chair, Department of Maternal and Child Health, Harvard School of Public Health

Ezra Davidson, Jr., M.D. (*Vice Chair*),[*] Associate Dean, Primary Care, and Professor of Obstetrics and Gynecology, Charles R. Drew University of Medicine and Science

Fred Battaglia, M.D.,[*] Professor of Pediatrics and of Obstetrics and Gynecology, Division of Perinatal Medicine, University of Colorado Health Sciences Center

Ronald Brookmeyer, Ph.D., Professor of Biostatistics, Johns Hopkins School of Public Health

Deborah Cotton, M.D., M.P.H., Professor of Medicine and Public Health; Director, Office of Clinical Research; and Assistant Provost of the Boston University Medical Center

Susan Cu-Uvin, M.D., Assistant Professor of Obstetrics and Gynecology, The Miriam Hospital, Brown University

Nancy Kass, Sc.D., Associate Professor and Director, Program in Law, Ethics, and Health, Johns Hopkins School of Public Health

Patricia King, J.D.,[*] Professor of Law, Medicine, Ethics, and Public Policy, Georgetown University Law Center

Lorraine Klerman, Dr.P.H., Professor, Department of Maternal and Child Health, School of Public Health, University of Alabama at Birmingham

Katherine Ruiz de Luzuriaga, M.D., Associate Professor of Pediatrics, University of Massachusetts Medical School

Ellen Mangione, M.D., M.P.H., Director, Disease Control and Environmental Epidemiology Division, Colorado Department of Public Health and Environment, Denver

Douglas Morgan, M.P.A.,[**] Assistant Commissioner, Division of AIDS Prevention and Control, New Jersey Department of Health and Senior Services, Trenton

Stephen Thomas, Ph.D., Director, Institute for Minority Health Research, and Associate Professor of Community Health, Department of Behavioral Sciences and Health Education, Rollins School of Public Health, Emory University

Sten Vermund, M.D., Ph.D., Professor, Department of Epidemiology, School of Public Health, University of Alabama at Birmingham

---

[*]Institute of Medicine member.
[**]Resigned April 1998, upon appointment to the Division of Service Systems, HIV/AIDS Bureau, Health Resources and Services Administration.

Liaison to the Board on Health Promotion and Disease Prevention

Robert Fullilove, Ed.D., Associate Dean for Community and Minority Affairs, Columbia University School of Public Health

Project Staff

Michael Stoto, Study Director
Donna Almario, Project and Research Assistant
Kathleen Stratton, Director, Division of Health Promotion and Disease Prevention
Donna Duncan, Division Assistant

Staff Consultants

David Abramson, Senior Research Analyst, Joseph L. Mailman School of Public Health of Columbia University
Barbara Aliza, Health Policy Consultant
Miriam Davis, Medical Writer and Consultant
Rebecca Denison, Executive Director, Women Organized to Respond to Life-threatening Diseases
Amy Fine, Health Policy and Program Consultant
Maria Hewitt, Analyst, Institute of Medicine

LIAISON PANEL

A. Cornelius Baker, Executive Director, National Association of People with AIDS

Guthrie Birkhead, M.D., M.P.H., Director, AIDS Institute Executive Office, New York State AIDS Institute (representing the Council of State and Territorial Epidemiologists)

Patricia Fleming, Ph.D., Chief, Reporting and Analysis Section, Surveillance Branch, Division of HIV/AIDS Prevention, Centers for Disease Control and Prevention

Michael Greene, M.D., Director of Maternal-Fetal Medicine, Vincent Memorial Obstetrics Division, Massachusetts General Hospital (representing the American College of Obstetricians and Gynecologists)

Leslie Hardy, M.H.S., Senior Policy Analyst, Office of the Assistant Secretary for Planning and Evaluation, Department of Health and Human Services

Karen D. Hench, R.N., M.S., Nurse Consultant, Maternal and Child Health Bureau, HIV/AIDS Bureau, Health Resources and Services Administration

Rosemary Johnson, Outreach Worker, Division of Gynecology and Obstetrics, School of Medicine, Johns Hopkins University

Michael Kaiser, M.D., Chief, Comprehensive Family Services Branch, HIV/AIDS Bureau, Health Resources and Services Administration

Joseph Kelly, Deputy Director, National Alliance of State and Territorial AIDS Directors

Miguelina Maldonado, M.S.W., Director of Government Relations and Policy, National Minority AIDS Council

Dorothy Mann, Executive Director, The Family Planning Council of Southeastern Pennsylvania (representing the AIDS Policy Center for Children, Youth and Families)

James McNamara, M.D., Chief, Pediatric Medicine Branch, Division of AIDS, National Institute of Allergy and Infectious Diseases, National Institutes of Health

Lynne Mofenson, M.D., Associate Branch Chief for Clinical Research, Pediatric, Adolescent, and Maternal AIDS Branch, National Institute of Child Health and Human Development, National Institutes of Health

Martha Rogers, M.D., Associate Director for Science, National Center for HIV, STD, and TB Prevention, Division of HIV/AIDS Prevention, Centers for Disease Control and Prevention

Shepherd Smith, The Children's AIDS Fund

Deborah Klein Walker, Ed.D., Assistant Commissioner, Bureau of Family and Community Health, Massachusetts Department of Public Health (representing the Association of Maternal and Child Health Programs)

Catherine Wilfert, M.D., Scientific Director, Elizabeth Glaser Pediatric AIDS Foundation (representing the American Academy of Pediatrics)

Pascale Wortley, M.D., Medical Officer, National Center for HIV, STD, and TB Prevention, Division of HIV/AIDS Prevention, Centers for Disease Control and Prevention

Deborah von Zinkernagel, R.N., S.M., M.S., Senior Policy Analyst, Office of HIV/AIDS, Department of Health and Human Services

Preface

The 1994 results of the AIDS Clinical Trials Group protocol number 076 (ACTG 076)—showing that the transmission of HIV from mothers to their children could be substantially reduced through the use of zidovudine (ZDV) by the mother during pregnancy and labor and in the newborn—represented one of the most important successes in the fight against AIDS. These findings led government agencies and professional organizations to propose and implement recommendations calling for counseling and testing all pregnant women for HIV, mostly on a voluntary basis. And as indicated in this report, this approach has been substantially successful. Yet despite the progress, more children than necessary continue to be born with HIV infection.

In response to a congressional mandate to "conduct an evaluation of the extent to which State efforts have been effective in reducing the perinatal transmission of the human immunodeficiency virus, and an analysis of the existing barriers to the further reduction in such transmission," this report addresses ways to increase prenatal testing, improve therapy for HIV-infected women and children, and generally reduce perinatal HIV infections. The report also considers the ethical and public health issues associated with screening policies as prevention tools, and their implications for prevention and treatment opportunities for women and infants.

The committee recognizes that screening and treating pregnant women is but one strategy among many to prevent perinatal transmission of HIV. The Institute of Medicine (IOM) has dealt with many issues in the primary prevention of HIV, as referenced in this report. The committee also emphasizes the connection between substance abuse and HIV infection in women as a factor in the perinatal transmission of HIV. More specific recommendations about the prevention and treatment of substance abuse are beyond the scope of this report. Likewise, one strategy for reducing perinatal transmission is to reduce the number of HIV-infected women who become pregnant unintentionally. The consequences and prevention of unintended pregnancy have also been examined recently by the IOM (IOM, 1995b). However, improved planning of pregnancy among HIV-infected women assumes that women know their HIV status. For many women, especially low income women, pregnancy may be a major opportunity for contact with the health care system. Thus access to care, the potential for ready implementation of screening along with other prenatal testing, and the availability of therapy to improve the outcomes of both mothers and infants in the face of HIV infection, all have led the committee to focus on this episode of care.

There are three additional issues related to HIV testing and perinatal transmission that are outside the committee's charge, and hence not dealt with in this report, except as they relate to preventing perinatal transmission. First, mandatory newborn testing, which is the law in New York State (see Appendixes C and L), and which could be the result of the Ryan White Comprehensive AIDS Resources Emergency (CARE) Act Amendments of 1996, has limited utility in preventing perinatal transmission of HIV. While there may be some benefits to the HIV-infected children that would otherwise not be identified (as discussed in Chapter 4), the public health goals behind newborn testing can be better served by improved efforts to prevent transmission, as outlined in this report.

Second, perinatal transmission of HIV is a major concern in many developing countries that do not have the resources to implement the ACTG 076 regimen. To address this, there have been efforts to test less expensive approaches through randomized trials in the affected countries, and these trials have been criticized on ethical grounds (Lurie and Wolfe, 1997). Because this issue is outside the committee's charge, which relates to preventing perinatal transmission in the United States, the committee has not addressed this issue.

Third, a number of states have recently instituted a policy of named HIV reporting, and others are considering doing the same. Although this approach has important surveillance benefits, it has been criticized on human rights grounds (Gostin et al., 1997; ACLU, 1997). Since it is not clear that instituting this policy has any impact on women's willingness to be tested as a routine part of prenatal care, the committee takes no position on named HIV reporting.

To carry out this report, the Institute of Medicine established a committee of 13 individuals, with expertise in pediatrics, obstetrics and gynecology, preventive medicine, women's health, and other relevant medical specialties; social and behavioral sciences; public health practice; epidemiology; program evaluation; health services research; bioethics; and public health law. In keeping with IOM policies, the committee members were chosen to encompass a variety of different perspective and areas of expertise on the issues. The committee met on five occasions between December 1997 and June 1998, sponsored two workshops, conducted five site visits, and commissioned a series of papers, as described in Chapter 1.

The committee was aided in its work by a liaison panel of 19 individuals representing federal agencies, professional organizations, and other groups interested and knowledgeable about perinatal transmission of HIV. The liaison panel members and their affiliations are listed after the committee members on pages v and vi. The liaison panel members participated in the first committee meeting and two workshops, contributed information to the committee, and had an opportunity to review and comment on the workshop summaries and site visit reports. The liaison panel members did not, however, contribute to or review the committee's conclusions and recommendations. The committee is very grateful for the information and ideas that the liaison panel members contributed to this project.

This report has been reviewed in draft form by individuals chosen for their diverse perspectives and technical expertise, in accordance with procedures approved by the National Research Council's (NRC) Report Review committee. The purpose of this independent review is to provide candid and critical comments that will assist the institution in making the published report as sound as possible and to ensure that the report meets institutional standards for objectivity, evidence, and responsiveness to the study charge. The review comments and draft manuscript remain confidential to protect the integrity of the deliberative process. We wish to thank the following individuals for their participation in the review of this report: Mary Ellen Avery, The Children's Hospital, Boston; Charles Carpenter, Boston University; Wendy Craytor, Alaska Department of Health and Social Services; James Curran, Emory University; Jill DeBoer, Minnesota Department of Health; Amitai Etzioni, The George Washington University; Fernando Guerra, San Antonio Metropolitan Health District; Luigi Mastroianni, Hospital of the University of Pennsylvania; C. Arden Miller, University of North Carolina at Chapel Hill; Nancy Padian, University of California at San Francisco School of Medicine; and Eugene Washington, University of California at San Francisco.

The committee is also thankful for the efforts of the individuals listed in the appendixes who helped to organize and participated in the committee site visits. We would especially like to thank those women, not named for reasons of confidentiality, who were willing to share their personal experience with prenatal HIV counseling and testing and in some cases treatment. Their stories, which appear in the appendixes as well as the body of the report, were extremely helpful to the committee. We would also like to express our gratitude to the individuals, also listed in the appendixes, who gave of their time to participate in the committee's workshops, especially those who were able to make presentations. The site visits and workshops were especially valuable in giving the committee access to the practical issues facing providers and patients dealing with perinatally transmitted HIV.

In addition to those who were able to attend the committee's activities in person, many individuals contributed information—ranging from data on prenatal testing in their state to their perspectives on the issues—by e-mail, fax, and phone. Some of this information is cited in relevant parts of the report, but it all was helpful in formulating our approach to the issues, and we are grateful for the effort that these individuals made.

Finally, the committee would like to thank sincerely the IOM staff and consultants who made its work possible. Barbara Aliza, Miriam Davis, Amy Fine, and Maria Hewitt served as consultants to the committee, attended workshops and site visits and summarized the results, prepared special analyses, and helped to draft sections of the report. Donna Almario was an unusually effective research assistant, and served simultaneously as the committee's project assistant, getting everyone to the right place, with the right information, at the right time. Finally, the committee is enormously grateful to Michael Stoto without whose energy and expertise the report would never have been completed in such a prompt fashion.

Marie C. McCormick
Chair

Contents

Reducing the Odds

Executive Summary

One of the most promising victories in the battle against AIDS was the finding, in 1994, that administration of the antiretroviral drug zidovudine (known as ZDV, and previously as AZT) during pregnancy and childbirth could reduce the chance that the child of an HIV-positive mother would be infected by about two-thirds (Connor et al., 1994). The "ACTG 076 results," referring to the AIDS Clinical Trials Group protocol number 76, quickly led the Public Health Service (PHS) to develop guidelines about counseling and testing of pregnant women for HIV infection (CDC, 1995b).

The 1995 PHS guidelines called for counseling all pregnant women about the risk of AIDS, the benefits of HIV testing, and voluntary testing. The approach was endorsed by the American College of Obstetricians and Gynecologists, the American Academy of Pediatrics, and other professional groups. The essence of the PHS guidelines also has been adopted by most states, either by policy or by legislation. Medical practice has changed in line with these recommendations, with an increasing proportion of women tested for HIV during prenatal care. As a result of these and other changes, there has been a substantial reduction—approximately 43% from a peak in 1992 to 1996—in the number of newborns diagnosed with AIDS. A reduction of this magnitude in only a few years certainly represents great progress, yet it is far less than the ACTG 076 findings can offer.

Two years after the publication of the ACTG 076 findings, Congress addressed perinatal transmission issues in the Ryan White Comprehensive AIDS Resources Emergency (CARE) Act Amendments of 1996 (P.L. 104-146). Depending on a determination by the Secretary of Health and Human Services about these practices, Ryan White CARE Act formula funds to the states could become contingent upon mandatory HIV testing of newborns.

1

The proportion of women . . .

- who are HIV-infected
  - who become pregnant
    - who do not seek prenatal care
      - who are not offered HIV testing
        - who refuse HIV testing
          - who are not offered the ACTG 076 regimen
            - who refuse the ACTG 076 regimen
              - who do not complete the ACTG 076 regimen
                - whose child is infected despite treatment

FIGURE 1   Chain of events leading to an HIV-infected child.

P.L. 104-146 also calls on the Institute of Medicine (IOM) to "conduct an evaluation of the extent to which State efforts have been effective in reducing the perinatal transmission of the human immunodeficiency virus, and an analysis of the existing barriers to the further reduction in such transmission." In its analysis, the committee has found it helpful to consider a chain of factors affecting perinatal transmission, as illustrated in Figure 1.

PUBLIC HEALTH SCREENING PROGRAMS

Disease screening is one of the most basic tools of modern public health and preventive medicine. As screening programs have been implemented over the years, a substantial body of experience has been gained. In practice, when screening is conducted in contexts of gender inequality, racial discrimination, sexual taboos, and poverty, these conditions shape the attitudes and beliefs of health system and public health decision makers as well as patients, including those who have lost confidence that the health care system will treat them fairly. Thus, if screening programs are poorly conceived, organized, or implemented, they may lead to interventions of questionable merit and enhance the vulnerability of groups and individuals. Through the experience with public health screening programs, a series of characteristics of well-organized public health screening programs has evolved (Wilson and Jungner, 1968).

The committee's summary of the relevant characteristics is as follows:

1. The goals of the screening program should be clearly specified and shown to be achievable.
2. The natural history of the condition should be adequately understood, and

treatment or intervention for those found positive widely accepted by the scientific and medical community, with evidence that early intervention improves health outcomes.

3. The screening test or measurement should distinguish those individuals who are likely to have the condition from those who are unlikely to have it.

4. There should be adequate facilities for diagnosis and resources for treatment for all who are found to have the condition, as well as agreement as to who will treat them.

5. The test and possible interventions should be acceptable to the affected population.

DESCRIPTIVE EPIDEMIOLOGY OF THE PERINATAL TRANSMISSION OF HIV

In 1997, women accounted for 21% of AIDS cases in adults, and the proportion of all cases that are among females continues to grow. At least two-thirds of AIDS in women can be attributed to injection drug use either directly or through sex with drug users. Although a subset of women with HIV have injected drugs or have had sex with a known injection drug user, an increasing proportion of women have become infected through sexual activity with men whose risk behaviors were unknown to them. AIDS is more prevalent in African-American and Hispanic women, in women in the Northeast and the South, and in women in large cities. Approximately 6,000 to 7,000 HIV-infected women give birth every year. Trend data show a relatively steady national rate of HIV prevalence in childbearing women between 1989 and 1994, the last year for which data are available.

Perinatal transmission accounted for at least 432 AIDS cases in the United States in 1997. The number of perinatally acquired AIDS cases rose rapidly in the late 1980s and early 1990s, peaked around 1992, and subsequently declined by approximately 43% by 1996. Such data on perinatal AIDS cases reflect the number of children born with HIV infection in previous years, and more recent data are not available because of reporting delays. Changes in the number of perinatal AIDS cases, therefore, are not direct estimates of the impact of prevention activities on perinatal transmission of HIV.

Pediatrics AIDS cases are concentrated in eastern states, and especially in the New York metropolitan area. In 1996, three states alone—New York, New Jersey, and Florida—reported 330 cases. This represents 49% of the diagnosed cases, even though only 15% of children are born in those states (CDC, 1996b; Ventura et al., 1998). In contrast to the concentration of perinatal AIDS cases in the Northeast, they are far less common in most geographical areas. In 1997, 39 states had fewer than ten perinatally transmitted AIDS cases (CDC, 1997c).

NATURAL HISTORY, DETECTION, AND TREATMENT OF HIV INFECTION IN PREGNANT WOMEN AND NEWBORNS

Perinatal transmission can occur antepartum (during pregnancy), intrapartum (during labor and delivery), and postpartum (after birth), but most mother-to-infant transmission appears to occur intrapartum. The ACTG 076 protocol showed that antiretroviral therapy could reduce perinatal transmission to 8% in some populations (Connor et al., 1994), and subsequent studies have suggested that rates of 5% or lower are possible.

To maximize prevention efforts, women must be identified as HIV-infected as early as possible during pregnancy. Early diagnosis of HIV infection allows the mother to institute effective antiretroviral therapy for her own health. This treatment is also capable of significantly reducing perinatal transmission. HIV-infected pregnant women can also be referred to appropriate psychological, social, legal, and substance abuse services. Babies born to HIV-positive mothers can be started on ZDV within hours of birth, as in the ACTG 076 regimen. Mothers who know they are HIV-positive can be counseled not to breast-feed their infants.

In terms of preventing perinatal transmission, newborn HIV testing has fewer benefits than maternal testing. When maternal serostatus is unknown, however, newborn HIV testing permits early identification and evaluation of exposed infants, allows for initiation of *Pneumocystis carinii* pneumonia (PCP) prophylaxis in the first months of life to prevent life-threatening bouts of PCP infection, may prevent transmission through breast-feeding or in future pregnancies, and could lead to mothers being treated for their own infection.

THE CONTEXT OF SERVICES FOR WOMEN AND CHILDREN AFFECTED BY HIV/AIDS

Women and children in the United States, including those at risk for or with HIV/AIDS, receive their health care from a variety of sources. Their care is financed by a mixture of public and/or private insurance and public funds. Its content and quality are influenced by public and professional organizations. Its oversight and regulation are achieved through a combination of national, state, and local authorities. Major modifications in Medicaid and welfare programs, the increasing number of uninsured, and the growing presence of managed care in both the public and the private sectors, are having a significant impact on the health care system, affecting not only the availability of quality services, but access to those services as well.

The federal government, with support from state and sometimes local governments, as well as foundations, charitable agencies, and other groups, has established special programs to provide HIV- and AIDS-related care to women and children. All states and territories have an AIDS program funded by the

Centers for Disease Control and Prevention (CDC) and Health Resources and Services Administration (HRSA). Moreover, an array of federal, state, and local laws, regulations, policies, institutions, and financing mechanisms shapes the services in any given locality and determines who has access to those services.

The complex patterns of medical care, financing mechanisms, program authority, and organizations that influence care make it difficult to institute uniform policies for reducing perinatal HIV transmission. In addition, the multiple lines of funding responsibility and accountability have made it extremely difficult to educate providers and convince them of the necessity of testing all pregnant women, as called for in the PHS counseling and testing guidelines (CDC, 1995b).

The resulting structure of the health care system presents a number of barriers to the treatment of HIV-positive women, which include—using the prevention chain as a framework—

- financial and access barriers that may discourage women from seeking prenatal care,
- time constraints that may discourage physicians from counseling pregnant patients about the importance of testing,
- prenatal care sites that may not have the staff to overcome the language and cultural barriers that may cause women to refuse testing, and
- financial and logistical problems that may make testing and treatment difficult.

IMPLEMENTATION AND IMPACT OF THE PUBLIC HEALTH SERVICE COUNSELING AND TESTING GUIDELINES

Since the publication of the ACTG 076 findings in 1994, there has been a concerted national effort to bring the benefits of HIV testing and appropriate treatment to as many women and children as possible. Reviewing the results of these efforts, the committee must make a qualified response to its congressional charge to assess "the extent to which state efforts have been effective in reducing the perinatal transmission of HIV." The committee interprets this charge to include the efforts of national as well as state and local health agencies, and professional organizations at both levels. The data reviewed indicate that, on the whole,

1. there have been substantial public and private efforts to implement the PHS recommendations,
2. prenatal care providers are more likely now than in the past to counsel their patients about HIV and the benefits of ZDV and to offer and recommend HIV tests,
3. women are more likely to accept HIV testing and ZDV if indicated, and
4. there has been a large reduction in perinatally transmitted cases of AIDS.

The number of children born with HIV, however, continues to be far above what is potentially achievable, so much more remains to be done. There is substantial variability from state to state in the way that the PHS guidelines have been implemented, but no evidence to suggest that any particular approach is more successful than others in preventing perinatal HIV.

RECOMMENDATIONS

Universal HIV Testing, with Patient Notification, as a Routine Component of Prenatal Care

To meet the goal that all pregnant women be tested for HIV as early in pregnancy as possible, and those who are positive remain in care so that they can receive optimal treatment for themselves and their children, **the committee's central recommendation is for the adoption of a national policy of universal HIV testing, with patient notification, as a routine component of prenatal care.**

There are two key elements to the committee's recommendation. The first is that HIV screening should be *routine with notification.* This means that the test for HIV would be integrated into the standard battery of prenatal tests and women would be informed that the HIV test is being conducted and of their right to refuse it. This element addresses the doctor–patient relationship, and can reduce barriers to patient acceptance of HIV testing. Most importantly, this approach preserves the right of the woman to refuse the test. If it is followed, women would not have to deal with the burden of disclosing personal risks or potential stereotyping; the test would simply be a part of prenatal care that is the same for everyone. Routine testing will also reduce burdens on providers such as the need for costly extensive pretest counseling and having discussions about personal risks that many providers think are embarrassing. A policy of routine testing might also help to reduce physicians' risk of liability to women and children, where providers incorrectly guess that a woman is not at risk for HIV infection.

The second key element to the recommendation is that screening should be *universal,* meaning that it applies to all pregnant women, regardless of their risk factors and of prevalence rates where they live. The benefit of universal screening is that it ameliorates the stigma associated with being "singled out" for testing, and it overcomes the problem that many HIV-infected women are missed when a risk-based or prevalence-based testing strategy is employed (Barbacci et al., 1991).

Making prenatal HIV testing universal also has broad social implications. First, if incorporated into standard prenatal testing procedures, the costs of universal HIV screening are low, and the benefits are high. Assuming that the marginal cost of adding an ELISA test to the current prenatal panel is $3 per woman and the prevalence of HIV in pregnant women is 2 per 10,000, the committee's calculations in Appendix K show that the cost of routine prenatal testing is $15,600 per HIV-positive woman found. Even if the cost of the test is $5 and the prevalence 1 per 10,000, the cost per case found is $51,100. Taken in the context of the cost of caring for an HIV-infected child, even though not all women found to be HIV-positive will benefit, these figures indicate the clear benefits of routine prenatal HIV testing.

Second, universal screening is the only way to deal with possible geographic shifts in the epidemiology of perinatal transmission. Although perinatal AIDS cases are currently concentrated in eastern states, particularly New York, New Jersey, and Florida, there have been shifts in the prevalence of HIV in pregnant women, including an increase in the South in the early 1990s. Changes in the regional demographics of drug use can also lead to changes in the distribution of HIV infection in pregnant women. Given the uncertainty of these trends, the committee considered universal testing the most prudent method to reduce perinatal transmission despite possible regional fluctuations.

Third, it would help to reduce stigmatization of groups by calling attention to a communicable disease that does not have inherent geographic barriers or a genetic predisposition. Focusing on the communicable disease aspect may allow national education programs that would otherwise be difficult, discouraging infected individuals from hiding themselves and thus not benefiting from care, and discouraging a "blame the victim" mentality.

Incorporating Universal, Routine HIV Testing into Prenatal Care

The following changes in health systems and public policy are needed by state health departments, health systems, and professional organizations to bring about the major change called for in the committee's central recommendation. The committee believes it is also important that these approaches be evaluated carefully, and that successful models be disseminated widely in the professional community.

Education of Prenatal Care Providers

One way to achieve the goal of universal HIV testing in prenatal care is for federal, state, and local health agencies, professional organizations, regional perinatal HIV research and treatment centers, AIDS Health Education Centers, and health plans to increase efforts to educate prenatal care providers about the value of testing in pregnancy. In particular,

The committee recommends that health departments, professional organizations, medical specialty boards, regional perinatal HIV centers, and health plans increase their emphasis on education of pre-

natal care providers about the value of universal HIV testing and about avenues of referral for patients who test positive.

Improved Provider Practices

A variety of specific clinical policies facilitate HIV testing, such as inclusion of HIV tests in the standard prenatal test panel and no longer requiring counseling as a prerequisite for HIV testing. In particular,

The committee recommends that professional organizations update their clinical practice guidelines to facilitate universal HIV testing, with patient notification, as a routine component of prenatal care.

In addition to their direct influence on clinical practices, guidelines of this sort issued by professional organizations have an important role to play in determining the standard of care.

In addition,

The committee recommends that all health care plans and providers develop, adopt, and evaluate clinical policies to facilitate universal prenatal HIV testing.

Clinical policies to implement the committee's recommendation for universal, routine testing with patient notification might include, for example, the inclusion of an HIV test on the checklist of clinical tests for which blood is drawn at the first prenatal visit, standing orders, and procedures to ensure that positive test results are delivered in a timely and appropriate way.

Performance Measures and Contract Language

Health care plans and providers increasingly are being held accountable for the services they provide through performance indicators in such areas as cost, quality of care, and patient satisfaction. In order to take advantage of this approach,

The committee recommends that health care plans and providers adopt performance measures for a policy of universal HIV testing, with patient notification, as a routine component of prenatal care.

To implement this recommendation, groups that develop performance measures, such as the National Committee for Quality Assurance (NCQA), should develop and adopt specific performance indicators for prenatal testing. Given the committee's emphasis on universal HIV testing as a routine component of prenatal care, the proportion of women in prenatal care actually tested would be an appropriate performance measure. Health care plans must, however, ensure patient confidentiality and guard against coercive testing when patients refuse to be tested.

Another approach to integrating public health goals and clinical practice is the development of contract language for managed care plans. In particular,

> **The committee recommends that health care purchasers adopt contract language supporting a policy of universal HIV testing, with patient notification, as a routine component of prenatal care.**

If universal HIV testing with patient notification is to become a routine component of prenatal care, contracts should not allow health insurers to deny benefits under "pre-existing conditions" or similar clauses based on the client's HIV status.

Improving Coordination of Care and Access to High-Quality HIV Treatment

Prenatal HIV testing can achieve its full value only if women who are found to be positive receive high-quality prenatal, intrapartum, and postnatal care for themselves and their children. Thus,

> **The committee recommends efforts to improve coordination of care and access to high-quality HIV interventions and treatment for HIV-positive pregnant women.**

Without linkage to specialty care for HIV-positive women, the committee's recommended policy of universal HIV testing, with patient notification, as a routine component of prenatal care would violate one of the fundamental criteria for public health screening programs, that is, there should be adequate facilities for diagnosis and resources for treatment for all who are found to have the condition, as well as agreement as to who will treat them.

Addressing Concerns about HIV Testing and Treatment

To enhance acceptance of HIV prenatal testing as a routine component of prenatal care, providers should understand the constellation of reasons why some pregnant women refuse HIV testing. Thus,

> **The committee encourages the development of outreach and education programs to address pregnant women's concerns about HIV testing and treatment.**

Resources and Infrastructure

Development and dissemination of policy goals will not, in and of themselves, achieve universal testing and optimal treatment—a comprehensive infrastructure is needed. Maintaining this infrastructure requires federal funding, a regional approach, and an ongoing surveillance program.

Federal Funding

Successful perinatal HIV centers consistently rely upon federal funding for research and for services through HRSA's Ryan White program to maintain the infrastructure they need to succeed. The efforts called for in the earlier recommendations in this chapter will require similar or higher levels of investment. Thus,

The committee recommends that federal funding for state and local efforts to prevent perinatal transmission, including both prenatal testing and care of HIV-infected women, be maintained.

The administration and Congress should examine current budgets thoroughly for adequacy, particularly in light of the expanded programs recommended by the committee. Maintaining current program levels is the minimum requirement. The Ryan White CARE Act Amendments of 1996 (section 2625), for instance, authorized $10 million per year in grants to the states to carry out a series of outreach and other activities that would assist in making HIVcounseling and testing available to pregnant women. Congress, however, never appropriated funds for this purpose. Doing so now would go a long way toward building the infrastructure needed to lower perinatal transmission rates.

As discussed in Chapter 1, The Ryan White CARE Act Amendments of 1996 set up a decision-making process that could result in states losing significant amounts of AIDS funding unless they demonstrate substantial increases in prenatal HIV testing or a substantial decrease in HIV transmission rates, or institute mandatory newborn testing. If the national goal is to prevent HIV transmission from mothers to children, the federal government should support prenatal testing and other state-based prevention efforts. The Ryan White CARE Act Amendments of 1996, paradoxically, could actually undermine them.

Regional Approach

HRSA currently funds a system of "HIV Programs for Children, Youth, Women and Families" through Title IV of the Ryan White CARE Act. Federal research funds in these and other centers also provide for both direct care and an infrastructure to support it. Many of these programs serve as de facto regional centers for specialized treatment of HIV-infected women and affected children, and to a lesser extent, for coordination of prevention activities. There is, however, no coordinated, regional approach. Thus,

The committee recommends that a regional system of perinatal HIV prevention and treatment centers be established.

The regional centers would help to assure optimal HIV care for all pregnant women and newborns, directly to those referred to the centers, and indirectly by working with primary care physicians who retain responsibility for the medical care of HIV-infected women. Moving beyond current practices, the regional centers would also help to develop and implement strategies to improve HIV testing in prenatal care, as discussed above.

Defining the organization, funding, and operations of the recommended regional approach is beyond the scope of this report. To advance this plan, HRSA's Bureau of HIV/AIDS and its Maternal and Child Health Bureau, which together have authority and funding to deal with prenatal care and HIV treatment, should convene a national working group to implement this regional approach. The members of the working group should include representatives of CDC for their prevention authority, National Institutes of Health (NIH) because many of the existing centers receive significant research funding, and Health Care Financing Adminstration (HCFA) because of its oversight of Medicaid. State and local health authorities, representatives of managed care organizations, and representatives of the prenatal care providers should also be involved.

Surveillance

Surveillance systems are needed to support policy development and program evaluation regarding perinatal transmission of HIV. Thus, in order to support the previous recommendation about performance measures, and to generally guide prevention efforts,

The committee recommends that federal, state, and local public health agencies maintain appropriate surveillance data on HIV-infected women and children as an essential component of national efforts to prevent perinatal transmission of HIV.

The universal testing approach that the committee recommends, as well as the call for health plan performance measures, should facilitate the development of appropriate public health surveillance systems.

Other Approaches to Preventing Perinatal HIV Transmission

Although the committee's charge was focused on prenatal HIV testing and appropriate care, other ways to prevent perinatal transmission of HIV should also be considered. In particular, the committee calls attention to the following areas.

Primary Prevention of HIV Infection

Since perinatal transmission begins with infected mothers and their partners, primary prevention of HIV can contribute markedly to preventing perinatal transmission by lowering the number of HIV-infected women and their male partners. There are many established approaches to primary prevention: HIV/AIDS education programs, behavioral interventions, partner notification, treatment and prevention of sexually transmitted diseases, and community programs. Beyond more general HIV prevention efforts, prevention and treatment programs targeting drug users appear to be especially vital for preventing perinatal HIV transmission.

Averting Unintended Pregnancy and Childbearing Among HIV-Infected Women

Pregnancies that are intended—consciously and clearly desired—at the time of conception are in the best interest of the mother and the child (IOM, 1995b). If a woman is infected with HIV, unintended pregnancy and childbearing clearly have special significance. For these reasons, preconception counseling represents an important opportunity to identify HIV-infected women who are considering pregnancy. Some women who know they are HIV-infected choose to become pregnant, especially now that the ACTG 076 regimen is available, but others become pregnant unintentionally. More women learn their HIV status through the course of their pregnancy. Nevertheless, improved knowledge of the consequences of unintended pregnancy (including HIV transmission) and the ways to avoid it, as well as access to contraception, can help to ensure that all pregnancies are intended (IOM, 1995b), and this would reduce, to some extent, the number of children born with HIV infection. The committee does not want to restrict reproductive choice (Faden et al., 1991), but notes that interventions for such women who choose to terminate unintended pregnancies can also be beneficial in reducing the number of children born with HIV infection.

Increasing Utilization of Prenatal Care

Roughly 15% of HIV-infected pregnant women, many of whom are drug users, receive no prenatal care. Efforts to increase the proportion of women, especially drug users, who receive prenatal care should therefore be a high priority. *Prenatal Care: Reaching Mothers, Reaching Infants* (IOM, 1988) recommends activities to (1) remove financial barriers to care; (2) make certain that basic system capacity is adequate for women; (3) improve the policies and practices that shape prenatal services at the delivery site; and (4) increase public information and education about prenatal care.

Enhanced HIV Prevention in Correctional Settings

Correctional settings—prisons and jails—offer a unique opportunity for prevention activities targeted to hard-to-reach women at risk for, or already infected with, HIV. The prevalence of HIV infection among incarcerated women is far higher than in the community at large: 4% of female state prison inmates nationwide are known to be HIV-positive; in nine states the proportion exceeds 10%. Women are more likely than men to be incarcerated for drug-related offenses, so female inmates are more likely than male inmates to be infected or at risk for HIV infection. Many interventions could be introduced in correctional settings either for primary prevention of HIV transmission or, particularly, for prevention of perinatal transmission among HIV-infected pregnant women. Interventions should focus on HIV testing and treatment, drug testing and treatment, prenatal care, and efforts to ensure continuity of care for HIV-positive patients who leave the correctional setting.

Development of Rapid HIV Tests

Because reporting of conventional HIV tests takes about one to two weeks, an accurate rapid test, with results available in hours, might have applications in prenatal, labor, and delivery settings to prevent perinatal transmission in some groups of patients. Women and newborns identified with a rapid test late in pregnancy or intrapartum could receive the intrapartum or postpartum component of the ACTG 076 regimen, respectively. In the prenatal setting, a rapid test might be especially valuable for women who are unlikely to return for test results. According to the committee's site visits and workshops, these women are more likely to be adolescents, drug users, undocumented immigrants, and/or homeless. In the labor and delivery setting, a rapid test might be valuable for women who have not been tested previously or have not received prenatal care. The prevalence of HIV infection is elevated in women who have not received prenatal care, and the labor and delivery setting offers the last opportunity to interrupt HIV transmission through administration of intrapartum therapy and advice to avoid breast-feeding. Since this is not an ideal time to obtain consent to testing and to discuss the implications of a positive result, program design and implementation would need to address these issues.

CONCLUSIONS

If the promise of the ACTG 076 findings, that perinatal transmission of HIV can largely be prevented, is to be fulfilled, the United States needs to adopt a goal that all pregnant women be tested for HIV, and those who are positive remain in care so they can receive optimal treatment for themselves and their children. In order to meet this goal, **the United States should adopt a national policy of universal HIV testing, with patient notification, as a routine component of prenatal care.** Adopting this policy will require the establishment of, and resources for, a comprehensive infrastructure. This infrastructure must include (1) education of prenatal care providers; (2) the development and implementation of practice guidelines and the implementation of clinical policies: (3) the development and adoption of performance measures and Medicaid managed care contract language for prenatal HIV testing; (4) efforts to improve coordination of care and access to high-quality HIV treatment; (5) interventions to overcome pregnant women's concerns about HIV testing and treatment; (6) and efforts to increase utilization of prenatal care, as described above.

1

Introduction

One of the most promising victories in the battle against AIDS was the finding, in 1994, that administration of zidovudine (known as ZDV, and previously as AZT) during pregnancy and childbirth could reduce by about two-thirds the chance that the child of an HIV-positive mother would be infected (Connor et al., 1994). Because 6,000 to 7,000 HIV-infected women give birth every year, and others have to carefully consider whether they should get pregnant, the potential impact of these findings was monumental. The "ACTG 076 results," referring to the AIDS Clinical Trials Group protocol number 76, quickly led the Public Health Service (PHS) to develop guidelines for treatment of pregnant women (CDC, 1994)[1] and, in 1995, guidelines about counseling and testing of pregnant women for HIV infection (CDC, 1995b).

The 1995 PHS guidelines called for universal counseling of pregnant women about the risk of AIDS, the benefits of HIV testing, and voluntary testing. The approach was endorsed by the American College of Obstetricians and Gynecologists, the American Academy of Pediatrics, and other professional groups. The essence of the PHS guidelines also has been adopted by most states, either by policy or by legislation. Medical practice has changed in line with these recommendations, with an increasing proportion of women tested for HIV during prenatal care. As a result of these and other changes, there has been a substantial reduction—approximately 43% from a peak in 1992 to 1996—in the number of newborns diagnosed with AIDS. A reduction of this magnitude in only a few

---

[1]Updated guidelines were issued in 1998 (CDC, 1998d).

years certainly represents great progress, yet it is far less than the ACTG 076 findings can offer.

Two years after the publication of the ACTG 076 findings, Congress addressed perinatal transmission issues in the Ryan White Comprehensive AIDS Resources Emergency (CARE) Act Amendments of 1996 (P.L. 104-146). This legislation set forth a series of conditions regarding routine practices leading to a determination by the Secretary of Health and Human Services that could make Ryan White CARE Act formula funds to the states contingent upon mandatory HIV testing of newborns. Nationally, more than $500 million (the 1998 appropriation for the Title II program, which supports health care and support services, continuation of health insurance, pharmaceutical treatments, and other services through the states) is at stake in this decision (HRSA, 1998a).

THE RYAN WHITE CARE ACT AMENDMENTS OF 1996

According to P.L. 104-146, the Secretary of Health and Human Services is required by October 1998 to determine whether HIV testing of all infants born in the United States whose mothers have not undergone prenatal HIV testing has become "routine practice." This is an important determination; if it is affirmative, all Ryan White funding to the states after April 2000 becomes contingent upon states demonstrating one of the following:

1. a 50% reduction (or a comparable measure for states with less than ten cases) in the rate of new AIDS cases resulting from perinatal transmission, comparing the most recent data to 1993 data;

2. at least 95% of women who have received at least two prenatal visits prior to 34 weeks of gestation have been tested for HIV; or

3. a program for mandatory testing of all newborns whose mothers have not undergone prenatal HIV testing.

To determine whether HIV testing of infants as described above has become "routine practice," the Secretary is required to consult with states and other public and private experts as to whether the following are routine practice in the United States:

1. testing of infants whose mothers have not received prenatal HIV testing;

2. release of HIV test results of newborns to parents, legal guardians, or health care providers;

3. disclosure of HIV test results of pregnant women conducted by the state (such as anonymous seroprevalence surveys) to the pregnant women involved;

4. provision of appropriate HIV counseling in disclosing test results under (2) and (3) and

5. prevention of insurers from discontinuing coverage on the basis of HIV or having been tested for HIV.

ORGANIZATION OF THE REPORT

This report is intended primarily to address the particular questions posed in the Institute of Medicine's (IOM's) congressional mandate: "the extent to which State efforts have been effective in reducing the perinatal transmission of the human immunodeficiency virus, and an analysis of the existing barriers to the further reduction in such transmission." The committee also intends this report to be useful to national, state, and local policy makers, as well as health care providers and public health practitioners who want to give the most effective and appropriate care to all women and children, and to do everything possible to prevent perinatal transmission of HIV. In the interest of a full and complete analysis, the report therefore takes up other issues raised by the Ryan White CARE Act Amendments of 1996.

To this end, the report aims to provide a complete analysis of (1) the impact of current approaches to reducing perinatal transmission, as well as the barriers to further reducing such transmission; (2) ways to increase prenatal testing, improve therapy for women and HIV-infected children, and generally reduce perinatal HIV infections; and (3) the ethical and public health issues associated with screening policies as prevention tools, and their implications for prevention and treatment opportunities for women and infants.

Despite the focus of the Ryan White CARE Act Amendments on newborn screening, the congressional mandate for this IOM study does not call for an evaluation of that option. As a result, the committee has not made any recommendations about mandatory newborn testing per se, but notes the limited role it can play in preventing transmission of HIV from mother to child, the focus of this report.

In its analysis, the committee has found it helpful to consider a chain of factors affecting perinatal transmission, as illustrated in Figure 1.1. Although precise data are not available for all of these proportions, the committee found this to be a helpful organizing framework, and it is used throughout this report. The chain is intended for heuristic purposes and is not a complete representation of all of the possible paths to HIV infection or interventions. Pregnancy termination is possible, for instance, at many stages in the chain. Women who are not tested as part of prenatal care may be tested during labor and receive some benefit from treatment, and children whose HIV status is detected after birth can be kept from breast-feeding.

Following this introduction, Chapter 2 provides historical and other background information on population-based screening and surveillance, HIV testing generally, prenatal and newborn screening for other conditions, and special considerations needed when the condition in question is concentrated in minority

The proportion of women . . .

- who are HIV-infected
  - who become pregnant
    - who do not seek prenatal care
      - who are not offered HIV testing
        - who refuse HIV testing
          - who are not offered the ACTG 076 regimen
            - who refuse the ACTG 076 regimen
              - who do not complete the ACTG 076 regimen
                - whose child is infected despite treatment

FIGURE 1.1   Chain of events leading to an HIV-infected child.

communities. Chapter 3 provides relevant information on the descriptive epide-miology of HIV and AIDS in women and newborns. Chapter 4 summarizes the scientific and clinical information about the detection and treatment of HIV infection in pregnant women and newborns, and includes a summary of current official clinical screening and treatment guidelines. The committee accepted these as they stand, and did not attempt to make clinical recommendations. Chapter 5 described the current context of services for women and children affected by HIV and AIDS.

The committee's conclusions and recommendations are concentrated in the final two chapters. Chapter 6 reviews the implementation and impact of the PHS voluntary prenatal screening recommendations in terms of (1) their implementa-tion in official guidelines and statements of medical professional organizations, as well as in state law and regulations; and (2) actual testing rates and provider practices. This chapter concludes that although extensive efforts have been made to implement the recommendations, and there have been major successes, there are still substantial gaps in the number of women who are not tested for HIV, largely because either they receive no prenatal care or their prenatal care provid-ers do not advise them to be tested.

The final chapter begins with the committee's central recommendation—that HIV testing, with patient notification, should be a routine and universal compo-nent of prenatal care—and a series of more specific recommendations related to the establishment of this approach in prenatal care. The infrastructure must in-clude, for instance, education of prenatal care providers; the development and implementation of practice guidelines, clinical policy performance measures, and Medicaid managed care contract language for prenatal HIV testing; efforts to improve coordination of care and access to high-quality HIV treatment; interventions to overcome pregnant women's concerns about HIV testing and treatment; and efforts to increase utilization of prenatal care, as described above. The chapter also includes recommendations regarding the resources and infrastructure needed to implement these approaches, and for preventing perinatally transmitted HIV through means other than prenatal testing and treatment.

THE COMMITTEE'S APPROACH

The committee's analyses and recommendations are based on a wide variety of quantitative and qualitative information. The committee began by reviewing the major official reports and scientific and medical articles relating to perinatal HIV diagnosis and treatment, HIV testing and screening, and related subjects from the United States and abroad. Prominent among these are government and medical association practice guidelines for testing and treatment of pregnant women, infants, and others, as well as a variety of scientific articles dealing with diagnosis and treatment of HIV, the consequences of HIV testing, and ethical issues. The committee also reviewed a 1991 IOM report on prenatal and newborn HIV screening (IOM, 1991). Although the report's conclusions are outdated because of developments in the intervening seven years, its analytical and ethical framework remain useful.

The committee has also reviewed a variety of statistical reports on HIV/AIDS trends, especially relating to women and perinatal transmission, from the Centers for Disease Control and Prevention (CDC) and other sources. For information on laws, regulations, and the implementation of perinatal transmission prevention efforts at the state level, the committee relied upon a survey and analysis of relevant state policies and laws prepared by CDC and the Georgetown Law Center (Gostin et al., in press). In addition, the committee reviewed information from many state health departments and HIV/AIDS programs on the implementation and effect of the voluntary testing guidelines.

To further add to the knowledge base for this report, the committee commissioned background papers in the following areas: a history of prenatal and newborn HIV testing in New York State; a history and analysis of screening for sickle cell disease; a report on the context of services for women and children affected by HIV/AIDS; and a report of the experiences of an HIV-positive peer counselor for pregnant women and new mothers. In addition, the committee solicited and received informal reports from a large number of knowledgeable individuals.

Finally, the committee organized a series of workshops and field visits to discuss the issues with the people affected by and concerned with the current and proposed policies: women who are HIV-infected or at risk of HIV infection, health care providers, and state and local policy makers. In particular, the committee convened workshops in Washington, D.C., on February 11 and April 1, 1998. Groups of committee members and staff made site visits to New York City and Newark, New Jersey; to Birmingham and rural Greene County, Alabama;

and to San Antonio, Texas, in April and May 1998. The findings from these field visits are summarized in the appendixes of this report. The committee organized a discussion of these issues with practitioners at the Florida HIV Conference in Orlando in April 1998 and at the Summer 1998 Correctional HIV Consortium Educational Update in Atlanta in June 1998. Committee members and staff also attended other national and local meetings at which perinatal transmission issues were discussed, and had numerous discussions with knowledgeable individuals.

2

Public Health Screening Programs

Disease screening is one of the most basic tools of modern public health and preventive medicine. Screening programs have a long and distinguished history in efforts to control epidemics of infectious diseases and targeting treatment for chronic diseases. Women in prenatal care routinely receive tests for complete blood count and blood type, diabetes, syphilis, and other conditions. Newborn children are routinely tested for errors of inborn metabolism and other problems. Although most of these outcomes are rare, a positive test result triggers interventions that benefit both mother and child, and these efforts have been responsible for substantial improvements in health and well-being.

As these screening programs have been implemented over the years, a substantial body of experience has been gained. In practice, when screening is conducted in contexts of gender inequality, racial discrimination, sexual taboos, and poverty, these conditions shape the attitudes and beliefs of health system and public health decision makers as well as patients, including those who have lost confidence that the health care system will treat them fairly. Thus, if screening programs are poorly conceived, organized, or implemented, they may lead to interventions of questionable merit and enhance the vulnerability of groups and individuals.

This chapter was prepared to provide background information on the terminology and generally accepted principles that should guide public health screening efforts, and to provide a historical and social context for implementation of HIV screening programs. The chapter begins with a discussion of screening as a public health paradigm, reviews a series of historical examples of perinatal screening programs in this context, and summarizes some of the issues associated with HIV testing in the United States.

SCREENING PROGRAMS: A PUBLIC HEALTH PARADIGM

In the public health paradigm, "testing," "screening," "case finding," "surveillance," and "counseling" are relevant to understanding what constitutes a screening program. In the context of this report, *testing* is the application of a test or measurement to selected individuals for the purpose of identifying a disease or medical condition. The individuals might be selected for testing because there is a clinical reason or risk factors that suggest the presence of the condition. *Screening* generally refers to the application of a test to all individuals in a defined population. Screening is commonly instituted for the purpose of *case finding*—identifying a previously unknown or unrecognized condition in apparently healthy or asymptomatic persons and offering presymptomatic treatment to those so identified. Screening is also sometimes done for *surveillance* purposes: to monitor the incidence or prevalence of a disease in a defined population over time, or to compare the incidence or prevalence among different populations. Surveillance is an important public health activity, and is necessary for monitoring the impact of, and allocating resources to, prevention programs. *Counseling* is the communication process by which individuals and their family members are given information about the nature, risks, burden, and benefits of testing, and the meaning of test results.

This report concentrates on HIV screening for the purpose of identifying and treating individual pregnant women for their own health and preventing transmission of HIV to their infants, that is, case finding. Testing of selected individuals and screening for surveillance purposes are important efforts, but not directly related to the committee's charge.

Principles of Public Health Screening

Through the experience with public health screening programs, a series of characteristics of well-organized public health screening programs has evolved (Wilson and Jungner, 1968). The committee's summary of the relevant characteristics is as follows:

1. The goals of the screening program should be clearly specified and shown to be achievable.

2. The natural history of the condition should be adequately understood, and treatment or intervention for those found positive widely accepted by the scientific and medical community, with evidence that early intervention improves health outcomes.

3. The screening test or measurement should distinguish those individuals who are likely to have the condition from those who are unlikely to have it. Tests can be judged in terms of their sensitivity (proportion of actual cases found by the test to be positive), specificity (proportion of non-cases found to be negative),

and positive predictive value (proportion of positive test results that are actual cases). Serious social, political, and economic problems tend to arise when screening tests fail to identify most of the people with the disease (false negatives), or identify far more people than actually have the disease (false positives).

4. There should be adequate facilities for diagnosis and resources for treatment for all who are found to have the condition, as well as agreement as to who will treat them. Psychological trauma and social disruption are most likely to result when screening programs identify people with a disease but fail to provide treatment.

5. The test and possible interventions should be acceptable to the affected population. For instance, a screening program that required a spinal tap of all participants, or had pregnancy termination as the only option, might not be acceptable to some groups. Programs in which there are concerns about the use of patient information or even the primary motives (using the test as a means of discrimination designed to deny civil rights, for instance) might also be judged unacceptable.

6. The cost of case finding, diagnosis, and treatment or intervention should be economically balanced in relation to the medical cost savings that might result from the screening program. Screening programs need not be cost-saving, but their costs must be reasonable in relation to the anticipated benefits, and to other opportunities for public health programs.

Various legal and ethical principles should also apply to public health screening programs (Faden et al., 1991). As a general principle, the least burdensome approach (from a legal and ethical viewpoint) that meets public health goals should always be preferred.

Programs must conform, first of all, to the requirements of the United States and state constitutions, common law, and statutory provisions. Targeted screening programs, for instance, must avoid problems of denial of equal protection inherent in focusing upon particular groups for testing. Moreover, the means to achieve otherwise acceptable social objectives must be narrowly tailored to avoid interference with the exercise of other important liberties, such as privacy. Screening programs must also comply with existing legal requirements concerning informed consent and confidentiality, duties to treat, and standards of professional negligence (Faden et al., 1991).

Moral considerations not protected by laws must also be taken into account. Three broad principles—beneficence, autonomy, and social justice—guide these considerations. Beneficence relates to the need to balance the benefits of public health measures (chiefly the protection from disease) against the harms (which could be physical or involve the loss of privacy or autonomy). Respect for autonomy emphasizes the importance of individual freedom and choice, both for political life and for personal decisions. Justice relates to the fair distribution of benefits and burdens of a public health program. None of these principles can be seen as consistently more important than the others, but the degree to which they are satisfied must be balanced in every instance (Faden et al., 1991).

Spectrum of Screening Programs

Although screening programs are commonly thought of as either voluntary or mandatory, there is in fact a continuum of approaches that can be taken. Faden and colleagues (1991) characterize five types of programs: (1) completely mandatory, (2) conditionally mandatory, (3) routine without notification, (4) routine with notification, and (5) non-directive patient choice.[1]

In a *completely mandatory* program, a government agency requires citizens to undergo a screening test and sanctions those who do not comply. In public health screening programs, either providers or patients can be compelled to take action and suffer the consequences of not doing so. In addition, mandatory programs differ in the degree to which they are enforced, and the nature of the sanction for not complying. Enforcement and sanctions typically vary according to the agency upon which the mandate falls. State health departments can more easily enforce a policy requiring hospitals to test individuals than one requiring individuals to be tested because hospitals are subject to regulation, receive government funding, and regularly report a variety of performance measures.

In a *conditionally mandatory* program, either government or a private institution makes access to a designated service or opportunity contingent upon participation in the screening program. A prenatal care provider, for instance, could require women to undergo certain tests as a condition of receiving prenatal care.

Individuals in a *routine without notification* program are routinely and automatically tested unless they expressly ask that the test not be done.

Participants in a *routine with notification* program are informed that a certain test is a standard part of prenatal care, and that they have the right to refuse before the testing is done. Most women will be tested unless they explicitly opt out. Written informed consent is not necessary, but providers might want to document patient refusals in order to protect themselves from malpractice liability.

In a *non-directive patient choice* program individuals are provided information about the test, and the choice about whether to be tested is left to them. Patients actively must choose to be tested, and if they do not opt to be tested, the default is that no testing will occur. This type of program is the model typically employed in the context of genetic counseling where it is labeled "non-directive counseling." This also is the model used by HIV anonymous test sites.

While routine with notification and routine without notification programs,

---

[1]Faden and colleagues (1991) called the last option "voluntary," but the committee chose to call it "non-directive patient choice" to stress the more active role of the patient inherent in this type of program.

like the patient choice model, are voluntary, in that women have the right to choose not to be tested, women are much more likely to be tested under either of the "routine" models. In routine programs, the default is that all women will be tested, implying that the health care team believes that the test is an important part of good medical care. In the routine without notification program, women are not likely to know that they are being tested. In a routine with notification program, the woman must be explicitly informed of the test, and that she has the opportunity to opt out.

This list of categories is not mutually exclusive, nor a strict rank ordering, and some policies can reflect a combination of these approaches. As documented in Chapter 6, the current law in California and New Jersey, for instance, requires prenatal care providers to offer an HIV test to all women, but leaves it to the women to decide whether they want to be tested. In Texas, providers are required to test all women in prenatal care and their newborns unless a woman objects in writing, and to notify them about the testing and their right to refuse.

EXPERIENCE WITH SELECTED PUBLIC HEALTH SCREENING PROGRAMS[2]

Pregnant women are routinely tested for many conditions. The American Academy of Pediatrics and the American College of Obstetricians and Gynecologists, for instance, recommend that the following tests be performed early in pregnancy: hematocrit or hemoglobin, urinalysis, urine testing to detect asymptomatic bacteriuria, determination of blood groups and CDS (Rh) type, antibody screen, determination of immunity to rubella virus, syphilis screen, cervical cytology (as needed), antibodies to hepatitis B virus surface antigen, and HIV (with the women's consent) (AAP and ACOG, 1997). Newborns are routinely tested for phenylketonuria (PKU), a condition that can lead to mental retardation without dietary interventions, and other inborn errors of metabolism (Acuff and Faden, 1991). These tests are well accepted, and seen to clearly benefit the women and her child. Some prenatal and postnatal testing programs, however, have been more controversial.

The first prenatal screening program mandated by law was for syphilis in the 1930s and 1940s. In early 1960s, many states mandated newborn screening for PKU. Screening for other inborn errors of metabolism (congenital hypothyroidism, galactosemia, homocystinuria, histidenemia, maple syrup urine disease, and tyrosinemia) followed in the 1970s. In the early 1970s, many states initiated mandatory screening for sickle cell disease, a disease that had limited treatment options, in a variety of populations. Later in the same decade, maternal serum

alpha-fetoprotein tests were introduced, on a voluntary basis, to help detect neural tube defects. Today, specific tests mandated or recommended as standards of
practice vary substantially across state lines. Mandatory prenatal and newborn
testing for substance abuse is increasingly common.

In order to understand the context and appreciate the issues and challenges
involved in making policy recommendations for HIV screening of pregnant
women, the committee has focused on the historical experience with five selected
conditions: (1) syphilis, (2) phenylketonuria, (3) sickle cell disease, (4) neural
tube defects, and (5) substance abuse. These examples were chosen because they
illustrate issues relevant to the perinatal transmission of HIV: they involve maternal and child health issues, infectious diseases, a variety of risks and benefits, and
minority populations.

Syphilis

Early in the twentieth century, syphilis was more common than all other
sexually transmitted diseases (STDs), and congenital syphilis was the leading
cause of spontaneous abortions and stillbirth. Approximately one million women
of childbearing age had syphilis. As a result 25,000 fetuses per year died before
birth and 60,000 were born with syphilis (U.S. PHS, 1940). Prenatal syphilis
testing was available as early as 1906, but was not mandated by law due to
"onerous treatment options and the stigma of being shown to have the disease"
(Acuff and Faden, 1991). Indeed, even being tested for syphilis was stigmatizing,
and many physicians were reluctant to embarrass women in their care by suggesting it.

In 1936, Thomas Parran, the U.S. Surgeon General, established a program
for controlling syphilis that included mandatory premarital and prenatal blood
tests. Two years later, a *New York Post* editorial entitled "13,000 Babies" described stillborn and affected babies in New York (*New York Post*, 1938). *Post*
staff reported that "although public prenatal clinics were requiring blood tests for
syphilis, only half of New York City's practicing obstetricians were routinely
testing their private patients." By the end of 1945, as a result of this campaign, 36
states had passed prenatal syphilis screening laws. Under these laws, birth certificates had to record whether the test had been done prenatally and to explain why
those who were not tested were not—women and physicians could refuse on
religious or other grounds. Although these laws were passed before the introduction of antibiotic treatment, they resulted in a rapid decline in congenital transmission through case finding (Acuff and Faden, 1991), contract tracing, and the
difficult and less effective therapies available at the time. Perhaps the most important aspect of these screening programs was that by making testing routine,
they overcame the resistance of physicians to risk offending patients by suggesting a test for syphilis.

Phenylketonuria

Phenylketonuria (PKU) is a hereditary metabolic disorder, in which a deficiency of an enzyme results in the accumulation of the amino acid phenylalanine, resulting in severe mental retardation. It occurs in approximately 1 per 12,000 to 15,000 live births. In most infants diagnosed with PKU, mental retardation can be prevented by restricting dietary phenylalanine, starting before four weeks of age. In 1961, a simple heel-stick test for the condition was developed, and voluntary screening in conjunction with educational programs was initiated soon after in Massachusetts. By 1963, all Massachusetts maternity hospitals had voluntarily enrolled in PKU screening programs and were screening all newborns for PKU. Later that year, Massachusetts became the first state to enact a mandatory screening law.

Although the American Academy of Pediatrics and other professional groups opposed a legislative approach, 43 states have enacted mandatory screening laws, and the rest have set up active testing programs without statutory support. The existing statutes do not punish noncompliant parents. PKU screening is thus an example of a mandatory screening program, with the onus of compliance on maternity hospitals. In 1975, Maryland repealed its compulsory PKU screening law, replacing it with a statute and regulations requiring parental informed consent (Holtzman, 1984). After this change, 99.9% of parents offered newborn screening accepted it (Faden et al., 1982).

Although the PKU program has prevented retardation in thousands of infants, it has been argued that it was introduced prematurely from a medical point of view. Critics of the programs say that the public was led to believe that there was a higher degree of certainty about the results of PKU tests than was the case (NAS, 1975). As a result, some, but probably only a small percentage, of infants identified by the test were incorrectly identified and treated as having PKU. Others have criticized the statutes for not providing either adequate quality assurance mechanisms or adequate funding to care for infants identified as having PKU. The concerns about PKU testing, therefore, are in terms of the third and fourth principle of public health screening described above.

Sickle Cell Disease

Sickle cell disease (SCD) is an autosomal recessive hemolytic anemia occurring most frequently in African Americans, but also in persons of Mediterranean origin and others. Sickle cell disease, the homozygous condition, is estimated to occur in as many as one in 400 African-American newborns, and approximately 8% of African Americans are carriers of the sickle cell trait, the heterozygous condition. At least 10% of SCD cases in the United States occur in non-African Americans.

Little attention was given to sickle cell screening until the 1970s, when Dr. Roland Scott, in a letter to the *New England Journal of Medicine*, called for mass premarital carrier screening (Scott, 1970). Scott argued that although it was more prevalent in African Americans than cystic fibrosis, PKU, and other conditions of concern, little public health effort was directed at SCD. Scott noted that there was no cure for SCD, but suggested that it could be the first hereditary illness to be controlled by genetic counseling (that is, by encouraging carriers not to marry or have children). Scott's appeal was echoed in a public awareness campaign, and in 1971, President Nixon singled out SCD for special attention in a health message to Congress, calling for an increase in federal spending on sickle cell research, education, and screening.

Also in 1971, Connecticut passed the first sickle cell screening legislation, which other states quickly followed. These laws were typically introduced by African-American legislators and passed by unanimous vote. Screening was typically mandatory for some groups, but the legislation did not always specify which populations should be targeted; some included newborns, preschool children, individuals seeking marriage licenses, or inmates. Some laws called for carrier screening and some for disease screening.

Initial supporters of SCD screening were spurred on by the success of PKU screening, but the clear difference between SCD and PKU was not fully appreciated until later. There was no intervention for SCD at this time other than counseling to avoid marriage or pregnancy (prenatal SCD screening was not feasible). In addition, questions about whether and how programs should be targeted led to the potential for stigmatization. Some states explicitly targeted only African Americans. The New York statute required urban schoolchildren to be screened, but not rural children. The lack of attention to the eugenic implications of informing someone that he carries sickle cell trait led to charges of racism and growing opposition to screening programs. Most of the laws that were passed in the 1970s lacked confidentiality provisions, and, as a result, there were many documented cases of job discrimination, especially in the military, even for those having asymptomatic sickle cell trait. Eventually, the National Sickle Cell Anemia Control Act, passed in 1972, said federal funds could be used for screening only if programs were voluntary.

Studies published in the 1980s demonstrated that a prophylactic regimen of penicillin in infants significantly reduced the morbidity and mortality of SCD, and in 1987 a National Institutes of Health (NIH) consensus conference called for universal (not targeted) newborn screening for hemoglobinopathies (NIH, 1987). As a result of this recommendation and increased federal funding, 29 states have reinstituted non-targeted newborn screening programs.

The experience with SCD screening in the 1970s illustrates the difficulties that can arise when the goals of screening programs are not clearly specified, when there is no treatment that improves health outcomes, and when the intervention is not acceptable to the target population because of stigma and discrimination. Current screening efforts, consistent with the NIH consensus statement, have addressed each of these problems and, as a result, are more acceptable on public health and ethical grounds. The change in approach to SCD screening over time, as new facts and treatment opportunities emerge, illustrates that programs must have the flexibility to change over time, as the situation changes.

Neural Tube Defects

Neural tube defects (NTDs) are major birth defects affecting the brain and spinal column. These defects range from uniformly fatal to severely disabling conditions, and include spina bifida. In 1973, it was reported that maternal serum alpha-fetoprotein (MSAFP) levels are elevated in pregnancies where the fetus is affected with an open neural tube. Alpha-fetoprotein (AFP) is a normal fetal protein that is usually present in maternal serum, so a higher than normal level indicates that the fetus is leaking fetal protein, usually, but not always, from an open neural tube. Follow-up tests such as amniocentesis and ultrasonography are required to confirm the diagnosis. By 1977, several companies had developed MSAFP kits, but the American College of Obstetricians and Gynecologists (ACOG) and other groups opposed their use because of the test's inherently high false positive rate. Others opposed the program because, since there is no identifiable high-risk groups for NTDs, all pregnant women would have to be screened. In addition, some individuals find the screening program unacceptable because the only option for preventing the birth of a child with an NTD is to terminate the pregnancy. Another concern was that some areas did not have the amniocentesis and ultrasonography facilities necessary to follow up a positive MSAFP test result. There are concerns, therefore, relating to the third, fourth, and fifth public health screening principles.

In 1985, ACOG, apparently driven by a concern about malpractice litigation, issued a strongly worded alert to its members advising them to investigate the availability of the tests in their area, familiarize themselves with the procedure and follow-up tests, advise every prenatal patient of the availability of the test, and document this discussion and the patient's decision. ACOG did not, at this time, change its recommendation that the test not be used routinely. Two years later, ACOG, citing greater understanding of MSAFP and improvement in follow-up tests, and new findings about the association of MSAFP with Down's syndrome, concluded:

> MSAFP screening for neural tube defects detection should now be undertaken in United States communities having expertise in ultrasound, genetic counseling, and amniocentesis. In communities in which these facilities are limited, it is still prudent to inform pregnant women of the availability of MSAFP screening. . . . Those communities not having appropriate facilities should attempt to

develop a full scale MSAFP program, collaboration with an existing program, at a regional level [Simpson and Nadler, 1987].

MSAFP is thus a non-directive patient choice screening program, with strong incentives to providers to inform women about its availability.

Prenatal and Newborn Screening for Substance Abuse

State policies on prenatal and newborn screening for substance abuse are evolving rapidly in the context of a discussion of changing state policies regarding drug use (Chavkin et al., 1998). Overall, states are moving away from a therapeutic approach focusing on treatment and oversight to criminal prosecution. Between 1992 and 1995, the number of states with mandatory drug or alcohol testing of pregnant women increased from one to six, and the number of states with mandatory drug or alcohol testing of neonates increased from zero to four.[3] An increasing number of states have a practice of reporting positive toxicology results. The number of states with such practices for pregnant women increased from 7 to 31, and for neonates from 18 to 33, over the same period. Furthermore, in 1995, 12 states mandated treatment for pregnant women found to be using drugs, and 13 mandated treatment for women with children. No states had mandatory treatment policies in 1992.

Many of these screening programs are being introduced in prenatal care as a result of substance abuse laws and policies, without clear public health goals and without providing treatment to improve health outcomes. In addition, the common intervention, removal of the child from the mother's care, is not acceptable to the affected population. Some of these programs are targeted to minority groups, and thus are stigmatizing. More basically, perinatal substance abuse screening programs illustrate the problems that arise when a screening program is set up to deal with a problem that all agree about (e.g., "crack babies") but the implications are not carefully thought through (Jos et al., 1995).

To date there has been little outcry about prenatal and newborn substance abuse screening programs, perhaps because the interests of the affected women are not well reflected in policy decisions, but the history of other screening programs suggests that this approach may not serve public health goals well.

HIV TESTING AND SCREENING IN THE UNITED STATES

As described in Chapter 4, the primary HIV/AIDS screening tests used in the United States identify antibodies to the HIV virus, indicating that an individual has been exposed to the virus and has mounted an immune response. As such,

---

[3]The District of Columbia is counted as a "state" in this paragraph.

HIV tests do not indicate whether "seropositive" individuals (those who test positive for HIV) have AIDS, a later stage in HIV disease. Also, infected individuals may not test positive for HIV for a period of weeks after infection. Thus there is a distinction between "HIV-infected," "seropositive," and "AIDS." When applied to newborns, standard HIV tests react to maternal antibodies, which are present in all children of HIV-infected mothers, up to 18 months after birth, whether the child is HIV-infected or not. Newborns who test positive for HIV antibodies are said to be "HIV-affected."

Serum HIV tests first became available in the United States in 1985 and were originally used to protect the safety of the blood supply by excluding blood from HIV-positive donors (IOM, 1995c). At the time, there was great concern about the safety of the blood supply, so the improved ability to accurately detect infected individuals (especially compared to the surrogate measures that were the best tools before this time) made serum HIV tests attractive public health measures. Tests also became available at this time for individuals, but stigma and discrimination associated with homosexuality, drug use, and AIDS itself, coupled with the fact that there were no measures available to alter the disease process in HIV-infected individuals, limited their acceptability. Some assumed that the primary purpose of testing was to facilitate the adoption of risk reduction behaviors. Over time, however, it became clear that knowledge of HIV status was insufficient to stimulate behavior change in all affected persons, and that many other factors contribute to decisions about risk reduction behaviors (Coates et al., 1988).

It was not until the discovery of effective interventions such as ZDV and *Pneumocystis carinii* pneumonia (PCP) prophylaxis in the late 1980s that HIV testing carried medical benefits for the individuals tested. Soon afterwards, some professionals advocated moving beyond testing solely as a means to stop the spread of HIV. Rhame and Maki (1989), for instance, reported that HIV testing had benefits for infected persons and the general public health. As an example, they noted that early detection of HIV status was one means to counteract denial, facilitate early treatment, and ultimately improve the health status of people infected with HIV. More generally, Rhame and Maki (1989) note that more general HIV testing would

1. reduce the reluctance of those at risk to pursue testing;
2. undermine the existence of the we/they mentality and stigma associated with HIV disease;
3. motivate risk reduction behaviors;
4. serve as the basis for partner notification programs; and
5. facilitate the identification of candidates for clinical research.

In a review of the factors associated with the acceptability of voluntary HIV testing in the United States, Irwin and colleagues (1996) concluded that the factors associated with high acceptance rates include (1) the person's perception of HIV risk; (2) acknowledging risk behaviors; (3) confidentiality protections; (4) presenting counseling and testing as "routine" rather than optional; and (5) the provider's belief that counseling and testing will benefit the client. Factors associated with low acceptance rates included prior HIV testing, fears about coping with results, and explicit informed consent.

While the benefits of testing appear clear and relevant to the current situation where effective treatment is available, serious cautions must be acknowledged. According to Quinn (1998), testing could have a paradoxical effect on public health. For example, tremendous fear about AIDS, its existence within stigmatized groups, and the perception that AIDS was a death sentence contributed to discrimination against those with AIDS or even those perceived to be at risk for HIV infection. Being tested per se was viewed as a sign that one was at risk. Additionally, among ethnic and racial minority populations, there were concerns that the benefits of early detection might have resulted in further stigma and discrimination (see below), outweighing the benefits of treatment. Thus, recommendations for broader testing might serve to drive those at highest risk underground.

When HIV testing programs were first instituted, HIV-positive individuals were subject to discrimination, and in some cases, even those known to have been *tested* for HIV were assumed to be at high risk. Presently, most HIV testing is voluntary and intended to benefit the person being tested, yet there is mandatory testing in certain situations such as the armed forces and prisons. Both the Congress and state legislatures continue to consider legislation mandating HIV testing for other defined populations. Considering these events, the affected communities have lingering concerns about HIV testing. This history explains why HIV testing was, and still is, thought by many to differ from other clinical testing and public health screening programs, part of a phenomenon often labeled "AIDS exceptionalism" (Bayer, 1991).

As this report was being prepared in 1998, an increasing number of states are requiring positive HIV test results to be reported to state health departments with names or other personal identifiers (Gostin et al., in press). The purpose of most of these requirements is to improve surveillance, as people with HIV infection are living longer and AIDS cases per se have become increasingly less informative about the HIV epidemic (Gostin et al., 1997). Legislation enacted in New York in June 1998, however, includes a provision that would require that HIV-positive individuals be asked about their sexual partners so that health department officials could trace contacts. AIDS activists have expressed concern about the potential loss of privacy that would come from linking surveillance and contact tracing activities, and suggested that these provisions would discourage people from being tested and seeking treatment (Perez-Pena, 1998).

Meeting in January 1998, AIDS activists, public health officials, and others considered the important changes that had occurred in recent years in terms of new diagnostic tests, improved treatment opportunities, and progress in behavioral science and the prevention of HIV risk behaviors, and concluded that their thoughts about HIV testing had not kept pace. The group's consensus is that knowledge of HIV status is desirable because it allows individuals to make informed treatment and prevention decisions. From this starting point, the group agreed on three themes that should guide current HIV testing activities:

1. HIV testing is a tool that should be linked to both prevention and care;
2. HIV testing should be expanded in a variety of settings, guided by public health principles; and
3. Testing strategies must address issues of stigma and social risk.

Although not stated in these terms, the consensus report essentially calls for an end to AIDS exceptionalism, balanced with efforts to reduce the need for a special approach in the first place (Kaiser Family Foundation, 1998b). Making testing more routine, in itself, can also help to reduce the stigma associated with testing per se.

Newborn HIV Screening

Newborn HIV screening was introduced in the late 1980s for the purpose of surveillance, not case finding, when public health officials in some states and at the Centers for Disease Control and Prevention (CDC) realized that blood samples routinely taken from all newborns for PKU testing also could be tested for HIV. Because these tests detected maternal antibodies, they revealed the mothers' and not the babies' HIV status. Since no known treatment for HIV-positive children or means to prevent transmission existed at that time, anonymous or "blind" testing was considered acceptable, and, since it was blind, women would not refuse to be tested based on known or perceived HIV risks, so prevalence data would be unbiased. This survey, known as the Survey of Childbearing Women (Davis et al., 1995), was thus extremely valuable for surveillance purposes, and indeed was the only truly reliable national surveillance data on HIV prevalence in any defined population (NRC, 1989).

In the mid-1990s New York State legislators and others argued, in the interest of the HIV-positive children whose status was not known to their parents or guardians, that the results should be "unblinded," as described in Appendix L, and CDC soon discontinued the Survey of Childbearing Women nationally. New York statutes now require notification of parents and health care providers of all infants with positive HIV tests, so what was a surveillance activity became a case finding program. As described in Chapter 1, the Ryan White Comprehensive AIDS Resources Emergency (CARE) Act Amendments of 1996 could, under certain conditions, obligate other states to institute similar programs. Such mandatory newborn screening approaches have been criticized as providing only limited benefits to the children found to be positive (compared to prenatal diagnosis of the mother), unable to prevent transmission from mother to child, and seriously intruding on the privacy and autonomy of the mothers, whose HIV status is actually being determined.

New York's "Baby AIDS" law illustrates the need for flexible policies that can accommodate new scientific and clinical information. According to Appendix L, by the early 1990s, PCP prophylaxis had been shown to be effective in preventing pneumonia in HIV-infected newborns. The New York City Child Welfare Administration's policy, however, made it difficult to test children in foster care for HIV, even if it was suspected that they were infected. Given these circumstances, and the lack of evidence at that time that transmission could be prevented, "unblinding" the results made sense, as a response the foster care situation in New York City. By the time that the idea of unblinding the heel-stick test results overcame political opposition and became law, the AIDS Clinical Trials Group protocol number 76 (ACTG 076) results had already shown transmission could be prevented. The law, thus, may have been an appropriate response to the situation before 1994, when it was first conceptualized. With its focus on newborn rather than prenatal testing, however, the law does not reflect current public health and clinical preventive approaches.

Community Response to HIV Testing

The advocacy of articulate, politically sophisticated organizations in the gay community has had a tremendous impact on AIDS policies. With the shift in the epidemic toward African-American and Hispanic populations in recent years, current support for protections against discrimination and voluntary measures to control the epidemic may be seriously eroded. These minority groups have limited advocacy organizations and resources needed to protect their rights. As the epidemic continues to affect people living in poverty and people who have historically been disenfranchised, there is an increased risk that testing can and will be used to discriminate against people infected with, or even thought to be infected with, HIV and will further isolate people with AIDS. Thus, policy decisions must incorporate strong protections for those who are already suffering from discrimination.

The potential for such regressive policies is underscored by the epidemiology of perinatal HIV transmission, characterized by its disproportionate impact on African-American and Hispanic women, and the devastation to their lives, their families, and their communities. These women must be the focus of increased prevention and treatment efforts. The interaction of race, gender, and social class will continue to be critical factors to be addressed as new policies are developed, implemented, and evaluated.

Much of the voiced African-American opposition to HIV testing programs must be understood in the context of historical perceptions of mistrust and fear toward the public health and medical research establishment. This underlying distrust and fear is grounded in a history of medical neglect and significant violations of human subjects in research, especially in the Tuskegee Study of Untreated Syphilis in the Negro Male (Jones, 1993; Gamble, 1993, 1997). A formal apology for this treatment, issued by President Clinton in 1997, should help to create a new, more favorable atmosphere on these issues (Thomas and Quinn, 1997).

Without adequate protection such as anonymous testing, case reporting without name identifiers, voluntary partner notification, and strong confidentiality regulations, those people at greatest risk who already feel significant distrust of the public health/government system may not seek HIV testing services. Consequently, there may continue to be a growth in numbers of unknowingly infected individuals, higher mortality rates than among those whose infection is detected early, tremendous budgetary strains on the health care delivery system, and more HIV-infected babies. This situation could spark public support for repressive policies against those suspected to be HIV-infected (Stoddard and Reiman, 1990; Lovvorn and Quinn, 1997).

CONCLUSIONS

Public health screening programs have helped to control epidemics of infectious disease and to target treatment for chronic diseases. The examples in this section, especially congenital syphilis and MSAFP, illustrate the tangible public health benefits of perinatal screening efforts. In practice, however, when screening is conducted in contexts of prevalent gender inequality, racial discrimination, sexual taboos, and poverty, these conditions shape the attitudes and beliefs of health system and public health decision makers as well as patients, including those who have lost confidence that the health care system will treat them fairly. Thus, if screening programs are poorly conceived, organized, or implemented, they may lead to interventions of questionable merit and enhance the vulnerability of groups and individuals.

3

Descriptive Epidemiology of the Perinatal Transmission of HIV

In 1997, at least 432 cases of perinatally transmitted AIDS were reported in the United States (CDC, 1997c). This number, however, represents only a small fraction of the number of individuals affected by this problem. First, these AIDS cases represent children born with HIV infection in 1997 and earlier years. Most of the AIDS cases resulting from children born with HIV infection in 1997 have not yet been diagnosed or reported. Second, although only a fraction of childbearing women with HIV pass the infection on to their children, each of the 6,000 to 7,000 HIV-infected women who gives birth each year requires treatment to prevent transmission as well as for her own infection. Finally, each of the millions of women who become pregnant each year must confront the possibility that she might be infected and could pass the virus on to her child.

To evaluate the progress that has already been made in implementing the Public Health Service (PHS) counseling and testing guidelines for pregnant women (CDC, 1995b), and to identify additional approaches to preventing perinatal transmission, it is important to understand recent trends and current characteristics of women and children with HIV infection and AIDS. To that end, this chapter describes the advantages and difficulties in current surveillance data systems, and presents descriptive information on the epidemiology of perinatal transmission.

HIV/AIDS SURVEILLANCE DATA

The impact of the HIV/AIDS epidemic can be seen in a variety of ways. Where available, data on new HIV infections and individuals infected with HIV are preferable, but data of this sort are often not available because, in many individuals, HIV is undetected or unreported. The HIV/AIDS epidemic, therefore, is often viewed through the imperfect lens of AIDS cases. AIDS is a clinically observable syndrome that is clearly defined and required to be reported in every state. Many individuals with new HIV infections have not progressed in their disease to the point that AIDS can be diagnosed, so AIDS statistics reflect HIV infections that occurred up to a decade or more in the past. Thus, five different type of epidemiological data can shed light on trends and patterns in perinatal transmission of HIV: (1) reported cases of AIDS in women, (2) reported cases of AIDS in children, (3) reported HIV infections in women (where available), (4) estimates of the prevalence of HIV in childbearing women based on the Survey of Childbearing Women (SCBW) (see below), and (5) reported HIV infections in newborn children. Data on HIV infections in children are typically available only in states with mandatory HIV reporting. These states monitor perinatally exposed children to see if they convert from HIV-positive due to maternal antibodies to HIV infection and AIDS status. Each type of data has its strengths and weaknesses, but taken together it is possible to construct a relatively complete picture of the perinatal HIV epidemic in the United States.

AIDS case reports, the source of the first two data series mentioned above, are gathered by state, territorial, and local health departments and reported to the Centers for Disease Control and Prevention (CDC) to form a national AIDS surveillance system. Standard CDC records for each case include information on age at diagnosis, sex, race and ethnicity, state of residence (and metropolitan area, if relevant), mode of exposure to HIV (including maternal risk for pediatric cases), month of AIDS diagnosis, date reported to CDC, and other information. The national data are made available in terms of biannual tabular reports (CDC, 1997c), an AIDS Public Information Data Set (APIDS) (CDC, 1997a), and other reports from CDC (see, for example, CDC, 1996a, 1997e; Wortley and Fleming, 1997). Many states also routinely produce HIV/AIDS surveillance reports.

Even though nearly all current pediatric AIDS cases are the result of perinatal transmission, information on reported AIDS in children provides only limited insight into the problem. First, many children infected with HIV perinatally do not develop AIDS until they are substantially older. There seems to be a bimodal distribution; approximately 48% of HIV-infected children develop AIDS by three years of age, and thereafter less than 3% per year develop AIDS (Pliner et al., 1998). Diagnosed AIDS cases thus reflect perinatal transmissions in births years earlier. Second, once diagnosed, AIDS data are subject to reporting delays. Overall, only 55% of cases are reported to CDC within three months of diagnosis, but 20% are reported more than one year after diagnosis (CDC, 1997a). Reporting delays are longer for pediatric cases (an average of six months) than for adult cases (which average three months). Published data are sometimes adjusted for reporting delays (CDC, 1997a), but by their nature these adjustments cannot be precise.[1]

HIV data for women and children are more problematic. As of December 1997, HIV cases are reportable in only 30 states (in 3 of these states for children only). These states reported only 28% of all prenatally acquired AIDS cases through September 1997 (CDC, 1997e). Even in these states, the data count only individuals who have been tested, not all HIV-infected individuals.

Between 1988 and 1994, most states anonymously tested newborn heel-stick blood samples for HIV in a program called the Survey of Childbearing Women (SCBW) (Davis et al., 1995). Because newborn blood carries maternal HIV antibodies, data from this survey reflect the prevalence of HIV in childbearing women. As described in Chapter 2, this survey was discontinued, but some states have continued to test newborn blood in the same way and report the results (see Appendix D). In addition, Byers and colleagues (1998) have been able to project the data from this survey to more recent years, yet the lack of recent data complicates the assessment of the impact of the PHS counseling and treatment guidelines.

HIV AND AIDS IN WOMEN

In 1997, women accounted for 21% of AIDS cases in adults, and the proportion of all cases that are female continues to grow. Most of these cases are attributed to injection drug use (32%) or heterosexual contact (38%). Since most of the women in the second category attribute their infection to sex with an injection drug user (29%) or sex with an HIV-infected partner with unknown risk (64%) (CDC, 1997c), at least two-thirds of AIDS cases in women can be directly or indirectly attributed to injection drug use. Although a subset of women with HIV have injected drugs or have had sex with a known injection drug user, an increasing proportion of women have become infected through sexual activity with men whose risk behaviors were unknown to them.

In 1997, 60% of AIDS cases reported in women were in African-American, non-Hispanic women, and 20% were in Hispanic women (CDC, 1997e). AIDS incidence rates are highest in African Americans (58.8 per 100,000 women) and Hispanics (21.5 per 100,000 women), compared to 3.0 per 100,000 in white, non-Hispanic women. AIDS is more prevalent in women in the Northeast (22.3 per 100,000 women in 1995) and the South (11.1 per 100,000 in 1995). While AIDS in women is also more common in large cities—74% of 1995 cases were in metropolitan areas with more than one million population—the greatest increases

---

[1]Furthermore, the published data are restricted in order to protect confidentiality. In particular, the APIDS system suppresses table cells with three or fewer cases in a state or MSA (metropolitan statistical area), even if data are aggregated over multiple areas. In addition, the most recent *HIV/ AIDS Surveillance Report* (CDC, 1997c) contains cases reported to CDC through December 1997, while the latest APIDS release (CDC, 1997a) includes cases reported through December 1996.

in incidence between 1991 and 1995 were in women in the South and younger women, those who were 14 to 18 years old in 1988 (Wortley and Fleming, 1997).

Approximately 6,000 to 7,000 HIV-infected women give birth every year (Byers et al., 1998). According to the SCBW, overall, 17 per 10,000 women giving birth are infected with HIV (Davis et al., 1995). Trend data show a relatively steady national rate of HIV prevalence in childbearing women between 1989 and 1994, the last year for which data are available. There are, however, important regional variations. In the Northeast, where the epidemic started and peaked earliest, a 25% decline occurred in the number of HIV-infected childbearing women between 1990 and 1994. In the South, where the epidemic started later, there was a 25% increase between 1989 and 1991, and a level trend thereafter. The West and Midwest had stable and relatively low rates (Appendix D).

Estimates of the proportion of children born to HIV-infected women who are themselves infected with HIV vary, ranging from 14% to 33% in studies performed in the United States and Europe before the ACTG 076 (AIDS Clincal Trials Group protocol number 76) results became known. More recent estimates of the transmission rate, reflecting partial implementation of the ACTG 076 protocol, range from 3% to 10% (see Chapter 4).

PERINATALLY TRANSMITTED AIDS

Taking into account changing prevalence and transmission rates, perinatal transmission of HIV accounted for a cumulative total of 7,335 AIDS cases and an unknown number of HIV-infected children in the United States as of December 1997 (CDC, 1997c). There were 473 cases of pediatric AIDS (i.e., under age 13 at time of diagnosis) reported in 1997, and a total of 8,086 since the beginning of the epidemic (CDC, 1997c). Of the 473 cases in 1997, 432 (91%) were born to mothers with or at risk for HIV infection, as shown in Table 3.1. The breakout by mother's risk indicates that 107 (25%) of the known perinatally transmitted cases had mothers who used injection drugs, and an additional 60 (14%) of the mothers had sex with an injection drug user. Drug use is probably responsible for a substantial proportion of the cases born to the 249 (58%) mothers with HIV infection whose risk is not specified or who had sex with an HIV infected person whose risk is not specified. Injection drug use, therefore, is associated with between 39% and 72% of perinatally acquired AIDS.

The number of reported perinatally acquired AIDS cases rose rapidly in the late 1980s and early 1990s, peaked around 1992, and subsequently declined by approximately 43% by 1996 (see Figure 3.1). In 1997, 473 cases of pediatric AIDS were reported (CDC, 1997c).[2] This decline was due to a number of factors.

---

[2]The 1997 figure is not adjusted for reporting delays, so is not comparable to the numbers in Figure 3.1.

TABLE 3.1 Pediatric AIDS Cases by Exposure Category, Reported in 1997 and Cumulative Total through December 1997

Exposure Category	1997 No.	(%)	Cumulative No.	(%)
Hemophilia/coagulation disorder	1	(0)	233	(3)
Mother with/at risk for HIV infection	432	(91)	7,335	(91)
Injecting drug use	107		2,936	
Sex with injecting drug user	60		1,340	
Sex with bisexual male	7		159	
Sex with person with hemophilia	2		28	
Sex with transfusion recipient	—		24	
Sex with HIV-infected person, risk not specified	102		1,033	
Receipt of blood transfusion, blood components, or tissue	7		154	
Has HIV infection, risk not specified	147		1,661	
Receipt of blood transfusion, blood components, or tissue	2	(0)	374	(5)
Risk not reported or identified	38	(8)	144	(2)
Total	473	(100)	8,086	(100)

SOURCE: CDC, 1997c.

First, CDC calculations based on the SCBW and other data show that between 1992 and 1995, there was a 17% decline in the number of births to HIV-infected women (Byers et al., 1998). Much of the rest has been attributed to increased testing and adherence to the ACTG 076 regimen and better prenatal and intrapartum care. Declines that occurred before the publication of the ACTG 076 findings have been attributed to broader use of ZDV (zidovudine) by women, regardless of pregnancy (see Appendix D).

Because good seroprevalence data are lacking for children, we must use AIDS case reports to understand changes in perinatally transmitted HIV. Reflecting the racial and ethnic composition of women with AIDS, perinatally transmitted cases were concentrated in African-American (60%) and Hispanic (24%) children in 1997.[3] These proportions have remained relatively stable for a decade. The disparity appears greater, however, when the numbers of African-American, Hispanic, and other births are taken into account. In 1996, perinatal AIDS incidence rates (perinatal AIDS cases as a proportion of births) were roughly four times higher for African Americans than for the entire population

---

[3]Here and elsewhere in this chapter, white, other, and unknown races are combined because of small numbers.

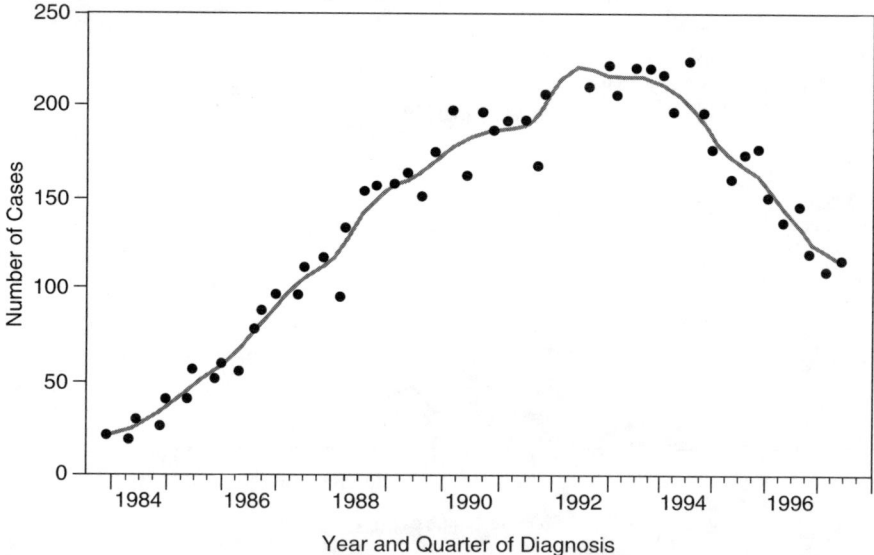

FIGURE 3.1   Number of perinatally acquired AIDS cases, by quarter year of diagnosis, 1984 through 1997. Estimates are based on cases reported through September 1997, adjusted for reporting delay and unreported risk but not for incomplete reporting of diagnosed AIDS cases. Points represent estimated quarterly incidence, and the line represents "smoothed" incidence. SOURCE: CDC, 1997e.

(65 versus 16 per 10,000 births), and higher than average among Hispanics (19 per 10,000 births). The incidence rate for whites and others is substantially lower than average (3 per 10,000 births), leading to a 32 to 1 differential between African-American and white incidence rates (CDC, 1996b; Ventura et al., 1997).

Figure 3.2 shows trends in the number of perinatal AIDS cases, by race and ethnicity, from 1979 through 1996. The number of African-American children with AIDS grew through 1992 and fell by about 42% between 1992 and 1996. The number of cases in Hispanic children was relatively flat from 1987 through 1992 and fell by 43% between 1992 and 1996. The number of perinatal AIDS cases in white children fell by 50% between 1992 and 1996.

Trends by age at diagnosis (Table 3.2) show that the largest declines are among children diagnosed as infants, with substantial declines also among children diagnosed at ages one to five years. For older children, similar levels of decline have not been observed (CDC, 1997d). These findings are consistent with the expectation that efforts to prevent perinatal transmission would be reflected earliest in infants because older children were born before antiretroviral therapy was used widely in pregnancy (Appendix D).

Pneumocystis carinii pneumonia (PCP) is the most common AIDS-defining condition in children. Since recommendations regarding PCP prophylaxis were

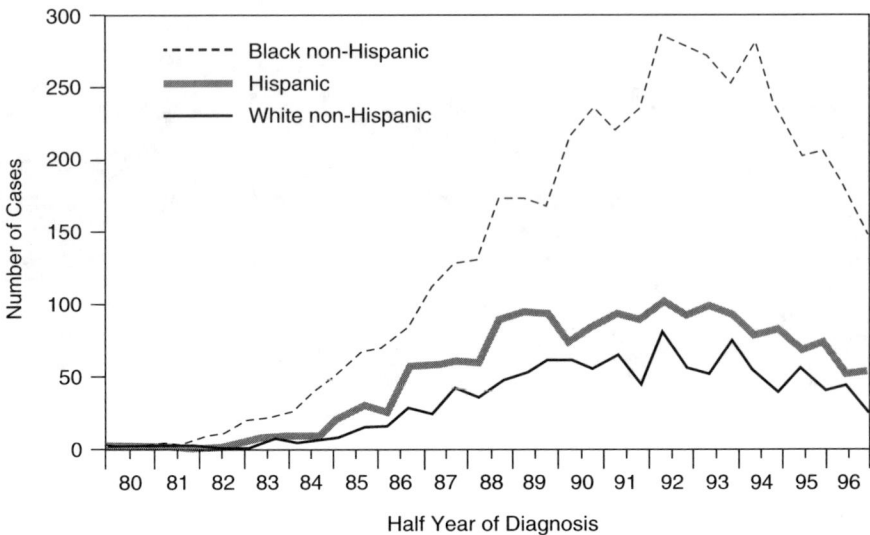

FIGURE 3.2 Number of perinatally acquired AIDS cases, by race and half year of diagnosis, 1979 through 1996. Estimates are based on cases reported through September 1997, adjusted for reporting delay and unreported risk but not for incomplete reporting of diagnosed AIDS cases. SOURCE: Lindegren et al., 1998.

evolving during the same period that dramatic declines occurred in perinatally acquired pediatric AIDS cases, it is useful to look at whether declines in pediatric AIDS reflect more than declines in PCP. CDC surveillance findings show substantial declines not only in PCP, but also in other opportunistic infections for which specific prophylaxis was not available, indicating that the decline in pediatric AIDS cases is not being driven solely by changes in PCP, but appears to reflect true declining perinatal HIV transmission rates.

Pediatric AIDS cases are concentrated in eastern states, and especially in the New York metropolitan area. In 1996, three states alone—New York, New Jersey, and Florida—reported 330 cases. This represents 49% of the diagnosed cases, even though only 15% of children are born in those states (CDC, 1996b; Ventura et al., 1998). In contrast to their concentration in the Northeast, perinatal AIDS cases are less common in most geographical areas. In 1997, 39 states had fewer than ten perinatally transmitted AIDS cases (CDC, 1997e).

Figure 3.3 displays pediatric AIDS incidence rates (perinatal AIDS cases as a proportion of births) by state for 1996 as an illustration of this great variability, ranging from 30.9 per 10,000 births in the District of Columbia to zero in 14 states. The District of Columbia, Florida (6.3 per 10,000), New York (6.1 per 10,000), New Jersey (4.3 per 10,000), Connecticut (3.8 per 10,000), and Maryland (3.0 per

TABLE 3.2   Estimated Number of Children with Perinatally Acquired AIDS, by Selected Characteristics, Year of Diagnosis, and Percentage Change from 1992 to 1996,United States, 1992–1996[a]

Characteristic	Year					% Change 1992 to 1996
	1992	1993	1994	1995	1996	
Race/Ethnicity[b]						
White, non-Hispanic	133	126	92	95	67	−50%
Black, non-Hispanic	566	531	522	415	331	−42%
Hispanic	195	195	166	146	111	−43%
Age at AIDS Diagnosis						
<5 years	733	693	613	459	360	−51%
≥5 years	168	169	179	202	156	−7%
Region[c]						
Northeast	361	379	315	265	212	−41%
South	362	315	332	243	223	−38%
Midwest	60	74	54	67	30	−50%
West	67	58	65	60	35	−48%
Metropolitan Statistical Area						
>500,000 pop.	748	732	675	558	450	−40%
50,000–500,000 pop.	102	75	75	62	41	−60%
<50,000 pop.	51	53	42	39	22	−57%

[a]Diagnosed through 1996 and reported through September 1997 adjusting for reporting delays and unreported risk.

[b]Numbers for other racial/ethnic groups were too small for meaningful analysis.

[c]Northeast = Connecticut, Maine, Massachusetts, New Hampshire, New Jersey, New York, Pennsylvania, Rhode Island, and Vermont; South = Alabama, Arkansas, Delaware, District of Columbia, Florida, Georgia, Kentucky, Louisiana, Maryland, Mississippi, North Carolina, Oklahoma, South Carolina, Tennessee, Texas, Virginia, and West Virginia; West = Alaska, Arizona, California, Colorado, Hawaii, Idaho, Montana, Nevada, New Mexico, Oregon, Utah, Washington, and Wyoming; and Midwest = Illinois, Indiana, Iowa, Kansas, Michigan, Minnesota, Missouri, Nebraska, North Dakota, Ohio, South Dakota, and Wisconsin.

SOURCE: CDC, 1997e.

10,000) have the highest incidence rates. Illinois (1.4 per 10,000), California (0.9 per 10,000), and Texas (0.5 per 10,000) have incidence rates lower than the national average of 1.7 per 10,000 (CDC, 1996b; Ventura et al., 1998).

Reviewing the data by metropolitan statistical areas (MSAs) suggests that perinatal AIDS cases were even more concentrated than the state analysis suggests. In fact, two of the three MSAs with the greatest number of perinatal AIDS cases (New York City and Newark, New Jersey) are in the New York metropoli-

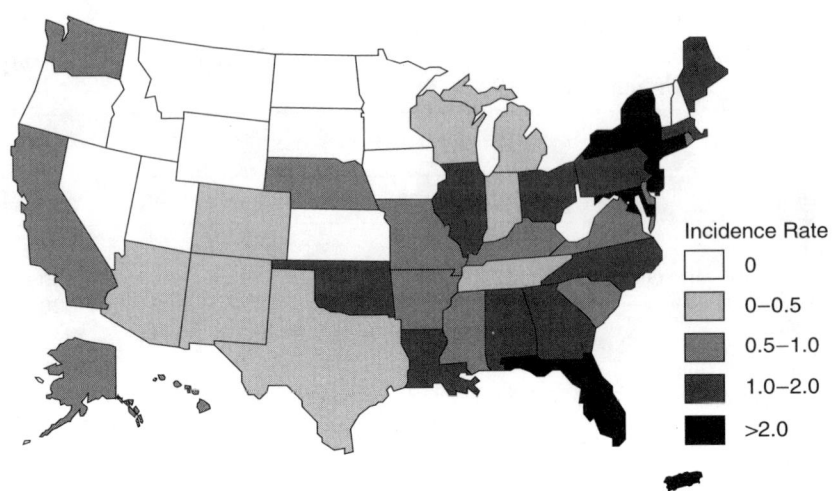

FIGURE 3.3   Annual incidence rates for perinatal AIDS, 1996, by state. SOURCE: calculated from CDC, 1996b; Ventura et al., 1998.

tan area. These two MSAs alone account for 38% of all perinatal AIDS cases in the United States. Data on the distribution of AIDS cases within New York City suggest that the concentration varies substantially by neighborhood (NRC, 1993), and this patchwork pattern is likely to be found for perinatal AIDS cases as well.

Perinatal transmission cases are similarly less common in most metropolitan areas. Out of the 253 MSAs for which AIDS data are available, only 66 (26%) have had more than ten reported perinatal cases from the beginning of the epidemic through the end of 1996. Only 24 MSAs (9%), have 50 or more cumulative cases each.

4

Natural History, Detection, and Treatment of HIV Infection in Pregnant Women and Newborns

In the United States the transmission of HIV from mother to infant (known as perinatal or vertical transmission) accounts for almost all new HIV infections in children (CDC, 1997c). Prior to the widespread use of antiretroviral therapy, transmission rates ranging from 14% to 33% were reported in the United States and Western Europe (Report of a Consensus Workshop, 1992). In the developing world, rates as high as 43% have been reported (Datta et al., 1994).

Recent improvements in the understanding of the timing and pathogenesis of perinatal HIV infection have allowed the development of effective strategies to prevent perinatal HIV transmission. The prenatal identification of HIV-seropositive women is crucial for the successful implementation of these strategies. In addition, it allows for optimal medical management of HIV-infected women and their infants. Improved detection and treatment of HIV infection in pregnant women has greatly reduced perinatal HIV transmission in the United States. In addition, advances in the early diagnosis and treatment of HIV-infected infants have markedly improved the clinical outcome following perinatal infection.

TIMING OF HIV TRANSMISSION

HIV transmission from mother to infant can occur antepartum (in utero), intrapartum (during labor or delivery), or postpartum (through breast-feeding) (Report of a Consensus Workshop, 1992). Available data suggest that at most 25% to 30% of perinatal HIV transmission occurs in utero (Rogers et al., 1989; Ehrnst et al., 1991; Luzuriaga et al., 1993). Evidence of infection in aborted first trimester fetal tissues has been reported (Sprecher et al., 1986), though potential contamination with maternal blood has not always been excluded. The intrauterine transmission of HIV is also suggested by the occasional isolation of HIV from amniotic fluid and cells. Finally, the isolation of HIV from, or the detection of the HIV genome in, blood samples obtained at birth from some HIV-infected infants also suggests intrauterine HIV transmission (Rogers et al., 1989; Ehrnst et al., 1991; Luzuriaga et al., 1993). The proportion of infants infected during each trimester of pregnancy is unknown.

Indirect evidence suggests that 70% to 75% or more of vertical HIV transmission can occur during delivery (Ehrnst et al., 1991; Luzuriaga et al., 1993; Rogers et al., 1994). Negative diagnostic studies in the first two days of life followed by the detection of infection after one week of age are compatible with intrapartum transmission (Luzuriaga et al., 1993). Increased risk of vertical HIV transmission has been correlated with increased duration of rupture of the membranes prior to delivery, particularly in the presence of acute chorioamnionitis (Landesman et al., 1996; Popek et al., 1997). A higher risk of transmission to the firstborn twin, particularly following prolonged labor (Duliege et al., 1995), also supports the concept of intrapartum transmission. The mechanism(s) of intrapartum transmission are unknown, but might include transplacental microtransfusion or infection through mucocutaneous exposure to maternal blood or cervical secretions. The establishment of infection following the inoculation of the simian homolog of HIV (simian immunodeficiency virus) into the conjunctival sac or oropharynx of newborn macaque monkeys also supports the mucocutaneous route of human neonatal infection (Baba et al., 1994).

Vertical HIV transmission can also occur through breast-feeding (Ziegler et al., 1985; Bulterys et al., 1995). HIV RNA and proviral DNA have been detected using the polymerase chain reaction (PCR) in breast milk; viral load appears to be particularly high in colostrum (Ruff et al., 1994). Large, prospective cohort studies suggest an increased risk of transmission associated with breast-feeding. In a meta-analysis, Dunn and colleagues (1992) have estimated that the proportion of transmission attributable to breast-feeding worldwide from an HIV-seropositive woman is 14% (95% confidence interval, 7% to 22%). The risk of breast milk transmission appears to be particularly high when maternal primary infection occurs within the first few months following delivery (Palasanthiran et al., 1993). For these reasons, HIV-seropositive women in industrialized countries are advised not to breast-feed their babies (AAP, 1995a). In July 1998, the World Health Organization recommended that HIV-infected women in developing countries be given information about the benefits and risks of breast-feeding, and an opportunity to make an informed choice about breast-feeding (WHO, 1998).

FACTORS ASSOCIATED WITH HIV MATERNAL–CHILD TRANSMISSION

The observed variability in reported transmission rates probably reflects the multiple factors that influence perinatal HIV transmission. Several studies have linked high maternal viral loads to increased risk of HIV perinatal transmission (Borkowsky et al., 1994; Weiser et al., 1994; Dickover et al., 1996; Cao et al., 1997; Thea et al., 1997). In aggregate, however, there is no identified absolute viral threshold value that can discriminate between transmitters and nontransmitters. Transmission may be observed across the full range of viral levels.

Maternal immune depletion also appears to correlate with vertical HIV transmission. Several cohort studies have documented an increased risk of vertical transmission with maternal AIDS or lowered CD4 T-cell counts (Study, 1994; Landesman et al., 1996). Maternal HIV specific immunity may also be important. A reduced risk of transmission has been reported from women with high titers of serum antibodies capable of neutralizing their own viral strains in vitro (Scarlatti et al., 1993). Others, however, have not found any association between maternal neutralizing antibody titers and transmission (Husson et al., 1995). Little is known regarding the potential role of maternal HIV cell-mediated immunity (e.g., HIV specific cytotoxic T-lymphocytes) in protection from transmission.

Recently, an abnormality in a cell surface receptor for HIV (CCR-5) was identified in uninfected adult individuals at high risk for infection through sexual or parental exposure (reviewed in D'Souza and Harden, 1996). Lymphocytes from these individuals were relatively resistant to infection with primary HIV isolates in vitro, suggesting that the defect in the co-receptor may have protected these individuals from infection. The frequency of the homozygous deletion is approximately 1% in Caucasians. It appears to be extremely rare in Asian and African populations. Heterozygous individuals do not appear to be protected from infection. Studies are currently in progress to determine to what extent mutations in infant CCR-5 alleles and other cellular HIV co-receptors may influence perinatal HIV transmission.

Other sexually transmitted infections may increase the risk of perinatal HIV transmission. An increased risk of vertical HIV transmission with maternal vitamin A deficiency has been reported (Semba et al., 1994). Duration of membrane rupture, hemorrhage during labor, chorioamnionitis, and invasive procedures during delivery have all been associated with an increased risk of perinatal HIV transmission (Minkoff et al., 1995; Landesman et al., 1996; Mandlebrot et al., 1996).

STRATEGIES TO PREVENT PERINATAL HIV TRANSMISSION

Recent advances in our understanding of the timing and pathogenesis of vertical HIV infection have led to the evaluation of a variety of strategies to prevent vertical HIV transmission, including the management of maternal co-infections, maternal nutritional intervention, bypassing the route of exposure, maternal and infant antiretroviral therapy, and vaccination.

The primary focus has been on the use of perinatal antiretroviral therapy to prevent vertical HIV transmission. Recently, a profound and significant reduction in vertical HIV transmission was observed in mother-infant pairs treated with zidovudine (ZDV; also known as AZT). Those receiving ZDV had a transmission rate of 7.6% compared to 22.6% for those who received placebo (Connor et al., 1994). In this study, therapy consisted of oral administration of ZDV five times per day during pregnancy, intravenous administration of ZDV to the mother during delivery, and six weeks of postnatal treatment of the infant with oral ZDV. The only observed short-term toxicity in ZDV treated infants was anemia, which was not clinically significant. While the risk of vertical HIV transmission in this study was directly correlated with maternal blood viral load and indirectly correlated with maternal CD4 count, the treatment effect was independent of maternal viral load and CD4 count (Sperling et al., 1996).

Studies conducted in the United States and Europe indicate widespread acceptance of the recommended ZDV regimen, and report resultant reductions in transmission rates to between 3% and 10% (Fiscus et al., 1996; Mayaux et al., 1997). In ACTG 185 (AIDS Clinical Trials Group protocol number 185), the ACTG 076 regimen was administered to women with advanced HIV infection and their infants; the perinatal HIV transmission rate was 4.8% (Mofenson, 1998).

The extent to which each component of the ACTG 076 regimen (i.e., the prenatal and intrapartum therapy of the mother and the postpartum therapy of the infant) contributes to this success is unclear. Receipt of only part of the ACTG 076 regimen may be associated with decreased risk of perinatal transmission (Birkhead et al., 1998). Several trials evaluating the efficacy of shorter and less intensive antiretroviral regimens are in progress. In Thailand, the use of short-course oral ZDV administered during the last two weeks of pregnancy and during labor and delivery resulted in a significant decline in HIV perinatal transmission. The estimated HIV transmission risks for placebo and ZDV groups were 18.6% and 9.2%, respectively, representing a 51% decrease in transmission risk (CDC, 1998a).

The most recent Public Health Service Task Force recommendations for the use of antiretroviral drugs among HIV-infected pregnant women in the United States have updated the 1994 guidelines, which were based on the findings of ACTG 076 (CDC, 1998d). Advances in the understanding of the pathogenesis of HIV infection have resulted in recent changes in the standard recommended antiretroviral therapy in HIV-infected adults. Combination drug regimens to maximally suppress the virus are now recommended (CDC, 1998e). Although considerations associated with pregnancy may affect decisions regarding the timing and choice of therapy, pregnancy is not a reason to defer standard combination antiretroviral therapy. It is recommended that offering antiretroviral therapy to HIV-infected women during pregnancy—whether primarily to treat HIV infection, to reduce perinatal transmission, or both—be accompanied by a discussion of the known and unknown potential benefits and risks of such therapy to the woman and infant. Optimal antiretroviral regimens should be discussed and offered to an HIV-infected woman and ZDV prophylaxis for perinatal transmission should be incorporated into those regimens whenever possible (CDC, 1998d).

Potential adverse effects of antiretroviral therapy on the mother and fetus should be discussed during counseling. Experience to date with the administration of antiretrovirals other than ZDV during pregnancy is quite limited. Table 4.1 summarizes the potential toxic effects of these drugs.*

Several programs have been developed to identify potential risks of antiretroviral therapy administered during pregnancy or early infancy. Animal models are often used to screen for potential toxicities and teratogenic properties of antiretroviral agents before these agents are evaluated clinically in humans. While the relevance of these models to human therapy is unproven, they may be useful in identifying agents of concern. Recently, severe congenital anomalies were identified in 3 of 13 infant monkeys born to mothers who had received Efavirenz, a non-nucleoside reverse transcriptase inhibitor, during pregnancy (DuPont-Merck, 1998). The doses used in this study were those anticipated to achieve plasma concentrations similar to those achieved in humans on standard recommended doses of the drug. Congenital anomalies were not observed in any of the 13 infants of mothers treated with the vehicle control. As a result of these studies, women receiving Efavirenz are advised to avoid pregnancy.

The Phase I evaluation of combination antiretroviral regimens, including protease inhibitors, in pregnant women and young infants is now under way through the ACTG. An ACTG Phase II/III trial evaluating the efficacy of nevirapine (a non-nucleoside reverse transcriptase inhibitor) in preventing perinatal HIV transmission is also under way. All ACTG protocol participants exposed to antiretroviral agents in utero or during infancy are encouraged to enroll in ACTG protocol 219, which will evaluate them at least through age 21 for potential long-term sequelae. Several pharmaceutical companies (Glaxo Wellcome, Inc.; Hoffmann-LaRoche, Inc.; Bristol-Myers Squibb Co.; and Merck & Co., Inc.), in cooperation with the Centers for Disease Control and Prevention (CDC), maintain a registry to assess the safety of ZDV, didanosine (ddI), lamivudine (3TC), saquinavir (SAQ), stavudine (d4t), and dideoxycytidine (ddC) during pregnancy. Providers are encouraged to enroll in this registry women who receive any of these drugs during pregnancy. The registry findings did not indicate any increase in the number of birth defects after receipt of ZDV alone. No consistent pattern of birth defects that would suggest a common cause has been observed. The number of cases reported through February 1997, however, was insufficient to reliably estimate the quantitative risk of birth defects after the administration of these agents, alone or in combination, to pregnant women and their infants.

---

*In July, 1998, a high rate of prematurity was reported in a study of infants whose mothers received antiretroviral therapy during pregnancy (Lorenzi et al., 1998). The small numbers of subjects and limited information about background rates of prematurity in this study limit the ability to attribute the prematurity to the antiretroviral therapy, and the PHS treatment recommendations (CDC, 1998d) have not been changed. Ongoing perinatal trials are being monitored intensively to evaluate potential relationships between antiretroviral use and adverse pregnancy outcomes.

TABLE 4.1 Potential Toxic Effects of Antiretrovirals

Antiretroviral Drug	FDA Pregnancy Category	Placental Passage	Long-Term Animal Carcinogenicity Studies	Side Effects
Zidovudine (ZDV)	C	In humans	Positive (rodent, noninvasive vaginal epithelial tumor)	Anemia, gastrointestinal (GI) upset, headache, myopathy
Zalcitabine (ddC)	C	In rhesus monkeys	Positive (rodent thymic lymphomas)	Pancreatitis, stomatitis, peripheral neuropathy
Didanosine (ddI)	B	In humans	Negative	Pancreatitis, diarrhea, peripheral neuropathy
Stavudine (d4T)	C	In rhesus monkeys	Not completed	Pancreatitis, peripheral neuropathy
Lamivudine (3TC)	C	In humans	Negative	Minimal toxicity
Nevirapine	C	In humans	Not completed	Rash
Delavirdine	C	Unknown	Not completed	Rash
Indinavir	C	In rats	Not completed	Nephrolithiasis, hyperbilirubinemia, drug interactions
Ritonavir	B	In rats	Not completed	GI upset, paresthesias, drug interactions
Saquinavir (SAQ)	B	In rats/rabbits	Not completed	GI upset
Nelfinavir	B	Unknown	Not completed	Diarrhea
Efavirenz (EF)			Congenital anomalies in 13 infant monkeys whose mothers received EF during gestation	Central Nervous System (anencephaly, microphthalmia, cleft palate)

SOURCES: CDC 1998c, 1998d, 1998e; Dupont-Merck, 1998

Since maternal sexually transmitted diseases or chorioamnionitis may increase the risk of vertical HIV transmission, efforts to prevent, detect, or treat these infections are important. Similarly, since active drug use may increase the risk of perinatal transmission (Landesman et al., 1996; Rodriguez et al., 1996) and may interfere with the ability of expectant women to seek and comply with appropriate medical care, efforts to improve access to drug treatment programs for pregnant women are also important.

As previously discussed, a majority of infants acquire HIV infection during delivery through mucosal exposure to maternal blood and/or vaginal secretions. Optimizing obstetrical practices (e.g., limiting the duration of rupture of membranes prior to delivery, avoidance of invasive procedures including scalp electrodes during delivery) might help to limit the risk of transmission. Cesarean section has been proposed as a means of reducing the risk of exposure, particularly if performed prior to the rupture of membranes. A meta-analysis suggested that cesarean section might protect against vertical HIV transmission (Rogers, 1997). In a recently reported study, cesarean section appeared to reduce the risk of vertical HIV-1 transmission; however, the benefit of cesarean section was only apparent when performed prior to the onset of labor and in mother-infant pairs who received ZDV (Mandelbrot et al., 1998). Virocidal cleansing of the birth canal prior to vaginal delivery has also been proposed as a means of reducing intrapartum HIV transmission, though a study in Malawi that evaluated chlorhexidine vaginal cleansing during labor did not find an overall reduction in transmission (Biggar et al., 1996). There was, however, a reduction in transmission if the chlorhexidine was administered to women whose membranes ruptured at least four hours prior to delivery (Biggar et al., 1996).

DIAGNOSIS OF HIV INFECTION IN WOMEN AND INFANTS

The HIV testing algorithm recommended by the Public Health Service (PHS) for pregnant women is comprised of initial screening with a Food and Drug Administration (FDA) licensed enzyme-linked immunosorbent assay (ELISA). Confirmatory testing of repeatedly reactive ELISAs with an FDA-licensed supplemental test (e.g., Western blot or immunofluorescence assay) must be done. The diagnosis of HIV infection in adults requires that both the ELISA and the confirmatory test be positive. According to the manufacturers, the third generation ELISAs are 100% sensitive (probability that the test will be positive if the individual tested is truly infected) in individuals infected long enough to have developed HIV antibodies and 99.9% specific (probability that the test will be negative if the individual tested is truly not infected). Despite these excellent performance characteristics, there may be a problem with false positive results in low-prevalence areas. For example, in a population of pregnant women where the prevalence of HIV is 0.03%, only 23% of samples with positive ELISA would be found to be truly positive by confirmatory Western blot test. In a high-prevalence area with 2% HIV infection, the positive predictive value of the ELISA would increase to 95% (see Appendix K).

To maximize prevention efforts, women must be identified as HIV-infected as early as possible during pregnancy. Early diagnosis of HIV infection allows the mother to avail herself of effective antiretroviral therapy for her own health, and that can significantly reduce perinatal transmission. Women who know their HIV status can be counseled not to breast-feed their infants. HIV-infected pregnant women can also be referred to appropriate psychological, social, legal, and substance abuse services.

Reporting of conventional ELISA and Western blot tests typically takes one to two weeks. At present, one rapid test (Single Use Diagnostic System HIV Test, Murex Corporation, Norcross, Georgia) is commercially available in the United States. As discussed in Chapter 7, an accurate rapid test would have utility among pregnant women in labor who do not know their HIV status. It would help identify HIV-infected pregnant women whose infants might still benefit from the intrapartum and postpartum components of the ACTG 076 regimen. Rapid tests can also be performed on newborns to ascertain their HIV exposure. The sensitivity and specificity of current rapid assays are comparable to those of ELISAs. Because the predictive value varies with the prevalence of HIV infection in the population tested, the positive predictive value of the test will be low in populations with low-prevalence, yielding many false positive results. A reactive rapid test must therefore be confirmed by standard testing. If a second rapid test is licensed, its performance would be independent of the current test, and the sensitivity and specificity of the pair would be sufficient for use in perinatal settings (CDC, 1998g). See Chapter 7 for further discussion.

Early diagnosis of HIV-infected infants is crucial for optimal medical management. Serologic methods are of limited utility for the early diagnosis of perinatal HIV infection. With efficient transfer of antibodies from an infected woman to her fetus during the third trimester of pregnancy, all infants born at or near term to an HIV-infected woman will be HIV-seropositive; uninfected infants may retain passively acquired antibodies through 18 months of age.

The detection of HIV proviral genome in peripheral blood mononuclear cells using the polymerase chain reaction (DNA PCR) is a highly sensitive, specific, rapid, and cost-effective screening test for vertical infection (Bremer et al., 1996; Luzuriaga et al., 1996). Using DNA PCR, 25% to 30% of infected infants may be identified at birth and the remaining 70% to 75% of infected infants can be identified by one month of age. According to the guidelines, the evaluation of the infants' infection status should begin within 48 hours of birth, with repeated evaluations at one to two weeks and at one, two, and six months (CDC, 1998c). Infants with single positive DNA PCR results should have a follow-up blood specimen drawn immediately for confirmatory studies (DNA PCR and viral isolation). The likelihood of infection is extremely low in those infants with negative DNA PCR studies through 6 months of age; subsequent serologic follow-up through 18 months of age is advised to document the loss of passively acquired maternal antibodies (CDC, 1998c).

Because transmission of HIV occurs primarily in utero and intrapartum, there is only limited utility in infant testing. When maternal serostatus is unknown, however, HIV antibody testing of the newborn is important for the identification of children at risk for perinatal HIV infection and early referral for appropriate medical evaluation and care. Control of viral replication and preservation of the developing immune system have been demonstrated in infants who initiated intensive combination antiretroviral therapy in early infancy (Luzuriaga et al., 1997). In addition, the initiation of prophylaxis against PCP at age four to six weeks has been recommended for all infants born to HIV-infected women; such prophylaxis should be continued until HIV infection has been excluded (CDC, 1995a).

SUMMARY

Perinatal transmission can occur antepartum, intrapartum, and postpartum. Several factors, including maternal and virologic factors, fetal factors, placental conditions, obstetric factors and breast-feeding, may influence the risk of perinatal transmission. Recent improvements in our understanding of the timing and pathogenesis of perinatal HIV infection have allowed the development of effective strategies to prevent perinatal HIV transmission. To maximize prevention efforts, women must be identified as HIV-infected as early as possible during pregnancy and offered effective antiretroviral therapy. Postnatal evaluation of the HIV at-risk infant, beginning immediately after birth, is important for early diagnosis and optimal medical management.

5

Context of Services for Women and Children Affected by HIV/AIDS

The committee's recommendations must reflect the complex health care system within which they might be implemented. Nations with a more integrated system of health care, universal health insurance, and/or a central organizational body that promulgates and enforces regulations might develop different approaches to the reduction of perinatal HIV transmission than those available in the United States. But in this country, women and children, including those at risk for or with HIV/AIDS, receive their health care from a variety of sources, depending in large part on their economic situation, the availability of providers, and their understanding of and comfort with the health care system in their community. Their care is financed by a mixture of public and/or private insurance and public funds; its content and quality are influenced by public and professional organizations; and oversight and regulation are achieved through a combination of national, state, and local authorities. These characteristics (see Table 5.1) and the fact that the health care system in the United States is undergoing rapid change, contribute to the challenges inherent in implementing the committee's recommendations.

This chapter first examines the community-level sites where women of childbearing age receive health care and how that care has been supplemented to meet the additional needs of women and children at risk for or with HIV/AIDS. This is followed by a review of the mechanisms for financing health care and of the organizations responsible for developing and implementing policies concerning maternity and HIV services. The chapter analyzes current trends in health care and social services to determine how they may affect access to services important for reducing the risk of perinatal HIV transmission and treating those already

TABLE 5.1 Sources of Care for Pregnant Women

Provider	Source of Funding for Service	Eligibility for Service	Oversight/Reporting by Provider	HIV Guidance
Practicing physicians and nurse practitioners	Patient fees; insurance; Medicaid	Determined by provider and/or MCO	State licensing authority: MCO	CDC; professional organizations; sometimes MCOs
Health department clinics (state and local)	Federal (especially MCHSBG), state, local governments; Medicaid; patient fees; sometimes insurance	Usually all within jurisdiction, with some limits based on income	Federal, state, and local governments or boards of health	CDC; state health departments; some local health departments
Community, migrant, and homeless health centers	Largely federal (BPHC); some state and local governments Medicaid; patient fees; insurance	May restrict to catchment area	Federal (BPHC), state, local governments; boards of directors	CDC; BPHC; state and local governments
Public and non-profit hospital outpatient facilities	Some state and local subsidies; Medicaid; patient fees; insurance	Public: usually all within community served Non-profit: usually no restriction	Public: governmental unit Non-profit: board of directors	
Family planning clinics, and women's health centers	Federal (especially family planning funds), state, local governments; Medicaid; patient fees	Usually no restrictions	Federal (Office of Population Affairs, DHHS), state, and local governments or boards of health; boards of directors	Office of Population Affairs (DHHS); CDC, state health departments, and some local health departments
Drug treatment facilities	Federal (especially SAMHSA), state, local governments	Few restrictions	Federal (SAMHSA), state, and local governments	SAMHSA
Prisons	Federal and state funds; ADAP for some county systems	All inmates	Federal, state, and county prison systems	Federal prison system; some state systems

NOTE: ADAP: AIDS Drug Assistance Program; BPHC: Bureau of Primary Health Care; CDC: Centers for Disease Control and Prevention; DHHS: Department of Health and Human Services; MCHSBG: Maternal and Child Health Services Block Grant; MCO: managed care organization; and SAMHSA: Substance Abuse and Mental Health Services Administration.

infected. This information provides the background for an understanding of the rationale for the committee's recommendations and should assist in their implementation. Appendix B contains more details on the issues covered here and full references.

COMMUNITY-LEVEL SOURCES OF CARE FOR WOMEN, CHILDREN, AND ADOLESCENTS

The current mix of service delivery structures available on the community level can be organized into two somewhat arbitrary categories—*public and private nonprofit providers* and *private providers*—neither of which is purely private nor exclusively public. Some private providers receive differing amounts of public funding for their patients, and many public and nonprofit providers use a combination of public and private providers to deliver services.

The majority of women of childbearing age and their children receive their health care, and, potentially, testing for and treatment of HIV/AIDS, in a private provider's office (Weisman, 1996). While most of these providers are physicians, including obstetricians, family physicians, internists, and pediatricians, a significant number of women receive care from nurse practitioners and nurse midwives. Private providers may be in a solo or group practice, and a large and growing percentage are affiliated with managed care organizations.

Some women and children are not served by private providers because they do not have health insurance, there are no private providers locally, or those available do not accept public insurance. These women and children rely on a variety of public and private, nonprofit facilities, often referred to as "the safety net." These facilities include clinics operated by state or local health departments, community or migrant health centers, public and private, nonprofit hospitals, and family planning clinics operated by Planned Parenthood affiliates and other private nonprofit groups. Safety net facilities may provide maternity, family planning, STD (sexually transmitted disease), nutrition, and other non-reproductive-related services to women, as well as well-child supervision and illness and specialty care to children. Many of those served in these facilities are at high risk for HIV infection because they are poor and come from disadvantaged communities with a high rate of HIV infection. Most adolescents receive their health care at community teen clinics, school-based clinics, community family practices, private family practices, and private pediatric practices (Blum et al., 1996). More than 900 school-based or school-affiliated health centers provide a range of preventive and primary care services to adolescents.

A number of other programs serving women of childbearing age and young children offer opportunities for reducing the risk of perinatal transmission of HIV. At any point in time, approximately 120,000 women are inmates in prisons and jails throughout the country and have access to limited care within these facilities. Increasingly, prisons and jails also contract with private or public providers in the community for primary and specialty care, often arranged through university medical centers and correctional health care companies, the latter on a capitated basis.

Community mental health centers and substance abuse treatment facilities offer specialized care to women and sometimes to children. Drug treatment is funded primarily through the Substance Abuse, Prevention, and Treatment Block Grant. States receiving this funding are required to set aside a minimum of 5% of the funds for treatment of pregnant women, and to give pregnant women priority in enrolling for treatment services. States are also required to provide primary care, prenatal care, and child care to the women served under the set-aside. In common with prison system, substance abuse treatment facilities often contract with community providers for primary and specialty health care services.

The Special Supplemental Nutrition Program for Women, Infants, and Children (WIC) offers food supplements, nutritional counseling, and referrals to maternity and child health care for pregnant women and children at approximately 10,000 sites, often at locations where they receive other care.

Many public and nonprofit providers receive funding to provide specific HIV- and AIDS-related care to women and children. In addition, there is a network of facilities to provide such care exclusively. These include HIV testing and counseling centers, community-based nonprofit AIDS service organizations, and clinic settings.

FINANCING HEALTH CARE SERVICES FOR WOMEN, CHILDREN, AND ADOLESCENTS

Health care for women of reproductive age and for children is financed by private and public insurance and by a wide range of other funding mechanisms that support community-based public and not-for-profit agencies. The number of Americans who do not have health insurance coverage continues to grow. Nearly 41 million persons under age 65 were without public or private health insurance in 1996. Approximately 19% of women of childbearing age (18–34 years) and 10% of children under 18 are uninsured (Kaiser Commission on Medicaid and Uninsured, 1998a). There are a number of reasons for this growth in the uninsured, not the least of which is the cost of coverage for the employer, the employee, and the individual purchaser.

The number of persons without health insurance coverage puts a strain on public and private, nonprofit community-level agencies that offer health care. If the patient has health insurance, these agencies receive reimbursement from the insurer, including Medicaid. If the patient does not have insurance, these agencies must cover patient care through grants and contracts and/or other types of support from multiple federal, state, and local sources, both public and private, including philanthropy.

Private Insurance

The majority of women of childbearing age (70%) and children (66%) have their health care paid for through private insurance (Kaiser Commission on Medicaid and Uninsured, unpublished). Private insurance is usually obtained through employment directly or as a dependent of an employed person. Private health insurance on an individual basis is much more expensive, and the percentage of women and children with private insurance has declined steadily over the past decade (EBRI, 1997).

A number of issues about private insurance coverage for HIV/AIDS remain unresolved at this time. These issues include whether health plans can exclude from coverage individuals who have received a diagnosis of HIV infection before coverage; whether an employer can restructure a health plan to reduce benefits for a specific type of illness after a claim has been filed; and whether specific services will be considered "medically necessary" and therefore covered under insurance plans (Gostin and Webber, 1998). In June 1998, the Supreme Court, ruled in *Bragdon v. Abbott*, that individuals with asymptomatic HIV infection meet the legal definition of having a physical impairment under the Americans with Disabilities Act (ADA). The impact of this ruling on discrimination in insurance, as well as in employment and services offered by business and government, remains to be seen (Kaiser Family Foundation, 1998a).

The Health Insurance Portability and Accountability Act (HIPAA), passed in 1996, addressed private insurance coverage for people with pre-existing conditions, including those with HIV/AIDS. The law prohibits group health plans, insurers, and managed care organizations from denying coverage because of pre-existing conditions if the person had been insured for an uninterrupted 12 months prior to the application. In addition, the law:

• limits to 12 months the time a person can be subject to a pre-existing medical condition exclusion if the individual had no previous health care coverage;
• guarantees the availability of individual health insurance policies for those who leave jobs and have maintained previous coverage;
• prohibits denial of coverage in group plans to persons in poor health; and
• requires insurers to sell plans to small employers and guarantees renewal for both small group and individual coverage.

Although the HIPAA provides protections for those affected by HIV, it does not address the cost of premiums that insurers may impose, an important issue related to access.

Public Insurance

Medicaid covers 32% of low-income women of childbearing age and 49% of low-income children under 18 (Kaiser Commission on Medicaid and Uninsured, 1998b). Medicaid is the second largest public financing mechanism for health care and the largest single payer of direct medical services for people with AIDS. Over 61.5% of women in care for HIV are insured by Medicaid (Rand, 1998). Medicaid also pays for the care of about 90% of children with AIDS (DHHS, 1998). In 1996 only 15% of women in care for HIV with an asymptomatic HIV diagnosis (CD4 count of 500 or above) had private insurance, 60% had public insurance (Medicaid and Medicare), and 25% had no insurance. As the disease progresses to AIDS (CD4 counts below 200), those with public insurance increased to 70% (Rand, 1998).

Under Medicaid, all states are required to cover maternity services through 60 days postpartum for pregnant women with incomes below 133% of the Federal Poverty Level (FPL) and, at state option, the income cut-off for pregnant women can be raised to 185% FPL (and the federal match still maintained). States are also required to cover infants born to Medicaid-eligible pregnant women through the first year of life. In addition, states must cover children through age 5 who live in families below 133% FPL, and children ages 6 to 13 whose family income falls below 100% FPL. Older children with family income below 100% FPL are to be gradually phased in until 18 year olds are covered in 2002. States have the option of expanding coverage for children beyond the minimum requirement, and as of October 1997, a total of 27 had chosen this option (Weil, 1997; Fine, 1997). Under the new, federal–state Child Health Insurance Program (CHIP), federal funds are available to states that choose to expand Medicaid coverage to children whose family incomes are up to 200% of poverty. Under CHIP, states may choose to expand Medicaid eligibility, or they may use the new federal funds to develop their own coverage programs for children.

The full range of services identified in a state Medicaid plan must be provided to all recipients, including those with HIV disease. In addition, some states offer optional services such as targeted case management, preventive health services, and hospice care. Not all physicians accept Medicaid as payment, however, because rates may be low, payment slow, and paperwork cumbersome. All public and private, nonprofit sites accept Medicaid payments, with the difference between the Medicaid reimbursement and the actual costs of the services provided at these sites often covered by grants, usually from the federal government to a community-based organization or to a state agency.

Medicaid currently covers all Food and Drug Administration (FDA) approved prescribed drugs, including those used for prophylactic treatment of AIDS-related opportunistic infections, and drugs for treatment of HIV disease and prevention of perinatal transmission. Although states are required to cover those drugs for people on Medicaid who participate in Medicaid's drug rebate contract, many states have imposed limitations by restricting the number of prescriptions a patient can purchase in a month, the number and terms of refills, a requirement for prior authorization, and a determination of "medical necessity." In June 1996, in response to reports that some managed care organizations did not include all FDA-approved drugs for HIV in their formulary, the Medicaid program issued a directive to states requiring that those which include drugs and cover the HIV population in managed care assure that those drugs are available in managed care formularies.

The federal Social Security program offers two types of benefits for which women and children with HIV/AIDS may be eligible. For persons with an employment history, Social Security Disability Insurance (SSDI) provides monthly benefits to those disabled with a medical condition that is expected to last a year or end in death and is serious enough to prevent them from doing substantial work. The monthly benefit depends upon how much was earned while working. After 24 months on SSDI, the recipient becomes eligible for Medicare. The Supplemental Security Income (SSI) program is intended for those with a disability who have not worked long enough to qualify for Social Security or whose benefits are low and resources limited. Children with disabilities who live in low-income families may qualify for the SSI Disabled Children's Program (SSIDCP). In most states, eligibility for SSI makes one eligible for Medicaid coverage.

Grants and Contracts

The range of funding mechanisms for primary and speciality care that existed prior to the HIV/AIDS epidemic has been supplemented by funding specifically for HIV/AIDS patients.

Primary and Specialty Care

Federal funds for primary and specialty care are authorized and appropriated by Congress and distributed primarily from the Department of Health and Human Services (DHHS) through the Maternal and Child Health Bureau (MCHB) and the Bureau of Primary Health Care (BPHC) of the Health Resources and Services Administration (HRSA); the Office of Population Affairs (OPA); the Centers for Disease Control and Prevention (CDC); and Substance Abuse and Mental Health Services Administration (SAMHSA). Federal money flows into the community either directly through grants to public and private providers in the community, or indirectly through state agencies, which then allocate funds in a manner specific to their mandate. State funding consists of matching contributions required by specific programs, shared funding, or supplemental funds used to expand service support. Local health agencies, especially ones serving large populations, may also fund primary and secondary health services. State and local health agencies frequently receive grants from private foundations for special initiatives.

HIV/AIDS

In addition to funding primary and specialty care, the federal, state, and sometimes local governments, as well as foundations, charitable agencies, and other groups, allocate funds exclusively to provide HIV- and AIDS-related care to women and children. The most important source of federal funding for HIV/AIDS care is the Ryan White Comprehensive AIDS Resources Emergency (CARE) Act, administered by HRSA's HIV/AIDS Bureau. In addition, CDC supports community programs.

Under the Ryan White CARE Act, funds are awarded to eligible metropolitan areas under Title I to provide outpatient health care, support services, and inpatient case management. Title II funds go to states for home- and community-based health care and support services, continuation of health insurance coverage, and drug treatment through the AIDS Drug Assistance Program (ADAP). Title III provides funds to community agencies for early intervention services. Title IV funds community-based agencies for coordinated HIV services and access to research for children, youth, women, and families, and funds a smaller program that focuses specifically on reducing perinatal HIV transmission. Title V funds a dental reimbursement program, education and training centers, and demonstration projects that address hard-to-reach populations.

A major source of concern for HIV/AIDS patients and their providers is the cost of the drugs used for treatment. Many private insurance polices cover these medications. Medicaid also covers pharmaceuticals, but may impose limits. The ADAP, operating under Title II of the Ryan White CARE Act, is the second largest source of funding for HIV/AIDS drugs after Medicaid and is the payment of "last resort" (i.e., ADAP funds may be used only after all other public and private insurance sources have been exhausted). The program provides funds to all 50 states, the District of Columbia, Puerto Rico, the Virgin Islands, and Guam to make protease inhibitors and other therapies available to the uninsured and underinsured individuals with HIV. Administered by the state AIDS directors, each state determines its own financial and medical eligibility criteria, the type and number of drugs covered, and their purchase and distribution.

The demand for ADAP funds has increased dramatically as the number of persons with HIV has grown and new therapeutic regimens have been developed. In 1996, 83,000 persons with HIV disease were served and $52 million in supplemental funds were appropriated to supplement the $53 million committed by states from their Title II awards. The FY 1997 ADAP budget had a 221% increase over FY 1996, with the majority of funds coming from federal sources (Doyle et al., 1997). Fifteen states have waiting lists for ADAP enrollment and/or for access to protease inhibitors (AIDS Policy Center for Children, Youth and Families, 1998). In 1997, four state programs did not cover protease inhibitors and two states covered only one. Five states did not cover any of the prophylactic drugs strongly recommended in the 1997 guidelines and only two states had the full complement recommended (CDC, 1997f; Doyle et al., 1997).

The CDC's Division of HIV/AIDS Prevention enters into cooperative agreements with states and territories to support more than 10,000 counseling and testing sites and health education and risk reduction activities. The Division of STD Prevention funds 3,000 STD clinics, the primary source of HIV testing in public facilities. CDC's Division of Adolescent and School Health supports the development and implementation of HIV-related school policies and curricula to prevent HIV infection.

As a result of these programs, all states and territories have an AIDS program funded by both state and federal governments. The bulk of funding for HIV/AIDS testing, counseling, and outreach services comes from HRSA and the CDC. Although some testing and counseling centers are run directly by the state, most other services are arranged through grants and contracts with community-based providers.

The National Institutes of Health (NIH) funds HIV clinical research in institutions across the country through three diverse clinical trials networks, the AIDS Clinical Trials Group (ACTG), the Pediatric AIDS Clinical Trials Groups (PACTG), and the Terry Beirn Community Programs for Clinical Research on AIDS (CPCRA). Although the primary purpose of these networks is research, they provide important opportunities for women and children affected by HIV who meet the protocol criteria to access health care services. The Ryan White Title IV program assists in linking women and children to NIH research protocols.

ORGANIZATIONS RESPONSIBLE FOR DEVELOPING AND IMPLEMENTING POLICIES

Most of the agencies that fund primary and specialty services and HIV/AIDS-specific services also exercise general or specific authority over those who provide these services, whether in the private or the public sector. Private providers are responsible to licensing boards, must follow Medicaid requirements if Medicaid-certified, must consider the recommendations of their professional organization regarding standards of care if they are to avoid litigation, and must respond to the standards of the hospitals or managed care organizations with which they are affiliated. State and local public and private, nonprofit agencies frequently have multiple sources of funds and must meet the requirements established by each of these funders, as well as state and local governing bodies and boards.

By law and custom, responsibility in health affairs is shared by federal, state, and local authorities. Federal and state entities often try to avoid issuing too many regulations or might be perceived by their respective constituents as "excessive" guidance. Many of these authorities "recommend" rather than "require." The degree to which responsibility or authority is shared among these authorities often shifts over time. The locus of responsibility for many public benefit programs has shifted during the 1990s, with some responsibility "devolving" from the federal to the state level and, in many states, to the local level. This shift has increased the variability that has always existed from community to community in the organization, structure, and funding of health care services, creating important challenges to mounting an effective effort to reduce HIV perinatal transmission.

Implementation of the committee's recommendations will require changes in the policies developed by federal, state, and local government groups, managed care organizations, and professional groups, as well as broad dissemination of those policies.

RECENT CHANGES IN HEALTH CARE AND SOCIAL SERVICES

Several recent changes in federal policies will affect women and children at risk for or already infected with HIV/AIDS.

Welfare Reform

The 1996 welfare reform legislation—the Personal Responsibility and Work Opportunity Reconciliation Act of 1996 (PRWORA)—mandated changes in a number of areas, including cash assistance, Medicaid, SSI, and access to federal means-tested benefits. PRWORA repealed the AFDC (Aid to Families with Dependent Children) program and replaced it with the Temporary Assistance for Needy Families (TANF) block grant, imposing limits on the amount of time a family can receive economic support, sanctioning those that do not comply with work requirements or requiring recipients to seek work or training first before applying for assistance, and restricting cash assistance to citizens and certain categories of legal immigrants. In addition, persons convicted of drug felonies are prohibited from receiving cash assistance. It is important to note that there has been a significant increase in the criminal prosecution of substance-abusing pregnant women over the past several years (Chavkin et al., 1998), thereby increasing the likelihood that these women will not be eligible for cash assistance during treatment.

PRWORA essentially bars many legal immigrants from receiving a range of federal means-tested benefits, including TANF, Medicaid, SSI, Food Stamps, and Social Service Block Grant services. It does, however, distinguish between "current" qualified immigrants—those residing in the United States on August 22, 1996—and "future" qualified immigrants—those arriving after that date. Current qualified immigrants are eligible for emergency Medicaid, may receive non-emergency Medicaid and/or TANF at the state's option, and may retain SSI if they were receiving benefits on August 22, 1996. Future qualified immigrants may receive emergency Medicaid only, are banned for five years from receiving

Medicaid and TANF benefits, and are ineligible for SSI until citizenship. Undocumented and "unqualified" immigrants are eligible for emergency Medicaid, but are barred from all other federal means-tested benefits.

Under PRWORA, Medicaid is maintained as a federal entitlement for low-income citizens. Medicaid eligibility is not linked with TANF; instead, families are eligible if they meet AFDC eligibility requirements that were in effect as of July 16, 1996.

Children with disabilities are also affected by PRWORA in that they must meet a narrower definition of disability to become eligible for assistance through the SSI Disabled Chidlren's Program (SSIDCP), a common entry point for Medicaid eligibility and enrollment. The Balanced Budget Act of 1997 restores Medicaid for children who were receiving SSI on August 22, 1996, but lost it due to changes in the welfare law.

These and other changes have a complex and significant impact on access to care and, therefore, primary and secondary prevention opportunities for reducing perinatal transmission. Most women with or at risk for HIV have low incomes, are uninsured, and/or often rely on government programs to support their access to health care. Women with HIV disease may become impoverished because the disease itself prevents them from working or because of the expenses associated with it. The traditional linkage of women with the Medicaid program often came with their enrollment in AFDC (the former welfare program). With reduced access to welfare due to changes in eligibility and the imposition of time limits and sanctions, women may not be aware of their potential eligibility for Medicaid or how to access the program. Although many states have attempted to ease access to Medicaid for those applying for TANF benefits by creating a single application for TANF and Medicaid, access has been made more complicated for those not eligible or interested in TANF benefits because separate routes to Medicaid have not been effectively established in many jurisdictions.

With access to both welfare and health care services restricted to certain categories of legal immigrants and unavailable for the undocumented, opportunities for prevention and treatment are more limited. Many undocumented women are fearful of accessing care because of Immigration and Naturalization Service reporting requirements. Recent reports indicate that, at least in some states, applications for Medicaid (and therefore presumably Medicaid enrollment) have dropped precipitously among households headed by non-citizens, even though many non-citizens and/or their children remain eligible (Lewis et al., 1998). Another potential problem is that even though transitional Medicaid is maintained under welfare reform, many women who move from welfare to work may eventually secure employment that places them above Medicaid income eligibility cut-offs, but do not provide private insurance. In some cases, newly found jobs may offer insurance but former welfare recipients may find it too expensive to cover themselves or their dependents.

Beyond any impact from welfare reform, there is also an ongoing problem of continuity of Medicaid coverage. Due to Medicaid recertification processes and/ or temporary or permanent changes in a recipient's eligibility status, about half of the Medicaid population is continuously enrolled for less than 12 months. This means that many women and children are without coverage for medical care for varying periods of time, an issue critical to continuity of care, counseling, testing for HIV, and the ability to comply with complex HIV drug regimens.

Access to care is also affected by the reduction in the disproportionate share hospital (DSH) payments enacted in the Balanced Budget Act of 1997. DSH payments compensate hospitals serving a large volume of uninsured and Medicaid patients. This program supports such safety net providers as outpatient HIV clinics at public and nonprofit hospitals across the nation. This legislation also provided states with the option of expanding access to Medicaid by creating a "buy-in" for persons whose income was under 250% of poverty and who would be eligible for SSI, but whose income was too high. This option has important implications for women with HIV (Families USA Foundation, 1997).

Managed Care

Managed care has become a major strategy to control health care costs in both the public and the private sectors. Although managed care arrangements can take different forms, they all include enrollment of individuals, contractual agreements between the provider and a payor, and varying degrees of gatekeeping and utilization control (Kaiser Commission on the Future of Medicaid, 1996). Because it is responsible for delivering care to a defined group of enrollees, managed care makes possible, for the first time, accountability for the quality of care of populations, including access to care and health outcomes (IOM, 1996a).

Enrollment in managed care arrangements has increased dramatically in both the public and the private sector over this decade. Not only has the percentage of employees enrolled in managed care plans increased from 48% in 1992 to 85% in 1997 (EBRI, 1998) but federal law now allows states to mandate the enrollment of Medicaid beneficiaries in managed care organizations (MCOs). Almost half of Medicaid recipients were enrolled in managed care in 1997 (HCFA, 1997). Women, children, and youth are moving most quickly into managed care. This population as a whole, particularly those with or at risk for HIV/AIDS, has unique and complex needs requiring a broad array of multidisciplinary medical and support services. For example, relationships have to be built between the MCOs and the type of providers that adolescents seek—teen clinics, school health clinics, community family practice sites, and family planning clinics.

Some of the problems encountered by persons with HIV enrolled in MCOs include reduced access to specialty care providers, including HIV specialists; reduced access to specific drug formularies and specific services; clinical decisions apparently made on the basis of cost; limitations placed on the information providers can provide; and insufficient time with providers. MCOs have difficulty setting appropriate capitation rates for those with HIV/AIDS. Also, many of the providers who do have experience in providing HIV/AIDS care do not have experience working within managed care environments (Kaiser Family Foundation, 1998b). More time is needed to gain experience providing HIV specialty services and to build systems that can monitor and evaluate the quality of care in the managed care setting and provide oversight. One strategy chosen by some states is to "carve out" or exclude specific services or populations from the managed care contract and allow them to be provided as they were before the affected individuals were placed in the managed care program. Some MCOs deal with HIV/AIDS care in this way.

Medicaid managed care arrangements compete with public providers and private community-based providers serving the uninsured and publicly insured. Before the advent of managed care, these providers were frequently the only ones who served the poor or near-poor patient. Reimbursement from Medicaid for eligible populations allowed these providers to cross-subsidize the uninsured or underinsured patient (Davis, 1997). Now, competition for Medicaid funds is threatening the ability of these providers to support services to those without adequate insurance coverage. In addition, "many public hospitals and . . . providers of care to the poor with a mission to render care to the uninsured are being sold to private, for-profit organizations without a comparable mission to provide uncompensated care" (Wehr et al., 1998).

Managed care contracts, like traditional insurance contracts, do not typically identify specific conditions, and services are limited to what the purchaser specifies. In 1996, 18 states covered counseling and testing for HIV in their Medicaid managed care contracts, usually in the context of family planning services only. Access to the ACTG 076 protocol was assured through specific language only in Florida, but specific clinical services are often not mentioned in these contracts (Wehr et al., 1998).

CONCLUSIONS

Improvements in the prevention and treatment of HIV/AIDS in women and children and the efforts to promote the application of these new procedures have taken place in the context of a health care system that is undergoing a revolution in structure and funding. Major changes in Medicaid and welfare programs, the growing number of uninsured, and the growing presence of managed care in both the public and the private sector, are having a significant impact on the health care system, affecting not only the availability of quality services, but access to those services.

An array of federal, state, and local laws, regulations, policies, institutions, and financing mechanisms shapes the services in any given locality and determines who has access to those services. The current mix of public and private services and funding streams not only varies significantly from state to state and community to community, but is undergoing rapid change and is financially vulnerable. The ability of public programs and private sector programs using public funds to provide care has been significantly challenged, not only by the growing number of uninsured and the reduction in public funding of health care services, but by the rapid growth of managed care arrangements.

The complex patterns of sources of medical care, financing mechanisms, program authorities, and organizations that influence care make it difficult to institute policies for reducing perinatal HIV transmission. Local, state, and federal agencies have made many efforts to inform providers and the public, and to promote counseling and testing of pregnant women wherever services are offered, especially in states and communities with a high incidence of HIV infection. But more needs to be done to maximize opportunities for prevention of perinatal transmission. The fact that our health care system is itself undergoing dramatic changes in structure, funding, and service delivery presents both challenges and opportunities.

The chain leading to perinatal transmission of HIV infection described in Chapter 1 (Figure 1.1) can be broken in a number of ways, including encouraging pregnant women to seek prenatal care, informing them about HIV testing and urging them to be tested, having all pregnant women tested, and providing treatment to those who test positive. The complexity of the U.S. health care system is often an impediment to the achievement of these goals. Among the many possible obstacles inherent in the current health care system are: financial and access barriers that may discourage women from seeking prenatal care; time constraints imposed by managed care that may discourage physicians from counseling pregnant patients about the importance of testing; prenatal care sites that may not have the staff to overcome the language and cultural barriers that may cause women to refuse testing; financial and logistical problems that may make testing difficult; and financial barriers to treatment of the HIV-positive woman. In addition, the multiple lines of funding responsibility and accountability have made it extremely difficult to educate providers and to convince them of the necessity of testing all pregnant women.

6

Implementation and Impact of the Public Health Service Counseling and Testing Guidelines

Since the publication of the ACTG 076 (AIDS Clinical Trials Group protocol number 76) findings (Connor et al., 1994) in 1994, there has been a concerted national effort to bring the benefits of HIV testing and appropriate treatment to as many women and children as possible. Federal and state public health agencies, as well as many professional organizations, have issued a series of guidelines, recommendations, and policies about HIV counseling and testing in prenatal care, and some states have passed laws regarding pre- and postnatal HIV testing. As a result of these efforts, and in direct response to the ACTG 076 findings themselves, many providers have changed their prenatal care practices. Despite these efforts, however, prenatal testing remains far from universal, and many HIV-infected women continue to receive substandard health care. Surveillance data, as discussed in Chapter 3, indicate substantial reductions in perinatally acquired AIDS cases since 1992, part of which have been attributed to prenatal HIV testing and treatment with zidovudine (ZDV). In response to the committee's congressional charge to assess "the extent to which state efforts have been effective in reducing the perinatal transmission of HIV," this chapter describes the efforts to implement the Public Health Service (PHS) guidelines, and attempts to estimate their impact.

The committee's analysis is based on a combination of statistical and anecdotal information drawn from the published literature, government reports, workshop presentations, and site visits. Although the information is not drawn from nationally representative studies, the committee believes that there is enough consistency in the information that is available to draw general conclusions.

DEVELOPMENT OF THE PUBLIC HEALTH SERVICE COUNSELING AND TESTING GUIDELINES

The development of the Public Health Service (PHS) counseling and HIV testing guidelines for pregnant women (CDC, 1995b), released on July 7, 1995, was triggered by the ACTG 076 results a year earlier. The guidelines called for universal counseling and voluntary testing of pregnant women, in lieu of a more targeted approach to either high-risk women or high-incidence states (the guidelines are reproduced in Appendix N). The rationale for universal counseling was that many HIV-infected pregnant women and newborns in low-risk groups and low-prevalence areas were not being tested and treated. The universal approach was seen by the PHS as a means of stimulating the development of a testing and treatment infrastructure in low-prevalence states and regions (Appendix C).

The adoption of voluntary, as opposed to mandatory, testing was recommended for a number of reasons: widespread support for the policy, particularly from patients for whom adherence to a demanding drug regimen is essential for prevention of transmission; a concern that mandatory testing might have served as a potential deterrent to prenatal care; the risks of testing positive (e.g., discrimination and domestic violence) might outweigh the benefits in some cases; and experience indicating that greater than 90% of women accept testing when offered (Appendix C).

IMPLEMENTATION OF THE PUBLIC HEALTH SERVICE GUIDELINES IN LAW, REGULATION, AND POLICY[1]

Based on a survey of state activities, Gostin and colleagues (in press) concluded that states have moved rapidly to implement the PHS counseling and testing guidelines (CDC, 1995b), mostly without mandatory or coercive actions. As of June 20, 1998, almost all states had taken steps to implement the PHS guidelines in law, regulation, or policy (see Box 6.1). Only three states (Idaho, Kansas, Vermont) have neither laws nor policies on counseling and testing of pregnant women. Most states have policies, recommendations, or guidelines to prevent perinatal transmission; 45 states have policies on counseling/testing of pregnant women; 38 have policies on treatment of pregnant women; and 22 have policies on testing, monitoring, or treatment of newborns. Only 19 states have adopted laws or regulations on HIV counseling and testing of pregnant women.

Four states (Michigan, Mississippi, Tennessee, Texas) have routine "opt-out" procedures, in which a woman will be tested unless she specifically objects.

---

[1]This section is based on Gostin and others (in press), reflecting data on 50 states and territories, but not the District of Columbia. To simplify the exposition, territories are counted as "states."

BOX 6.1   Sample State Laws and Regulations about Perinatal HIV Counseling and Testing

• In *Texas*, section 97.135 of the state health code, amended in 1996, requires prenatal care providers to distribute information about HIV provided by the Texas Department of Health, verbally notify women (and note in their medical records that notification was given) that an HIV test will be performed if the patient does not object, advise women that the test is not anonymous, and take a sample of blood and have it tested for HIV infection. In addition, physicians or others who attend births must test new mothers or umbilical cord blood for HIV within 24 hours of delivery for all births, unless the woman objects.

• As of January 1, 1998, the *Tennessee* HIV Pregnancy Screening Act of 1997 requires all providers who assume responsibility for prenatal care "to counsel pregnant women regarding HIV infection and, except in cases where women refuse testing, to test these women for HIV and to provide counseling for those women who test positive."

• *New Jersey* has had a law since 1995 requiring prenatal care providers to provide their patients with information about HIV and AIDS, inform them of the benefits of being tested for HIV, and present them with the option of being tested. The New Jersey Department of Health and Senior Services has no authority to enforce this law, but has undertaken a number of programs to educate providers and patients about its provisions.

• *California* statute requires every prenatal care provider to offer HIV information and counseling (the content of which is specified in the law), and to offer an HIV test, to every pregnant patient. The offering must include discussion of the purpose of the test, its risks and benefits, and the voluntary nature of the test. The law also requires that these activities be documented in the woman's medical record. The state has also developed and widely disseminated comprehensive clinician education and resource materials (including interactive teaching materials for use with patients) and has made a toll-free clinician help line available.

• Since 1996, the *New York* Department of Health (DoH) has had regulations requiring hospitals, diagnostic and treatment centers, health maintenance organizations, and birthing centers (all of which are regulated by the DoH) to provide HIV counseling and recommend voluntary testing to all women in prenatal care. According to DoH, universal HIV counseling and recommended voluntary testing is now the standard of medical care for all prenatal care settings, whether regulated or not. Pre-test counseling must be provided, and written informed consent for the HIV test must be recorded on a DoH-approved consent form.

Three states (Indiana, New Jersey, Rhode Island) have routine "opt-in" procedures, which require prenatal care providers to offer the test. Testing is voluntary with informed consent in the remaining 47 states. According to state policies or laws, prenatal HIV counseling is required in 22 states, is routine in 10 states, and is recommended in 18 states.

Most states have laws governing disclosure of HIV test results. Thirty-seven states require reporting to the state health department. Other states permit disclosure to the person's spouse, or sexual or needle-sharing partner (26 states); to foster agencies or families (9 states); or to the newborn's pediatrician (15 states). Eight states regulate disclosure to insurers.

Six states have adopted laws or regulations on HIV testing, monitoring, or treatment of exposed newborns. Only New York State strictly mandates newborn testing; Texas requires it, but allows mothers to refuse. At least six states have provisions permitting testing of infants or minors without parental consent. In two states, a doctor may test a newborn for HIV if he or she determines it is medically necessary.

Virtually all states have programs to disseminate educational information to health care institutions (40 states), to providers (41 states), and to pregnant women and the public (31 states). These efforts are aimed at specific socioeconomic (10 states), ethnic (17 states), and age (19 states) groups, and 20 states distribute information in languages other than English. Thirty-seven states incorporate PHS guidelines into state-sponsored HIV programs, mostly through education and training of counselors and health care providers. Eighteen states have reviewed their contracts with managed care organizations regarding HIV issues, and nine states report having required changes in the covered programs to implement the PHS guidelines.

Although the issue has not been carefully studied, the committee has identified no evidence that the existence of state laws or policies mandating HIV testing for either pregnant women or newborns has had any effect on offering or accepting tests, or on avoidance of prenatal or other health care. Indeed, in the course of its site visits, the committee heard many instances of providers and patients who were unaware or confused about perinatal HIV testing laws and policies in their states. If many people are unaware of the policies, they are unlikely to change behavior.

IMPLEMENTATION OF THE GUIDELINES BY PROFESSIONAL ORGANIZATIONS

Most organizations representing professionals who provide prenatal or newborn health care have adopted positions that support universal counseling and voluntary testing of pregnant women. The American College of Obstetricians and Gynecologists (ACOG) advocates (1) routine counseling of all pregnant women as part of prenatal care; (2) voluntary testing with consent; and (3) documentation of refusal of testing in the patient's chart. ACOG recommends that pre-test counseling include information about risk behaviors, vertical transmission, availability and effectiveness of therapy, and the potential social and psychological implications of testing positive. The group also recommends, on a voluntary basis, contacting sexual partners of HIV-positive patients, as well as sharing testing information with health care professionals, including pediatricians (ACOG, 1997; Hale and Zinberg, 1997).

The American Academy of Pediatrics (AAP) also calls for universal counseling and voluntary testing of pregnant women, and recommends testing of all newborns whose mothers either are HIV-infected or have unknown HIV status. The AAP's recommendations include these key points: (1) All pregnant women should receive routine HIV education and routine testing, with consent. Consent can take the form of the right of refusal in order to facilitate rapid incorporation of HIV testing into routine practice. (2) All testing programs should evaluate the percentage of women who refuse testing. In cases of poor acceptance rates, programs should analyze why and make changes. (3) Newborn testing should be performed, with maternal consent, when the mother's HIV status is unknown. If the newborn tests positive, the mother should be notified and should receive referral for her testing and treatment. (4) Results of maternal testing should be provided to the pediatric health care provider. (5) Comprehensive HIV-related medical services should be available to all infected mothers, infants, and other family members (AAP, 1995b).

The National Medical Association (NMA) position on HIV testing of pregnant women asserts that (1) health care professionals should offer counseling and voluntary HIV testing to all pregnant women on a confidential basis; (2) health care professionals should offer zidovudine (ZDV) therapy to all HIV-infected pregnant women and newborns without attempting to coerce treatment; (3) in HIV-infected women, amniocentesis, fetal scalp electrode placement, or measures that lead to prolonged rupture of the fetal membranes should be avoided, as should breast-feeding; and (4) confidentiality, while extremely important, should not extend to withholding test information from other health care workers, such as pediatricians, for whom the information has medical significance (Appendix C).

The American Academy of Family Physicians (AAFP) recommends universal HIV counseling and voluntary testing for all pregnant women, and has adopted as policy the section "Guidelines for Counseling and Testing for HIV Antibody" from the CDC statement "Public Health Service Guidelines for Counseling and Antibody Testing to Prevent HIV Infection and AIDS" (CDC, 1987). In addition, HIV education is part of state association meetings, and the two AAFP publications also cover HIV issues.

The American Medical Association (AMA) is the only professional organization that supports mandatory HIV testing of all pregnant women and newborns, but this policy is not without controversy. In June 1995, the AMA Council on Scientific Affairs reviewed the available scientific data available and recommended that the AMA adopt a policy encouraging physicians to give a high priority to educating all women about HIV infection, and calling for prenatal HIV testing to be voluntary and its acceptance the responsibility of the woman (AMA, 1995). In June 1996, however, the AMA House of Delegates adopted a policy acknowledging that "mandatory testing for HIV of newborns at birth is too late to prevent perinatal transmission of this virus," but concluding that "there should be mandatory HIV testing of all pregnant women and newborns with counseling and recommendations for appropriate treatment" (AMA, 1996). The House of Delegates reaffirmed this position in 1997 (AMA, 1997).

The American College of Nurse Midwives (ACNM) policy is that all women should be counseled on HIV risk behaviors and risk reduction strategies, and following counseling, all women should be offered HIV testing with informed consent. The group opposes mandatory testing as a condition of receiving care, and recommends that women be counseled in a non-directive manner regarding reproductive choices and pregnancy care. ACNM recommends that all HIV-infected women be counseled on the risks and benefits of ZDV therapy during pregnancy, and offered this medication. The college also recommends that all HIV-infected women receive prenatal and perinatal care that minimizes the risk of vertical transmission through utilization of non-invasive techniques, and that HIV-infected women with access to adequate formula supplies should be advised to avoid breast-feeding (ACNM, 1997). The Association of Women's Health, Obstetric and Neonatal Nurses (AWHONN) also supports voluntary HIV testing with appropriate counseling, maintenance of confidentiality, and freedom from discrimination based on HIV status (AWHONN, 1995).

The Association of Maternal and Child Health Programs (AMCHP), which represents state maternal and child health programs, has incorporated PHS guidelines into its policy on HIV counseling and testing (AMCHP, 1995), which supports early and routine counseling to enable all pregnant women and others of reproductive age to understand the risk of HIV infection and the benefits of early testing, identification, and treatment. In addition, the statement calls for voluntary testing with informed consent as the standard of practice.

The AIDS Policy Center for Children, Youth and Families (APCCYF), an advocacy organization for service providers supported by Title IV of the Ryan White Comprehensive AIDS Resources Emergency (CARE) Act, recommends that routine HIV counseling and voluntary, confidential HIV testing with informed consent be the standard of care for all pregnant women, and supports policies and procedures in all hospitals, clinics, and doctors' offices related to routine HIV counseling and voluntary, confidential HIV testing with informed consent, and follow-up for linkages to care (APCCYF, 1995).

IMPLEMENTATION OF COUNSELING AND HIV TESTING AND QUALITY CARE FOR HIV-INFECTED PREGNANT WOMEN

As indicated in Chapter 1, the committee has organized its analysis in terms of a chain of events needed to prevent perinatal transmission of HIV (Figure 1.1). In the following section, this chain is used to summarize the evidence about the implementation of the PHS counseling and testing guidelines (CDC, 1995b) in clinical practice. In particular, this section covers access to and utilization of prenatal care; counseling and offering HIV testing in prenatal care; acceptance of prenatal HIV testing; offering, accepting, and complying with ZDV treatment; and provision of quality health care for HIV-infected women.

Early Prenatal Care

As indicated in Chapter 4, to successfully reduce perinatal HIV transmission, HIV-infected women would ideally be identified early in pregnancy. Late or no prenatal care is thus a significant barrier to identification and treatment of HIV-infected pregnant women.

From 1970 to 1995, the percentage of women in the United States receiving prenatal care in the first trimester of pregnancy steadily increased from 68.0% to 81.3%, and the percentage of women receiving late (i.e., at seven to nine months gestation) or no prenatal care declined from 7.9% to 4.2% (NCHS, 1997). Relatively few women receive no prenatal care (1.7% in 1992), but rates increase with parity, are higher in African-American women, and are highest in large cities. In 1992, as many as 8.5% of women living in the largest American cities (i.e., the 22 urban areas with populations of 500,000 or more residents) received no prenatal care. Among African-American urban residents, 11.7% had received no prenatal care (compared to 7.0% of white urban women), but rates are over 20% in some urban areas (for example, 22.1% and 20.7% in Manhattan and Philadelphia, respectively) (DHHS, 1992). This trend is worrisome because HIV infection in women tends to be concentrated in large urban areas in the Northeast.

The prenatal care patterns of HIV-infected pregnant women have been assessed in at least three studies. Among the 1,311 HIV-infected pregnant women identified in CDC's State Enhanced Pediatric HIV Surveillance Program (STEP) in four states (New Jersey, South Carolina, Michigan, and Louisiana) from 1993 to 1996, 14% had no prenatal care, and another 23% started care in their third trimester. As many as 35% of drug using, HIV-infected women had no prenatal care (Appendix D; CDC, 1998f). In a study of HIV-infected pregnant Medicaid recipients giving birth from 1985 to 1990, 90% had initiated prenatal or HIV care by 34 weeks' gestation, but only 50% had initiated care by 14 weeks. Fourteen percent of these women received no care until the last few weeks of pregnancy (Turner et al., 1997). Similarly, 14% of HIV-infected women in several counties in Texas received late or no prenatal care (Shakarishvili et al., 1996). These studies would suggest that roughly 15% of HIV-infected women receive no prenatal care.

Counseling and Offering HIV Testing

PHS guidelines recommend that all pregnant women in the United States be offered and encouraged to accept voluntary HIV antibody testing early in pregnancy (CDC, 1995b). Some states go further, requiring that all women in prenatal care be offered an HIV test. Meeting this target requires that prenatal care providers be aware of the benefits of maternal HIV screening and adopt practices to ensure that all pregnant women are counseled and offered testing. A total of 22 recent studies (conducted from 1994 to 1997) of prenatal care providers' attitudes and practices regarding HIV counseling and testing have been identified, and are summarized in Table 6.1. These studies were conducted in 22 states, and all involved surveys of prenatal care providers. The specific methods of study varied somewhat (e.g., telephone versus mail administration of survey), as did the sampling (representative versus convenience samples) and the response rates (from 25% to 84%). Many of the studies were unpublished at the time of this review and therefore have not been subject to peer review. Because most of the literature on provider behavior is based on surveys that rely on self-reports, there is a possibility of biased reporting favoring compliance with recommended practice. It is difficult to draw a national picture from the results of these selected states, but there does appear to be significant variation across geographic areas and significant gaps between provider awareness and application of recommended practices.

Awareness of CDC's guidelines, state HIV testing laws, and the ACTG 076 results appears to vary among prenatal care providers:

• In 1997, 60% of prenatal care providers in Oregon were familiar with CDC's recommendations regarding perinatal HIV transmission (Rosenberg et al., undated abstract).

• In 1996, 92% of Michigan providers were aware of state HIV laws (Michigan Department of Community Health, 1997).

• In 1996, 93% of Wisconsin providers had read a position paper, attended continuing education programs, or implemented an HIV testing policy (Wisconsin AIDS/HIV Program, 1997).

• In 1996, 87% of Montana's obstetric providers were aware of CDC recommendations for testing pregnant women for HIV (Montana Department of Public Health and Human Services, 1996).

• In 1995, 75% of California obstetricians were familiar with state law regarding HIV testing (Segal, 1996).

• In 1995, 90% of North Carolina providers had heard of the ACTG 076 results, but fewer providers reported familiarity in later years in Colorado (75% in 1996) and Atlanta, Georgia (60% in 1997) (Newton and Bell, 1997; Walter et al., 1998; Nyquist, undated abstract).

Provider surveys, on the other hand, indicate substantial variability in clinical practices and significant gaps between recommended and reported practices:

• In 1997, 94% of providers in New Jersey said they offered HIV testing to all or most of their prenatal patients (Ching et al., 1997).

TABLE 6.1 Summary of Selected Recent Research on Prenatal Care
Providers' Attitudes and Behaviors Related to Perinatal HIV Testing

Investigator(s)	Study Period	Geographic Area	Methods
Newton ZB, Bell WC July 21, 1997 Report from Georgia Department of Human Resources	Spring 1997	Metropolitan Atlanta, Georgia	Survey of a convenience sample of 150 private practice OB/GYNs at nine hospitals in metropolitan Atlanta. No information on RR
Ching S, Paul S, Goldman K May 1, 1997 Abstract and graduate program fieldwork project write-up	1997	New Jersey	Mail survey of members of state medical association of OB/GYNs. RR 51% (160/315)
Bell LJ 1997 Reported in State Disease Prevention and Epidemiology Newsletter	July 1997	South Carolina	Mail survey of licensed obstetricians. RR 63% of practicing OBs
Rosenberg KD, Townes JM, Gonzales K, Modesitt SK, Fleming DW Abstract	January 1997	Oregon	Mail survey of 208 persons named as birth attendants on randomly selected birth certificates of children born in Oregon between January 1995 and July 1996. RR 80% (167/208). Analysis limited to 159 prenatal care providers
Partika N, Johnson J November 14, 1997 Unpublished report	July 1996 to June 1997	Hawaii	Mail survey of 326 OB/GYN and family practice physicians statewide. RR 33% (107/326). 61 reported caring for pregnant women in last year
Riley CW January 1998 Perinatal HIV Infection White Paper, Virginia Department of Health	1996	Virginia	Mail survey of 281 medical practices providing prenatal care in Virginia. 230 in sample were OB/GYN practices

Results	Comments
60% are aware of the ACTG 076 study, 72% report encounters with HIV+ patients. 77% have policy of routine offer of HIV test to all patients; 6% report testing by risk assessment or patient request. Only 15% report all patients are screened. 55% report lack of information makes implementing ACTG guidelines difficult	
94% report offering HIV testing to all or most pregnant patients, 90% discuss benefits of HIV testing with all or most, 77% report counseling all or most about HIV, 59% provide counseling, discuss benefits of HIV testing, and offer test to all pregnant patients. Gender, years of practice, and number of HIV patients not related to levels of implementation	New Jersey requires providers to provide HIV counseling, discussion of HIV test benefits, and a voluntary HIV test offer
97% routinely screen pregnant women for HIV. 90% report at least 75% of women accepting test. 21% of OBs test without informed consent	
60% familiar with the CDC recommendations, 63% encourage all pregnant patients to be tested, 33% encouraged testing only for those with known risk factors. HIV counseling and screening practices did not differ by provider type, location of practice, specialty, or number of births attended per year. Fewer than one-half of all pregnant women are estimated to have been tested	Responding providers attend approximately 40% of Oregon births
86% (53/61) offered HIV counseling and testing to most or all of their pregnant patients (76% to 100%). 47% (29/61) report that most or all pregnant women accepted HIV counseling and testing. 29% (18/61) report that less than 50% of women offered HIV counseling and testing accepted it. No explanations for the refusals was offered	
54% of practices report offering HIV tests to 76% to 100% of patients. Among OB/GYN practices, 99% report offering HIV test to 76% to 100% of patients. Less than half (48%) of practices report that 76% to 100% of patients accept HIV tests. 15% report that 10% or fewer patients accept the test. Physicians report that the most common reason women decline testing is that they think that they are not at risk or they have already been tested	As of July 1995, providers are required by law to counsel women seeking prenatal care about HIV and to offer voluntary testing

Continued

TABLE 6.1 *Continued*

Investigator(s)	Study Period	Geographic Area	Methods
Wisconsin AIDS/HIV Program April 1997 Unpublished report	1996	Wisconsin	Mail survey of 600 physicians (GP/FP, OB/GYN, other M.D. prenatal providers), and 400 nurse practitioners providing prenatal care, nurse midwives, and physician assistants specializing in family practice and OB/GYN. RR 75%. Analyses limited to 591 providing prenatal/obstetric care
Ohio Department of Health October 31, 1997 Unpublished report	Fall 1996	Ohio	Mail survey of systematic random sample of Ohio registered OB/GYNs. RR 68% of eligible physicians contacted (393/582)
Nyquist C Undated abstract	Fall 1996	Colorado	Mail survey of FPs, OBs, and nurse midwives (members of professional societies). RR 49% (634/1,301). 324 provide prenatal care (about one-third of OBs; two-thirds FPs).
Michigan Department of Community Health 1997 Report of Subcommittee on Perinatal HIV Reduction	October 1996	Michigan	Survey of 150 OB/GYNs attending a regional ACOG meeting. RR 25%. Survey of 25 M.D.s at the Michigan State Medical Society/Maternal and Child Health Subcommittee. RR 48%. Mail survey of 102 members of the American College of Nurse Midwives practicing in Michigan. RR 49%. A total of 100 providers included in analyses

Results	Comments
93% had read a position paper, attended continuing education, or implemented a policy regarding HIV testing of pregnant women. 93% agreed that all pregnant women in their community should be offered HIV testing. 74% offer HIV testing to all prenatal patients. 57% report a consent rate greater than 75% when they offer HIV testing. Since 1994, 72% of prenatal care providers report increased level of HIV testing	According to a 1993 survey, only 39% of prenatal care providers reported that they offered HIV testing to all of their pregnant patients
More than 93% offered HIV testing, and most offered it for all pregnant women. Vast majority said that some form of HIV counseling was available to at least some pregnant women, but 14% counsel only patients with positive tests and 9% offered no counseling. Percentage of women tested varied from 0 to 100%, with a median value of 60%	Barriers to counseling mentioned were lack of support staff and lack of time
75% stated familiarity with findings of ACTG 076. 90% screen pregnant women for HIV infection, 50% always test for HIV, 75% strongly agree/agree that "all pregnant women should be tested for HIV regardless of stated risk behaviors"	
92% of providers are aware of Michigan's HIV laws, 94% of midwives and 82% of OBs said that they were compliant all the time with the counseling aspects of the law. 68% of midwives and 55% of OBs said they were compliant with the laws in terms of routinely incorporating HIV testing in the care of pregnant patients	Michigan law requires all pregnant women be counseled about, and tested for HIV. HIV testing of pregnant women and their infants is voluntary. Written, informed consent for testing must be obtained prior to testing

Continued

TABLE 6.1 *Continued*

Investigator(s)	Study Period	Geographic Area	Methods
Allen D, Gortmaker SL, Cotton DJ, Gardner JD Unpublished report	1996	Massachusetts	Mail survey of all obstetricians and midwives regarding 1995 HIV counseling and testing policies and practices. RR 56%
Rubin T, HCFA IOM workshop presentation April 1, 1998	January 1996, follow-up December 1996	Delaware, Florida, New Jersey, Rhode Island	Mail survey of Medicaid participating providers of prenatal and obstetric care regarding counseling practices and use of the ACTG 076 treatment protocol. RR 24% to 40% across sites for first wave, 23% to 42% across sites for second wave
Montana Department of Public Health and Human Services STD/HIV Section Unpublished report	1996	Montana	Survey of 225 family practice and OB/GYN physicians providing OB care in Montana. RR 52%
Phillips KA, Morrison KR, Sonnad SS, Bleecker T 1997	1995	California, San Francisco Bay area	Mail survey of 180 primary care providers (OB/GYN, FP, or GP). Not limited to obstetric providers. RR 73% (121)
Sage A, Mahon B, Colford JM 1995 Unpublished report	February 1994	California	Mail survey of 700 OBs/ FPs and 300 certified nurse midwives (CNMs) with $5 incentive. RR 74% M.D.s, 82% CNMs. 430 provided prenatal care

Results	Comments
62% have explicit policy on counseling, and 75% use standardized approach to testing. "On average respondents reported counseling 67%, offering an HIV test to 73%, and testing 39% of patients"	Presence of clinical policies was predictive of counseling and testing
47% to 71% of those providing prenatal care treat HIV+ pregnant women (wave 1), 46% to 83% (wave 2). Roughly 70% of providers in both waves 1 and 2 routinely offer HIV tests and are familiar with the ACTG 076 protocol	Conducted as part of an evaluation of the HCFA Maternal AIDS Consumer Information Project. A follow-up survey in each state has been conducted
87% report awareness of CDC recommendations. 18% reported screening all pregnant patients and 55% screen less than one-fourth of pregnant patients for HIV. 62% reported that pregnant women are not screened because there is no perceived risk. Other barriers included women's fear of test results, fears about confidentiality, cost, and women's lack of awareness regarding treatment	
86% support voluntary testing, 61% support routine testing without explicit consent, and 55% support mandatory testing. Few providers state that they support policies targeting testing to women with risk factors, yet in practice, providers are much more likely to encourage testing for women with risk factors than those without risk factors—90% of providers are very likely to encourage pregnant women with risk factors to be tested; 34% encourage women without risk factors, and only 9% encourage women without risk factors	Following this study (as of January 1996), California providers are required by law to offer all pregnant women voluntary HIV testing and document this in the medical record
42% providers discuss HIV/AIDS with all pregnant patients, 44% recommend an HIV test for all patients. Providers tested a median of 18% of pregnant patients. Providers from high-prevalence areas were more likely than those in low-prevalence areas to discuss HIV/AIDS with all of their pregnant patients. Female providers and providers in HMOs were more likely than others to recommend testing and to test more patients	

Continued

TABLE 6.1 *Continued*

Investigator(s)	Study Period	Geographic Area	Methods
Segal AI 1996 Published paper	1995	California	Mail survey of ACOG fellows in California regarding attitudes toward HIV counseling and testing. RR 50%
Hamm RH, Donnell HD, Wilson F., Meredith K, Louise S, 1996 Published paper	October 1995	Missouri	Mail survey of 1,535 licensed OB/GYNs, GP/FPs delivering infants, advanced practice nurses reporting OB/GYN as an area of interest, and other nurses. RR 25% (303 providers offering pregnancy care included in analyses)
Mills WA, Martin DL, Bertrand JR, Belongia EA March 1998 Published paper	August through October 1995	Minnesota	Telephone survey of 83 OBs and 94 FPs randomly selected from the Minnesota Medical Association directory. All practiced obstetrics. RR 86% OBs, 95% FPs
Louisiana Morbidity Report 1995	August 1995	Louisiana	Mail survey of 167 OBs in urban and rural areas (all OBs in rural areas included in sample). RR 84%. Mail survey of 68 hospitals that provide labor and delivery services. RR 99%
Walter EB, Lampe MA, Livingston E, Royce RA 1998 Published paper	July 1995	North Carolina	Statewide mail survey of prenatal care providers (OB/GYN, FPs, nurse midwives, nurse practitioners). $1 incentive. RR 59% (594/1,010); 66% eligible providers (594/907). Analyses limited to 511 prenatal care providers

Results	Comments
74% understood California law regarding testing, 64% favor mandatory HIV testing. 66% thought voluntary testing would not effectively decrease transmission rates. 10% to 20% do not provide any level of HIV counseling or testing, 45% expressed competence and "comfort" to care for HIV+ patients	Supplementary comments provided suggest that OBs view HIV counseling requirements and confidential record keeping as logistically difficult, time consuming, and expensive
70% of OBs and 57% of FPs aware of 1994 PHS guidelines on use of ZDV; 90% or more of providers reported that all pregnant women should be offered HIV testing by their prenatal care provider. 68% of OB/GYNs, 55% of GP/FPs, and 69% of advanced practice nurses offer HIV testing to all pregnant women who are present for care	Barriers to comprehensive counseling reported by physicians are limited staff time and patient population at low risk/no need
89% of physicians agreed with a recommendation for universal HIV counseling and voluntary screening of pregnant women. In practice 49% screen high-risk patients only, 43% screen all patients, and 8% do not screen patients. Median percentage of prenatal patients screened was only 10%. Women were more likely than male physicians to screen their patients for HIV	Most physicians reported screening all patients for syphilis and hepatitis B. Percentages of patients screened for other STDs were considerably lower (e.g., gonorrhea, chlamydia)
69% of urban and 70% of rural OBs routinely test pregnant women for HIV. 43% of hospitals test pregnant women for HIV at the time of delivery if their HIV status is unknown. Based on estimates of percentage of patients tested at hospitals, 68% of pregnant women knew their status at the time of delivery	
90% of providers had heard of ACTG 076. Among providers with access to HIV testing, 82% had a policy to offer HIV testing to all patients. But actual testing practice for many is based upon risk assessment. 67% offer HIV tests to all women that they see for prenatal care. Women seen in private offices are less likely than those seen in public health departments to be tested during pregnancy	In 1994, 18% of HIV-exposed newborns were not identified and tested for HIV

Continued

TABLE 6.1   *Continued*

Investigator(s)	Study Period	Geographic Area	Methods
Hill B, Nevada State Health Division, HIV/ AIDS Program Office 1998 Personal communication	May 1995	Nevada	Mail survey of 139 board certified OB/GYNs. RR 58% (80/139)
Herczfeld ND 1995 Dissertation, Yale	Fall 1994	Connecticut	Mail survey of 200 FPs, 269 OB/GYNs, and 87 nurse midwives randomly selected from lists of licensed practitioners. RR 54% FPs; 53% OB/GYNs; 78% nurse midwives. 100 M.D.s and 62 nurse midwives provided prenatal or obstetric care

NOTE: RR = response rate.

- In 1997, 63% of Oregon providers said they encouraged all pregnant women to be tested (Rosenberg et al., undated abstract).
- In 1997, 97% of South Carolina's obstetricians reported routinely screening pregnant women for HIV (Bell, 1997).
- In 1996, 74% of Wisconsin providers offered HIV testing to all prenatal patients (Wisconsin AIDS/HIV Program, 1997).
- In 1996 to 1997, 86% of Hawaii obstetric providers offered HIV counseling and testing to 76% to 100% of their pregnant patients (Partika and Johnson, 1997).
- In 1996, 55% of Michigan obstetricians said they complied with the laws in terms of routinely incorporating HIV testing in the care of pregnant patients (Michigan Department of Community Health, 1997).
- In 1996, 54% of prenatal care practices in Virginia reported offering HIV tests to 76% to 100% of patients (Riley, 1998).
- In 1996, 50% of prenatal care providers in Colorado said they always tested for HIV (Nyquist, undated abstract).

In several states, the overwhelming majority of providers agreed in principle with offering HIV testing to all patients, but in practice 50% to 75% actually did so (e.g., Wisconsin, Colorado, Minnesota, North Carolina, and Connecticut) (Herczfeld, 1995; Nyquist, undated abstract; Wisconsin AIDS/HIV Program,

Results	Comments
OB/GYNs reported testing virtually all women for HIV (95%), syphilis (100%), and hepatitis B (100%). On average, OB/GYNs reported pre-test counseling for 62% of patients and post-test counseling for 45%	
90% of prenatal care providers agree that all pregnant women should be assessed for their risk of HIV infection, and 89% agree that HIV testing should be offered to all pregnant women in their community. 51% report offering HIV tests to all patients, 15% offer them to 76% to 99% of patients, 5% offer them to 51% to 75% of patients, 30% offer them to 50% or fewer patients. 61% report that legal requirements for informed consent discourage HIV testing, and 79% report that HIV testing should be an option on prenatal screening panels	

1997; Mills et al., 1998; Walter et al., 1998). Instead, actual testing practice was based upon providers' assessment of maternal risk or the providers' perceptions of maternal risk (Mills et al., 1998; Walter et al., 1998). Providers noted that barriers to offering their pregnant patients HIV counseling and testing included the lack of provider time, legal requirements for counseling informed consent, the need for confidential record keeping, a lack of perceived risk, and lack of awareness of effective treatment among pregnant women (Hamm et al., 1996; Segal 1996; Ohio Department of Health, 1997). The committee's workshop and site visits also provided evidence that some providers do not offer HIV tests because they feel that discussing or even bringing up the matter with some patients would be too "embarrassing."

Acceptance of Prenatal HIV Testing

Pregnant women's use of HIV tests has increased significantly since the release of the 1995 PHS guidelines (studies of HIV test use are summarized in Table 6.2). According to preliminary data from CDC's Behavioral Risk Factor Surveillance System (BRFSS), HIV test use among pregnant women increased from 50% to 75% between 1993 and 1996 (Alderton, 1998). The BRFSS involves surveys in all states and these estimates represent the most recent national

TABLE 6.2 Summary of Selected Recent Research on the Prevalence of
Perinatal HIV Counseling and Testing

Investigator(s)	Study Period	Geographic Area	Methods
Partika N, John A Burns School of Medicine, University of Hawaii Personal communication May 1998	April 1997 to March 1998	Hawai	Analysis of HIV testing data from Hawaii laboratories
Mitchell B 1998 Personal communication April 1998	January to June 1997	Texas	Analysis of birth certificate reports of HIV testing (prenatal and at delivery)
New York Department of Health, Maternal-Perinatal HIV Prevention and Care Program	February to October 1997	New York	Analysis of administrative data from the New York State program
Pettiti DB, Southern California Kaiser Permanente Medical Group Personal communication May 1998.	1994–1997	Southern California, Kaiser Permanente Medical Group	Analysis of health plan HIV testing data. Percent of women having prenatal screening panel who had HIV test
Simonds RJ, Rogers M IOM workshop presentation April 1, 1998 Unpublished preliminary data from CDC	1996	Alabama, Alaska, Florida Georgia, Maine, Michigan, New York, Oklahoma, South Carolina, Washington, West Virginia	Pregnancy Risk Assessment System survey of women with recent birth in 11 states (1,300 to 3,000 respondents per state). RR 75%. All 11 states asked "Did a provider talk to you about getting a HIV blood test" and 5 states asked "Did you have a blood test?" (New York, Oklahoma, West Virginia, Georgia, Florida). RR 71% to 80% across states

Results	Comments
An estimated 56% of women delivering live births were tested for HIV	
86% of women giving birth in Texas in the first half of 1997 were tested for HIV prenatally, 74% were tested at delivery, and 94% were tested either prenatally or at delivery. HIV test use was similar by age and race/ethnicity (83% among Hispanics; 89% among whites), but differed by type of prenatal care provider (90% for those cared for by a private physician; 76%, hospital clinic; 84%, public health; 59%, midwives; 88%, other; 22%, no provider)	Birth certificate data have not yet been validated with medical record reports, but comparisons of birth certificate and SCBW for HIV+ prevalence are comparable
48% pregnant women tested during pregnancy	
HIV test use among pregnant women rose from 55% in 1994, to 63% in 1995, 72% in 1996, and 85% in 1997. In 1997, there were an estimated 32,000 women who had a prenatal care screening panel	Variation in the HIV testing rate across Kaiser 6 service areas has decreased over time. In 1994, rates varied from 30% to 80%. In 1997, rates varied from 74% to 90%.
In 11 states, the proportion of women reporting that a provider talked to them about getting an HIV test ranged from 60% to 84% (median 75%). Among those offered testing, 75% to 86% of women accepted the HIV test (median 83%). Testing rates ranged from 59% to 77% (HIV test questions asked in five states). Acceptance was higher among African Americans, those with low educational attainment, those seen in public settings, and among those covered under Medicaid	

Continued

TABLE 6.2 *Continued*

Investigator(s)	Study Period	Geographic Area	Methods
Royce RA, Walter EB, Eckman A, Bennett B IOM workshop presentation, April 1, 1998	1996–1997	North Carolina	Pregnancy, Infection, and Nutrition Study. Prospective cohort study with 1,002 English-speaking women enrolled
Simonds RJ, Rogers M IOM workshop presentation, April 1, 1998	1996–1997	North Carolina; Miami, Florida; Brooklyn, New York; Connecticut	Perinatal Guideline Evaluation Project. Prenatal study in three sites (excluded North Carolina) involved in-person interviews with women in prenatal care regarding HIV-related communications with provider, content of HIV counseling, and factors related to acceptance of HIV test. Postpartum survey conducted in four sites
Simonds RJ, Rogers M IOM workshop presentation, April 1, 1998; CDC, 1998f	1993–1996	New Jersey, South Carolina, Louisiana, Michigan	State Enhanced Pediatric HIV Surveillance Program (STEP). Focus on HIV-infected women and what proportion are identified before delivery. Medical record abstraction. States match birth registries to surveillance data (extrapolations of SCBW data)
Alderton D, CDC, HIV/ AIDS Surveillance Branch Personal communication April 8, 1998	1993–1996	United States	Analyses of BRFSS surveys conducted by states. Surveys include question regarding use of HIV test and whether currently pregnant

Results	Comments

89% of women were offered an HIV test; of these, 75% got tested (overall, 68% were tested). 73% not offered test would have accepted test had it been offered, and 75% of all women would have been tested if all had been offered test. Testing rates were higher among women who perceived that their provider thought test important. Main reasons women were not tested: they did not believe they had HIV/AIDS (68%), because they had been tested recently (24%)

According to the postpartum survey, 87% to 100% of women were offered an HIV test across the four sites. Among those offered a test, an average of 93% accepted testing (63% acceptance in Connecticut; 95% acceptance in Miami). According to the prenatal survey, 72% to 93% of women accepted testing across the three sites (on average, 83%). Those most likely to be tested were younger, African-American, Hispanic, and had a provider strongly recommending the test. Major reasons women said they were not tested included "no perceived need," "previously tested," and "did not want to know"

Barrier to testing and treatment among HIV+ women is that 14% receive no prenatal care and 23% start prenatal care in third trimester. Among those with a history of drug use, about 35% had no prenatal care. Across sites, 68% of HIV+ women were identified prior to birth in 1993, 79% in 1995, and 81% in 1996

HIV test use (ever tested) among pregnant women increased from 1993 to 1996: 1993 (50%), 1994 (64%), 1995 (66%), 1996 (75%). In 1996, 71% of pregnant women had been tested in the last 12 months

Some HIV test use recorded in the BRFSS survey is associated with blood donation

Continued

TABLE 6.2 *Continued*

Investigator(s)	Study Period	Geographic Area	Methods
Royce RA, et al. IOM workshop presentation, April 1, 1998	Ongoing study	Central North Carolina	Prospective cohort study of 7,000 pregnant women attending public prenatal care clinics
Carusi D, Learman LA, Posner SF 1998 Published report	1996	San Francisco	Survey of a convenience sample of 247 antenatal patients at San Francisco General Hospital (English and Spanish speakers) regarding HIV testing policy (routine vs. voluntary testing)
Hewitt M 1998 See Appendix J	1995	United States	Analysis of 1995 National Survey of Family Growth. HIV test use assessed among women reporting a pregnancy or receiving pre- or postnatal care within the last 12 months. Test use limited to self-reported testing (excludes mentions of blood donation without mention of HIV test use)
Limata C, Schoen E, Cohen D, et al. 1997 Published report	1994, 1995	Northern California Kaiser Permanente Health Plan	Cross-sectional study of HIV test use among pregnant members of Kaiser Permanente Health Plan (31 facilities manage more than 30,000 pregnancies per year). Survey of facilities regarding HIV testing program
Hewitt M 1998 See Appendix J	1994	United States	Analyses of the 1994 National Health Interview Survey, AIDS Attitude and Knowledge Supplement. HIV test use examined by pregnancy status. Women delivering a baby in the last 13 months identified as "pregnant"

Results	Comments

Among the first 88 women interviewed, 86% reported receiving HIV counseling and 71% accepted prenatal HIV testing

72% accepted HIV tests. Test use was not associated with the presence of risk factors, self-perceived HIV risk, or demographic factors. Test acceptance was associated with patients' knowledge of medical intervention to reduce vertical transmission and their willingness to learn a positive HIV test result. Only 24% knew that perinatal transmission could be reduced with medication. 69% said prenatal HIV testing should be routine and 27% said that it should be done only after specific written consent.

Hospital serves a low-income, publicly insured or uninsured population

Nearly twice as many women experiencing a recent pregnancy as non-pregnant women reported HIV testing (60% vs. 31%). According to multivariate analyses, pregnant women most likely to be tested are those reporting HIV risk behaviors, formerly married, residents of the South, and those with low educational attainment

HIV test use increased from 50% in 1994 to 63% in 1995. Factors associated with test use in 1994 included ease and accessibility of HIV testing (immediate availability of consent form and test), a designated educator, and presence of a registered nurse on the counseling team

California legislation mandating HIV testing and offering information and counseling went into effect after this study was completed (January 1996). By early 1998, test use had risen to 80% (Schoen EJ, personal communication 1998).

Pregnant women as compared to non-pregnant women were much more likely to report HIV testing (58% vs. 33%)

Continued

TABLE 6.2 *Continued*

Investigator(s)	Study Period	Geographic Area	Methods
Webber MP, Schoenbaum EE, Bonuck KA 1997 Published report	1993–1994	Bronx, New York	Postpartum interviews with a convenience sample of 544 women at a public hospital
Walter EB, Elliott AJ, Regan AN et al. 1995 Published report	November 1993 to May 1994	Durham, North Carolina	Counselor offered HIV testing to all women delivering newborns
Lindsay MK 1993 Published report	1991–1993	Atlanta, Georgia	Prospective cohort study of HIV test use among >30,000 pregnant women registered for care at Grady Memorial Hospital
Healton C, Howard J, Messeri P, et al. 1996 Published report	1991	New York	Telephone survey of 136 women's health organizations (family planning programs and prenatal care assistance programs), telephone and in-person interviews with 98 HIV counselors, and in-person interviews with 354 women
Mason J, Preisinger J, Sperling R., et al. 1991 Published report	1989	New York City	Descriptive study of HIV education and counseling program within a hospital prenatal care program
Lindsay MK, Peterson HB, Willis S, et al. 1991c Published report	July 1987 to June 1990	Atlanta, Georgia	Prospective cohort study of HIV test use among 23,432 pregnant women registered for care at Grady Memorial Hospital

Results	Comments
79% of women were voluntarily tested for HIV. Strongest correlate of HIV testing was a history of drug use. Women with a drug risk were more than nine times as likely as others to have delivered without receiving any prenatal care	Study conducted prior to the publication of ACTG 076. Prevalence of newborn HIV in Bronx in 1994 was 1.4%
61% offered newborn testing accepted. In multivariate analyses, acceptance was higher among African Americans	
95% of women provided HIV counseling and follow-up services according to a protocol involving a multidisciplinary team accept HIV testing	Study hospital provides care for a predominantly African-American inner-city population
Slightly fewer than 60% of women agreed to be counseled, and of those, less than half consented to an HIV test at the counseling site. Women at the prenatal care programs were twice as likely as women at family planning programs to be tested (30% vs. 14%). Women were not tested mainly because they already knew their HIV status (31%) or did not want to know their HIV status (31%). Approximately two-thirds of women who were tested returned for their results and post-test counseling. Clients' recall of pre-test counseling content was relatively poor. Organization variables rather than client factors explained counseling and test use (young counselors, pre-counseling sentiments, presence of HIV primary care, heavy caseloads)	Investigators did not present information by pregnancy status. It is unclear whether family planning settings provided prenatal care
20% (297/1,453) of women participating in a prenatal group orientation session on HIV elected to be tested	Study hospital provides health care to predominantly minority women
Nearly all pregnant women receiving prenatal care (95%) consented to HIV testing	Study hospital provides care for a predominantly African-American inner-city population

Continued

TABLE 6.2 *Continued*

Investigator(s)	Study Period	Geographic Area	Methods
Cozen W, Mascola L, Enguidanos R 1993 Published report	1989	Los Angeles County	Results of pilot project to integrate voluntary HIV testing into prenatal care. Pre-test counseling offered in group settings ($n =$ 9,069). Compared a sign-on versus sign-off consent form
Lindsay MK, Adefris W, Peterson HB, et al. 1991a Published report	September 1989 to March 1990	Atlanta, Georgia	Prospective cohort study of HIV test use among 4,731 pregnant women registered for care at Grady Memorial Hospital
Lindsay MK, Feng TI, Peterson HB, et al. 1991b Published report	July 1987 to June 1988	Atlanta, Georgia	Prospective cohort study of voluntary HIV antibody testing within the University of Illinois Medical Center obstetric clinic
Barton JJ, O'Connor TM, Cannon MJ, et al. 1989 Published report	1987	Chicago, Illinois	Prospective cohort study of HIV test use and risk behaviors of 7,617 pregnant women (registered and unregistered) cared for at Grady Memorial Hospital

NOTE: RR = response rate.

estimates of HIV test use among pregnant women. These estimates refer to "ever" having been tested for HIV, but most testing occurred within a year of the currently reported pregnancy.

When offered an HIV testing on a voluntary basis, most pregnant women accept. According to preliminary results of 11 state-based surveys conducted in 1996 of women contacted following a recent live birth as part of CDC's Pregnancy Risk Assessment Monitoring System (PRAMS), from 60% to 84% of women reported that their provider talked to them about getting an HIV test, and

Results	Comments
76% of women accepted HIV testing. No difference in test acceptance by sign-off versus sign-on consent form	
Nearly all pregnant women receiving prenatal care (96%) consented to HIV testing. HIV test acceptors were more likely to be young, African American, and single, and less likely to have received education beyond high school. Nearly all women (98%) stated that they were not pressured into having HIV testing performed	Study hospital provides care for a predominantly African-American inner-city population
13% of pregnant women were without prenatal care (i.e., unregistered). Nearly all of these women agreed to be HIV tested, but test acceptance was lower than for women seeking prenatal care (87% vs. 96%). Women with no prenatal care had higher rates of self-reported HIV risk behaviors (14.3% vs. 9.9%) and had higher HIV-positive test results (1.4% vs. 0.44%) than women with prenatal care	Study hospital provides care for a predominantly African-American inner-city population
78% of women (585/751) counseled regarding HIV consented to testing	University obstetric unit serves inner-city, poor, predominantly African-American and Hispanic women

75% to 86% of pregnant women accepted HIV testing when it was offered (HIV testing rates ranged from 59% to 77%). Test acceptance was higher when providers strongly recommended testing, and among women seen in public settings, those with Medicaid coverage, African Americans, and those with low educational attainment (Appendix D).

Very high HIV test acceptance was recorded in postpartum surveys conducted as part of CDC's Perinatal Guideline Evaluation Project. Between 87% and 100% of women surveyed were offered an HIV test across the four study sites and 63% to 95% of women offered an HIV test actually had the test performed (Appendix D).

The evidence indicates that very high rates of HIV test acceptance are feasible within voluntary programs. Nearly nine of ten pregnant women (86%) are tested prenatally for HIV in Texas according to preliminary data from the state's 1997 birth certificates, which record whether a woman was tested prenatally and at delivery (Mitchell, 1998). Since 1995, Texas has required all prenatal care providers to test every pregnant woman for HIV, unless the woman refuses.

Other states that are monitoring perinatal HIV test use have relatively low prenatal testing rates. While virtually all newborns are tested following the implementation of New York State's mandated newborn HIV screening program, only 48% of pregnant women were tested prenatally in 1997 (Birkhead, 1998). According to analyses of laboratory data, an estimated 56% of pregnant women received prenatal HIV testing in Hawaii from April 1997 to March 1998 (Partika, 1998).

Providers Offering ZDV Treatment, Women Accepting and Complying with the Recommended ZDV Treatment Regimen

As discussed in Chapter 4, once an HIV-infected pregnant women has been identified, health care providers need to be familiar with PHS treatment recommendations (CDC, 1998d), offer the treatment to women, and monitor compliance and potential side effects of therapy throughout pregnancy, labor, and the postpartum period. The actual recommended ZDV regimen is complex insofar as it is fairly intensive, there is uncertainty regarding long-term effects, administration involves coordination across providers and sites (e.g., obstetric and pediatric personnel, outpatient and inpatient services), and may be associated with side effects and complications that require monitoring.

Compliance with the ACTG 076 regimen involves women taking an oral dose of ZDV five times daily[2] starting at 14 to 34 weeks of gestation and continuing throughout her pregnancy. During labor, providers need to ensure that ZDV is administered intravenously, and after birth, newborns need to be given an oral dose of ZDV syrup every six hours for the first six weeks of life, beginning eight to twelve hours after birth (CDC, 1994). This regimen was followed as part of the ACTG 076 trial, but clinicians need to use their judgment and consider calling upon experts for advice when their patients do not fit the profile of the women enrolled in the clinical trial (e.g., those with a history of extensive ZDV therapy before pregnancy). Providers also need to conduct special tests monthly to assess potential adverse effects of ZDV.

---

[2] More recent data indicate that transmission reduction can be accomplished with fewer daily ZDV doses (CDC, 1998e).

According to recent CDC and state-sponsored studies, more than 80% of HIV-exposed infants whose mothers' HIV infection was identified before birth are receiving at least some ZDV treatment (Table 6.3 shows summaries of studies of ZDV use). In a CDC-sponsored study involving 29 states that conduct surveillance of perinatally HIV-exposed children, by 1996 more than 80% of perinatally exposed children whose mothers were diagnosed HIV-infected before or at birth were treated with ZDV, during either the prenatal, the intrapartum, or the neonatal period. Roughly 70% of HIV-exposed infants had prenatal ZDV treatment (Appendix D). Analyses of blood specimens collected as part of the Survey of Childbearing Women (SCBW) showed increases in ZDV use from 1994 to 1995 and on average that, more than half of HIV-infected women giving birth in eight states in 1995 had received perinatal treatment with ZDV.

Evidence from three states suggests variations in success with providing ZDV treatment. As of 1997, 62% of HIV-infected women in New York State received ZDV treatment during pregnancy and 79% of HIV-exposed newborns received at least some ZDV treatment (prenatal, intrapartum, or neonatal) (Birkhead, 1998). In Michigan, as many as 93% of HIV-infected women used ZDV prenatally in 1996, and 90% of HIV-exposed babies were treated with ZDV (Michigan Department of Community Health, 1998). In New Jersey, prenatal ZDV use among women known to be HIV-infected increased from 8% to 47% between 1993 and 1996, and neonatal ZDV use increased from less than 1% to 64% between 1993 and 1996, according to heel-stick blood sample studies (Paul et al., 1998b). In 1995, HIV-infected women under age 30 were more likely than older women to have used ZDV, but race/ethnicity and volume of HIV-positive births in hospitals were not correlated to ZDV use (Appendix D).

Most women who are offered ZDV treatment initiate therapy. Side effects of treatment and the intense treatment regimen, however, contribute to treatment non-compliance. In a CDC-sponsored review of the medical charts of HIV-infected women and their babies in four states (New Jersey, South Carolina, Louisiana, and Michigan) in 1994–1995, very few (5%) women had chart-documented evidence of refusal of ZDV when offered. Relatively few (6%) women discontinued using ZDV during pregnancy, but this is likely an underestimate because non-compliance may not have been documented in the medical chart. Some have suggested that intensive nurse case management increases adherence to the ACTG 076 regimen and reduces perinatal transmission (Havens et al., 1997).

Barriers to use of ZDV among HIV-infected pregnant women include not having information about maternal HIV status, late onset of prenatal care, insufficient time to administer ZDV (e.g., short labor), and discontinuity in care (e.g., delivery at hospital not associated with prenatal care providers). Some evidence suggests that there are negative attitudes toward ZDV use among some HIV-infected women. In a series of face-to-face interviews with 71 HIV-infected women in New York City, many women viewed the drug as highly toxic with distressing and dangerous side effects, prescribed indiscriminately by providers

TABLE 6.3 Summary of Selected Recent Research on the Use of Zidovudine (ZDV) to Prevent Perinatal HIV Transmission

Investigator(s)	Study Period	Geographic Area	Methods
Birkhead GS, Warren BL, Charbonneau TT, et al. Abstract 1998	1997	New York	Newborn HIV testing program data from February 1 to October 31, 1997
Michigan Dept. of Health, 1998	1992–1997	Michigan	HIV/AIDS surveillance data reported through October 1, 1997
Lindegren ML IOM workshop presentation, April 1, 1998	1995–1996	New Jersey South Carolina Louisiana Michigan	STEP project
Lindegren ML IOM workshop presentation, April 1, 1998	1993–1996	29 HIV-reporting states	Surveillance data
Lindegren ML IOM workshop presentation, April 1, 1998	1994–1995	Florida, Louisiana, Michigan, Minnesota, New Jersey, Nevada Oregon, Texas	ZDV assays of HIV+ SCBW samples from eight states. Positive assay indicates administration of ZDV intrapartum or to newborn to prevent perinatal transmission. Method provides a minimum estimate of ZDV use (e.g., not all HIV+ women had been identified of giving birth)
Wiznia AA, Crane M, Lambert G, et al. 1996 Published report	February 1994 to August 1995	Bronx, New York	ZDV use among HIV+ pregnant women cared for at one hospital. All women were counseled regarding the results of the ACTG 076 trial

Results	Comments
62% (285/461) of HIV+ women received ZDV treatment during pregnancy and 79% received at least some ZDV treatment (i.e., during pregnancy, intrapartum, newborn within three days)	
93% of HIV infected women used ZDV prenatally in 1996, an increase from 13% and 30% in 1992 and 1993, respectively. 90% of HIV-exposed babies used ZDV in 1996, an increase from 6% and 14% in 1992 and 1993, respectively	
Very few (5%) women have chart-documented evidence of refusal of ZDV when offered. Relatively few (6%) women discontinue using ZDV during pregnancy (as documented in medical chart, so a minimum estimate)	
ZDV (either prenatal, intrapartum, or neonatal) use increased from under 20% prior to 1994 to more than 80% in 1996 among perinatally exposed/infected children whose mothers were diagnosed HIV+ before/at birth. Roughly 70% of HIV-exposed babies had prenatal ZDV treatment	
On average, more than one-half of all HIV+ women giving birth in eight states in 1995 received perinatal treatment with ZDV. ZDV use increased substantially between 1994 and 1995	
75% (37/49) of HIV+ pregnant women chose to use ZDV. Women refusing ZDV were more likely to report injection drug use as their HIV risk factor and to continue to use drugs during pregnancy. 67% (24/36) of women using ZDV received all components of therapy. Twelve women missed the intrapartum dose (because of short labor related to cocaine use). Overall, 52% (24/46) of women who completed their pregnancy took ZDV prenatally, intrapartum, and administered ZDV to their infants	Compliance might be improved by using outreach workers, integrating prenatal care with drug treatment programs, or expanding women's support structures

Continued

TABLE 6.3 *Continued*

Investigator(s)	Study Period	Geographic Area	Methods
Paul SM, Cross H, Costa SJ. et al. IOM workshop presentation, April 1, 1998	1993–1996	New Jersey	SCBW, enhanced pediatric surveillance
Fiscus SA, Adimora AA, Schoenbach VJ, et al. 1996 Published report	1993–1994	North Carolina	SCBW, pediatric surveillance

without regard to women's experience and perceptions, inadequately tested in women and minorities, promoted for the wrong reasons, and inappropriate while they were feeling well (Siegel and Gorey, 1997). Nevertheless, studies of pregnant women residing in high-prevalence areas suggest that most women would take ZDV if they were to test positive for HIV (Pemberton, 1997; Silverman et al., 1997).

Health Care for HIV-Infected Women

As Chapter 4 shows, HIV-infected women and their babies now have greatly improved chances of survival because of ZDV and other antiretroviral therapy. With prenatal and intrapartum ZDV therapy, the rate of perinatal HIV transmission has been dramatically reduced and new, more complex therapies promise even greater reductions in mother-to-child transmission. High-risk HIV care centers specializing in maternity and postpartum services for HIV-infected women and their babies have been developed in high-incidence areas of the country. These centers continue to test and improve upon therapeutic approaches. Equally important, the centers give the kind of comprehensive care that is essential to reaching the best possible outcomes for HIV-infected mothers and their infants.

While specialty clinics provide a model for quality perinatal HIV care, these services are clearly not uniformly available to infected women and their infants. The committee repeatedly heard testimony about a range of care-related problems women encounter once they have tested positive for HIV. Site visits in Alabama, New York and New Jersey, Florida, and South Texas, as well as testimony by providers and patients from the San Francisco Bay area (see Appen-

Results	Comments
Prenatal ZDV use among women known to be HIV-infected increased from 8% to 47% from 1993 to 1996. Known ZDV use in neonates increased from less than 1% in 1993 to 64% in 1996. According to a 1995 SCBW study, women under age 30 were more likely than older women to have used ZDV. Race/ethnicity and volume of HIV+ births in hospitals were not correlated to ZDV use	
The proportion of HIV-exposed children in North Carolina who were identified and tested increased from 60% to 82% from 1993 to 1994. After results of ACTG 076, ZDV was given to 75% of HIV+ women who delivered infants in North Carolina	

dix C through I), for instance, all point to a similar conclusion: testing does not necessarily lead to care, and even when it does, women are not necessarily receiving the quality treatment and services they need.

Getting Timely, Accurate, and Confidential Test Results

The committee repeatedly heard reports about the emotional difficulty of receiving positive HIV test results, even under ideal circumstances. For some women, however, the shock is intensified by the circumstances under which they are informed of their status. In Birmingham, Alabama, specialty care providers reported that some private providers test women without their knowledge and then relate positive results over the phone. By the time these women make their way to the specialty clinic, they are already distrustful of the health care system. Rebecca Denison, an HIV-positive mother who founded and is executive director of Women Organized to Respond to Life-threatening Diseases (WORLD) in Oakland, California, spoke of women who received calls from their physicians' offices telling them they had tested positive for HIV and that they should see a specialist since their own provider could not see them or "could not tell them what the test results mean." The problem of health care providers being ill-equipped to inform and counsel HIV-infected women was also noted in San Antonio, Texas, where a case was cited in which an obviously nervous medical resident could not answer questions about care options. In another instance cited in San Antonio, an HIV-positive woman and her husband were shown lab results that they could not understand, and were given a prescription for ZDV and a pamphlet to read, but the woman's physician could not answer essential questions or give needed support.

Some women who test positive never receive the news that they are infected, or receive the news many months into their pregnancies. In New York City, Newark, New Jersey, and San Antonio, committee members were told of women who test positive being lost to follow-up. This was of particular concern in managed care settings where hospital stays are abbreviated.

Finally, in San Antonio, committee members were told of situations where providers simply did not understand the nature of screening results or the need for retests to confirm ELISA results. As a result, women with positive ELISA tests were told they were definitely infected. In one case, a women asking for a retest was told, "The tests are accurate and there is no need for a retest."

Getting to High-Risk Specialty Providers

Even in some high-incidence areas, specialty providers are not available. In the entire East Bay of the San Francisco Bay area, for instance, there is no obstetrician or perinatologist specializing in the care of HIV-infected pregnant women. This includes high-incidence cities such as Oakland, Richmond, Berkeley, and Fremont. Women seeking specialty care must travel an hour across the bay to San Francisco. For women living in low-incidence and/or rural areas, the difficulty in reaching specialty care is even more pronounced. A Birmingham specialty clinic treats women from northern Alabama who travel four to five hours just to get their care.

Getting Appropriate Care from Non-Specialty Providers

The committee heard repeatedly about situations in which providers were not well informed about current care practices and therefore could not give HIV-infected women optimal or even adequate care during pregnancy. Keeping up with the latest therapies may be particularly problematic for primary care providers in low-incidence areas, or with low-incidence practices; however, the problem goes beyond these kinds of practices. Rebecca Denison from WORLD gave the following examples from women she has counseled (see Appendix I).

• When "Kim" asked her doctor if he knew how to manage an HIV pregnancy he said, "Oh, yes. Don't worry. We use gloves during the delivery with everyone." This same doctor, who knew she was HIV-positive, asked her three times, "Now, tell me again why you're not planning to breast-feed?"

• "Natalie" had an undetectable viral load on a combination of two drugs when she found out she was pregnant. An obstetrician with no experience with HIV told her to go off her drugs immediately because she was in her first trimester. Almost immediately her viral load went from undetectable to over 130,000 copies/mL.

• "Kelly" tested positive at age 22, during a planned pregnancy. With an hour of her diagnosis she was told, "We can schedule the abortion today." It was only after she terminated her pregnancy that she learned there would have been a good chance of the baby being born HIV-free.

• "Sheila" knew she was HIV-positive when she became pregnant by accident. Her doctor put her on ZDV and d4T, a combination that is contraindicated in any HIV-infected person, pregnant or not.

• "Sandra" delivered her baby in a high-incidence city to a doctor and medical team who knew she was HIV-positive. "They"—not just the doctor, but the entire medical team—forgot to administer intravenous ZDV.

In San Antonio, a case was cited in which a doctor assumed the pharmacy automatically stocked ZDV, which he planned to administer to a pregnant HIV-infected woman during labor. By the time he realized the pharmacy did not have ZDV readily available and ordered it from a specialty HIV clinic, it was too late. The woman delivered without benefit of intrapartum antiretroviral therapy.

Availability of Complex Therapies

In Birmingham and San Antonio, committee members were told that although high-risk centers provide triple or other multiple therapies, many other providers offer only ZDV. In some instances the reliance on monotherapy seems to reflect a resource shortage, and in others it reflects a concern among providers that multiple therapies are still experimental and that their use may be unethical and/or leave the provider subject to malpractice charges. In testimony at the April 1, 1998 Workshop, Denison noted the importance of continuing research protocols and of incorporating new findings into standard care for HIV-infected women (Appendix D).

Standards of Care

Even when women receive care from specialty clinics, they and their providers are often faced with difficult decisions about care options. For many basic obstetric procedures, there is no standard of care established for HIV-infected women. There are, for example, no standard recommendations or cost-benefit analyses on cesarean sections, amniocentesis, and fetal scalp monitoring for the HIV-positive mother and her infant.

Special Populations

There are extra barriers for some special populations to obtaining adequate care for HIV-infected pregnant women and their infants. These special populations include undocumented immigrants, some categories of legal immigrants, substance users, and adolescents. Chapter 7 reviews some of the systemic issues related to receipt of HIV-specific and other care for these populations.

Medicaid

While Medicaid provides crucial financing of prenatal care, labor delivery, and postpartum care for HIV-infected women, many states end coverage for all but the poorest women at six weeks postpartum. For an HIV-infected woman, the loss of Medicaid can have devastating effects on her own health and her ability to care for her infant. Providers in Birmingham noted that while specialty clinics thus far have been able to piece together financing for women's medication and treatment for women who are no longer eligible for Medicaid, it is not clear that clinics will be able to continue coverage in the future. A second Medicaid-related issue was raised at the San Antonio site visit, where the move to Medicaid managed care has left both providers and patients confused about care options for HIV-infected women. At issue is whether or not patients can switch to the high-risk HIV care center as a primary provider of maternity services.

Women, Infants, and Children Program

The Special Supplemental Nutrition Program for Women, Infants and Children (WIC) provides health education and supplemental foods for pregnant women and their infants. Like Medicaid, it is an important source of care for HIV-infected women and their babies. Denison, however, reports that WIC programs, which promote breast-feeding as the best alternative for infant nutrition, in some instances are not sufficiently sensitive to the needs of HIV-infected mothers.[3]

STRATEGIES TO REDUCE PERINATAL HIV TRANSMISSION

Inadequate prenatal care among women at high risk for HIV, health care providers' lack of adherence to PHS guidelines, and women's rejection of HIV testing and ZDV use all limit the ability to further reduce perinatal HIV transmission. This section of the report provides estimates of each potential barrier to HIV transmission reduction, and presents a simple model for assessing the implications of different intervention strategies.

If a hypothetical population of 7,000 HIV-infected pregnant women all obtained early prenatal care; if their providers were in complete compliance with PHS recommendations regarding counseling, testing, and ZDV treatment; and if the women all accepted HIV tests and ZDV treatment and all pregnancies resulted in a live birth, the committee estimates that 350 HIV-infected babies would be born (that is, the risk of transmission under optimal care is 5%). If, however,

---

[3]The Food and Nutrition Service of the Department of Agriculture is expected to finalize its guidelines related to HIV and breastfeeding and disseminate them to WIC sites in 1998.

prenatal care, provider behavior, or other factors affecting perinatal HIV transmission are not optimal, the number of HIV-infected babies increases. For the purposes of this illustration, the committee's assumptions about current practices are as follows: 85% of HIV-infected women seek prenatal care, 75% of women are counseled regarding HIV testing, 80% of women accept the test, 90% of HIV-infected women are offered ZDV, and 90% of women accept and comply with ZDV treatment when it is offered. Given this scenario, 1,172 babies would be born to the hypothetical cohort of 7,000 HIV-infected women, a 235% increase over the currently achievable state (i.e., from 350 to 1,172 HIV-infected babies).[4]

If we hold all but one condition constant, changing one parameter at a time, the impact of changes in the current environment can be assessed (for details, see Appendix K):

• Increasing receipt of prenatal care from 85% to 100% reduces the number of HIV-infected babies by 9% (i.e., from 1,172 to 1,070).
• Increasing the rate at which providers' offer HIV tests from 75% to 100% reduces the number of HIV-infected babies by 16% (i.e., from 1,172 to 979).
• Increasing women's acceptance of HIV tests from 80% to 100% reduces the number of HIV-infected babies by 12% (i.e., from 1,172 to 1,027).
• Increasing providers' offering of ZDV treatment from 90% to 100% reduces the number of HIV-infected babies by 5% (from 1,172 to 1,107).
• Increasing women's acceptance of ZDV treatment from 90% to 100% reduces the number of HIV-infected babies by 5% (i.e., from 1,172 to 1,107).

Given the current environment, the most effective single intervention to reduce perinatal transmission is to increase providers' offering of HIV tests (reduces perinatal HIV transmission by 16%). If providers were in complete compliance with the PHS guidelines (i.e., they offered HIV tests and ZDV treatment to all women), there would be a 24% decrease in the number of HIV-infected babies (from 1,172 to 893). Alternatively, if the current environment remained the same, but all HIV-infected women accepted HIV testing when offered, and accepted and complied with ZDV treatment, there would be a 19% reduction in the number of HIV-infected babies (i.e., from 1,172 to 947). If both providers and HIV-infected women had optimal rates (i.e., if all but prenatal care is set to 100%), there would be a 52% decline in the number of HIV-infected babies (i.e., from 1,172 to 560). Increasing the rate at which providers offer HIV tests from 75% to 100%, and increasing the proportion of women who accept it from 80% to 100%,

---

[4] The model assumes only two HIV transmission rates, 0.25 if women are not treated and 0.05 if they are treated. These transmission rates actually vary according to the HIV-infected woman's clinical state, and the onset and completeness of treatment. The model also assumes that testing rates for HIV-positive women are similar to those observed in the general population of pregnant women.

for instance, would reduce the number of HIV-infected babies by 33%—about 386 children per year.

This simplified model illustrates the need for multifaceted approaches to significantly reduce perinatal HIV transmission. Even with a multifaceted approach, however, it will be difficult to achieve significant further reductions in the number of HIV-infected babies. As shown in Appendix K, even if the gap were reduced by 50% (e.g., prenatal care increases from 85% to 92.5%), there would only be a 29% decline in the number of HIV-infected babies (i.e., from 1,172 to 830). Here it is assumed that 92.5% of HIV-infected pregnant women obtain early prenatal care, 87.5% of women are offered HIV testing, 90% of women accept testing, 95% of HIV-infected women are offered ZDV, and 95% of women accept and comply with ZDV therapy. To achieve a further 50% decline in the number of HIV-infected babies (i.e., from 1,172 to 580 infected babies) and be within reach of the currently achievable state (i.e., 350 infected babies), the gap between observed and achievable rates would have to close by 78% and rates for factors related to transmission would have to be very high (e.g., 96.7% of women receiving prenatal care).

CONCLUSIONS

Since the publication of the ACTG 076 findings in 1994, there has been a concerted national effort to bring the benefits of HIV testing and appropriate treatment to as many women and children as possible. In 1995, the PHS published guidelines focusing on universal counseling and voluntary testing of pregnant women (CDC, 1995b). In the ensuing years, professional organizations representing prenatal, obstetrical, and perinatal care providers developed practice recommendations consistent with this approach. Only the American Medical Association chose to adopt a more stringent approach, mandating HIV testing for all pregnant women and newborns. States have also moved rapidly to implement the PHS guidelines. Almost all have taken steps to implement the guidelines in law, regulation, or policy, in most cases without mandatory or coercive actions. Some states have chosen to require counseling about HIV, or the offering of an HIV test, in prenatal care. Texas chose to make HIV testing a routine part of prenatal care, with notification and opportunity for women to refuse.

As a result of these efforts, and in direct response to the ACTG 076 findings themselves, many providers have changed their prenatal care practices. As documented in Chapter 3, perinatal AIDS cases fell by about 43% between 1992 and 1997. This decline was due to a number of factors, including a 17% decline in the number of births to HIV-infected women, increased testing and adherence to the ACTG 076 guidelines, better prenatal and intrapartum care, and (for declines that occurred before the publication of the ACTG 076 findings) use of ZDV for women's own health.

Despite the efforts of government and professional organizations, however, prenatal testing remains far from universal, and many HIV-infected women continue to be inadequately treated for their disease because they do not seek prenatal care, because they are not tested for HIV, or because their treatment does not reflect current standards of care. Although there have been substantial improvements in prenatal care coverage in recent years for most women, some 15% of HIV-infected women, especially those who use drugs, receive late or no prenatal care. Prenatal care providers are generally aware of the need for HIV testing, but there are still significant variations across the country in the application of recommended practices. Even in areas where the overwhelming majority of providers agree in principle that HIV testing should be offered to all pregnant women, only 50% to 75% actually offer the test to all women in their practices. Citing a lack of time, resources, legal requirement for pretest counseling, and perceived risk, actual testing practice is often based on providers' assessments of maternal HIV risk, which are not very accurate. On the positive side, the available evidence suggests that when offered, 90% or more of women will accept an HIV test, and acceptance can be enhanced if providers strongly recommend the test and incorporate it into routine practice.

For women who are found to be infected, Ryan White Title IV centers provide excellent maternal and child HIV treatment and care for those who have access to them. Despite the complexity of the ACTG 076 regimen and other difficulties, most HIV-infected women do accept and comply with ZDV treatment. Yet testimony to the committee and its own site visits all point to the conclusion that testing does not necessarily lead to care, and even when it does, women are not necessarily receiving the quality treatment and services they need.

Given these results, the committee must make a qualified response to its congressional charge to assess "the extent to which state efforts have been effective in reducing the perinatal transmission of HIV." The committee interprets this charge to include the efforts of national as well as state and local health agencies, and professional organizations at both levels. The data reviewed indicate that, on the whole,

1. there have been substantial public and private efforts to implement the PHS recommendations;

2. prenatal care providers are more likely now than in the past to counsel their patients about HIV and the benefits of ZDV and to offer and recommend HIV tests;

3. women are more likely to accept HIV testing and ZDV if indicated; and

4. there has been a large reduction in perinatally transmitted cases of AIDS.

The number of children born with AIDS, however, continues to be far above what is potentially achievable. Much more remains to be done. There is substantial variability from state to state in the way that the PHS guidelines have been implemented, but no evidence to suggest that any particular approach is more successful than others in preventing perinatal HIV.

Starting with the current partial implementation of the PHS guidelines, the committee estimates that the most effective change would be to increase the number of women in prenatal care who are offered HIV testing by their providers and accept it. Increasing the rate at which providers offer HIV tests from 75% to 100%, and increasing the proportion of women who accept it from 80% to 100%, for instance, would reduce the number of HIV-infected babies by 33%—about 386 children per year. To reduce perinatally acquired HIV even further, efforts are needed to increase the availability and utilization of prenatal care, especially in women who use drugs; to improve the coordination and quality of health care for HIV-infected women; and to prevent HIV infection in women initially.

7

Recommendations

As discussed in the preceding chapter, there have been substantial public and private efforts since the publication of the AIDS Clinical Trials Group protocol number 76 (ACTG 076) results to implement the Public Health Service (PHS) recommendations for prenatal HIV testing. As a result, women are more likely than in the past to be offered and accept HIV testing in prenatal care and to use zidovudine (ZDV) if indicated. There has also been a large reduction in perinatally transmitted cases of HIV infection. The number of children born with HIV infection, however, continues to be far above what is potentially achievable, and the medical care that some HIV-infected women receive is, regrettably, substandard.

To improve this situation, the committee recommends a national policy of universal HIV testing, with patient notification, as a routine component of prenatal care, as detailed below. Following an analysis of this proposed approach, the committee offers in this chapter a series of more specific recommendations relating to HIV testing as a routine component of prenatal care, which are intended to support this central recommendation. The focus thus is on one element of the chain in Figure 1.1: to increase the number of pregnant women who are tested for HIV. This chapter also includes recommendations for improving treatment of HIV-infected women and their children; and for preventing perinatal transmission of HIV through means other than prenatal testing (earlier in the chain); and regarding the resources and infrastructure needed to implement these approaches.

UNIVERSAL HIV TESTING, WITH PATIENT NOTIFICATION, AS A ROUTINE COMPONENT OF PRENATAL CARE

Based on its review of the benefits and risks of prenatal HIV testing and appropriate interventions and treatment for HIV-infected mothers and their children, the committee believes that all pregnant women should be tested for HIV as early in pregnancy as possible, and those who are positive should remain in care so that they can receive optimal treatment for themselves and their children. In order to meet this goal, **the committee's central recommendation is for the adoption of a national policy of universal HIV testing, with patient notification, as a routine component of prenatal care.** *Routine with notification* means that the test for HIV would be integrated into the standard battery of prenatal tests, and that women would be informed that the HIV test is being conducted and of their right to refuse it. The HIV test can be readily added to the list of tests for which blood already is drawn, such as complete blood count, blood type, and syphilis.

Providers have reported that, in the context of prenatal care, pre-test counseling following standard HIV protocols (CDC, 1994) is too onerous and that, therefore, many of their patients remain untested. Eliminating the requirement for extensive pre-test counseling, while requiring the provision of the basic information to all patients, would likely increase the proportion of women tested for HIV. The committee therefore recommends that pre-test counseling consist primarily of notification that HIV testing is a regular part of prenatal care for everyone, and that women have a right to refuse it. Patients' explicit written consent to be tested should not be necessary, but some professional guidelines say that refusal should be documented in the patient's medical record to protect the provider from liability. This recommendation is not intended to diminish more extensive counseling when providers feel it is warranted.

Under the proposed policy, women found to be HIV-positive would receive extensive counseling and be referred for treatment for themselves and to prevent perinatal transmission. For the small proportion of women who test positive, PHS counseling and testing guidelines suggest that post-test counseling include information about the clinical implications of a positive test result; the benefit of, and ways to obtain, HIV-related medical interventions and treatment; the interaction between pregnancy and HIV infection; the risk for perinatal HIV transmission and ways to reduce this risk; transmission to partners; and the prognosis for infants who become infected (CDC, 1995b).

Refusal of the HIV test at the initial prenatal visit should not necessarily be taken as final, but providers should assess the clinical circumstances and, in some cases, counsel women at later prenatal care visits about the benefits of HIV testing. At its site visits, the committee learned of many cases in which pregnant women, later identified as HIV-positive, initially refused testing, but eventually agreed after repeated discussions with their providers. Patients who continue to refuse testing should never be coerced or denied services, and providers should understand that for some women a positive test may lead to severe consequences, such as discrimination, eviction from housing, and domestic violence. Also, there may be clinical indications for repeating the HIV test later in pregnancy.

The committee's de-emphasis of pre-test HIV counseling also should not be taken to undermine the need for health care professionals to counsel their patients in routine encounters about the risks of sexually transmitted diseases or methods for preventing them (IOM, 1997), or in practices where providers decide routine pre-test counseling is appropriate. Rather, providers should not allow the requirements for pre-test HIV counseling to become a barrier to testing itself.

Clinical policies to implement universal HIV testing, with patient notification, as a routine component of prenatal care, will have to be developed, as discussed below. These policies should be tailored to the needs of the patients served by the practice, and should include the protection of confidentiality.

The committee's recommendation is in concert with recent analyses and policy changes in other countries. In April 1998, for instance, an Intercollegiate Working Party for Enhancing Voluntary Confidential HIV Testing in Pregnancy in the United Kingdom recommended that "testing for HIV infection should be integrated within established antenatal testing such as for hepatitis B, rubella and syphilis." (Intercollegiate Working Party, 1998). A recent clinical trial in Scotland showed an increase in testing from 18% to 90% of pregnant women when the approach was switched from opt-in (non-directive patient choice) to opt-out (routine, with notification) (Simpson et al., 1998). In September 1998, Alberta Health will begin to promote a policy of routine HIV testing, as part of the standard battery of prenatal exams for all pregnant women in Alberta, Canada (Pilon, 1998).

Rationale for the Committee's Recommendation

The discussion of public health screening programs in Chapter 2 sets out a series of policy options ranging from completely mandatory to voluntary, and Chapter 6 shows how current laws and policies implement a wide variety of approaches to prenatal HIV screening. Rather than this patchwork approach, the committee believes that a policy of *universal, routine testing with notification* reflects an appropriate balance among public health goals, justice, and individual rights. This policy would increase HIV testing, and hence improve outcomes, by striking a balance in the doctor/patient interaction as well as in the broader society.

There are two key elements to the committee's recommendation. The first is that HIV screening should be *routine with notification*. This element addresses the doctor/patient relationship, and can reduce barriers to patient acceptance of HIV testing. Most importantly, this approach preserves the right of the woman to refuse the test. Women would not have to deal with the burden of disclosing personal risks or potential stereotyping because the test would simply be a part of prenatal care that is the same for everyone. Routine testing will also reduce burdens on providers such as the need for costly extensive pre-test counseling and having discussions about personal risks that many providers think are embarrassing. A policy of routine testing might also help to reduce physicians' risk of liability to women and children when providers incorrectly guess that a woman is not at risk for HIV infection.

The second key element of the recommendation is that screening should be *universal*, meaning that it applies to all pregnant women, regardless of their risk factors and of prevalence rates where they live. The benefit of universal screening is that it ameliorates the stigma associated with being "singled out" for testing, and it alleviates the problem of many HIV-infected women being missed when a risk-based or prevalence-based testing strategy is employed (Barbacci et al., 1991). The PHS guidelines (CDC, 1995b), many state laws and regulations, and professional society recommendations all already call for universal testing.

Making prenatal HIV testing universal also has broad social implications. First, if incorporated into standard prenatal testing procedures, the costs of universal HIV screening are low, and the benefits arc high. Assuming that the marginal cost of adding an ELISA test to the current prenatal panel is $3 per woman and the prevalence of HIV in pregnant women is 2 per 10,000, the committee's calculations show that the cost of routine prenatal testing is $15,600 per HIV-positive woman found.[1] Even if the cost of the test is $5 and the prevalence 1 per 10,000, the cost per case found is $51,100. Taken in the context of the cost of caring for an HIV-infected child,[2] even though not all women found to be HIV-positive will benefit, these figures indicate the clear benefits of routine prenatal HIV testing.

Second, universal screening is the only way to deal with possible geographic shifts in the epidemiology of perinatal transmission. Although perinatal AIDS cases are currently concentrated in eastern states, particularly New York, New Jersey, and Florida, there have been shifts in the prevalence of HIV in pregnant women, including an increase in the South in the early 1990s. Changes in the regional demographics of drug use can also lead to changes in the distribution of HIV infection in pregnant women. Given the uncertainty of these trends, the committee considers universal testing the most prudent method to reduce perinatal transmission despite possible regional fluctuations.

Third, it would help to reduce stigmatization of groups by calling attention to a communicable disease that does not have inherent geographic barriers or a genetic predisposition. Focusing on the communicable disease aspect may allow

---

[1]In other words, if 10,000 women were tested to identify two positive cases, the aggregate cost of the screening program would be $31,200, or $15,600 per HIV-infected woman found. This calculation includes the cost of confirmatory tests when necessary, but does not account for the unknown proportion of women whose HIV status was known before pregnancy or would have been detected through other means.

[2]The lifetime costs of treating perinatally acquired HIV infection have been estimated at $65,000 to $200,000 (Ecker, 1996; Gorsky et al., 1996; Myers et al., 1998). In addition, there may be reduced costs associated with early detection of HIV infection in the mother.

national education programs that would otherwise be difficult, discouraging infected individuals from hiding themselves and thus not benefiting from care, and discouraging a "blame-the-victim" mentality.

The committee prefers universal HIV testing, with patient notification, as a routine component of prenatal care testing to policies that require providers to counsel or offer HIV tests to all women in prenatal care. As noted in Chapter 2 for screening programs in general, and in Chapter 6 for prenatal HIV testing, there is no evidence that making a program "mandatory," in and of itself, leads to more testing. Routine testing with patient notification thus is likely to be at least as or more effective in meeting public health goals, and less onerous.

INCORPORATING UNIVERSAL, ROUTINE HIV TESTING INTO PRENATAL CARE

As documented in Chapter 6, prenatal care providers are generally aware of and agree with PHS and other recommendations for universal testing. Yet there is great variation among providers in the proportion of women actually tested. Provider and patient surveys (see Chapter 6), the committee's workshops and field visits, and the committee members' own experience have indicated the need for a number of changes in health systems and public policy focused on health care provider behavior. In this light, the committee makes the following general recommendations, although precise actions should vary across states and clinical practices, and according to current practices, the nature of the epidemic, and available resources.

The first condition for these recommendations to be successful, is strong leadership in the public health and medical community, especially at the local level. The committee is aware of the extensive efforts that have been made at the national and state level to develop guidelines, recommendations, laws, and regulations to implement the ACTG 076 findings. The committee's site visits, on the other hand, have revealed a number of instances in which local public health officials and leaders of the medical community have missed opportunities to educate themselves about and encourage prenatal HIV testing, monitor progress, or enforce existing laws or regulations (Appendixes E, F, and G). It is also important, the committee believes, that these approaches be evaluated carefully, and that successful models be disseminated widely in the professional community.

Education of Prenatal Care Providers

Although most prenatal providers are aware of and agree with the need for offering HIV tests to pregnant women, their awareness and attitudes do not always translate into action. In addition to the demands of pre-test counseling, lack of knowledge about HIV therapies and the lack of a referral network, for instance, may deter physicians in private practice from offering HIV tests. One way to achieve the goal of universal HIV testing in prenatal care is for federal, state, and local health agencies; professional organizations; regional perinatal HIV research and treatment centers; AIDS Health Education Centers (AHECs); and health plans to increase efforts to educate prenatal care providers about the value of testing in pregnancy. They also must ensure that providers are linked to sources of information and referral for women who test positive. In addition, academic and residency training programs in family medicine, pediatrics, obstetrics/gynecology should include the knowledge, skills, and techniques for prevention of perinatal HIV transmission.

In particular,

The committee recommends that health departments, professional organizations, medical specialty boards, regional perinatal HIV centers, and health plans increase their emphasis on education of prenatal care providers about the value of universal HIV testing and about avenues of referral for patients who test positive.

Through its workshops and site visits, the committee found many examples of existing provider education programs initiated by state and local health departments and professional organizations. Nearly all states have sent material about the ACTG 076 results and the PHS counseling and testing guidelines (CDC, 1995b) to prenatal care providers. Provider education programs have been designed to explain the risks of perinatal transmission, the importance of universal prenatal testing, the benefits of interventions, and the availability of referral sites. These efforts should be continued and enhanced.

California and New Jersey developed their education programs as a result of legislation mandating that providers counsel and offer voluntary HIV testing to all pregnant women (see Appendixes D and E). California recently devised and disseminated comprehensive clinician education and resource materials (including interactive teaching materials for use with patients) and made available a toll-free physician help line. Similar educational programs need to be developed and evaluated in other states. It has been difficult, however, to get physicians to participate, because many do not think that HIV is common enough in their practices to warrant the time (see Appendixes E and G).

It is important for provider education programs to overcome physicians' apparent tendency to offer HIV tests only to pregnant women who report, or in whom they suspect, HIV risk behaviors. Risk-based counseling and testing strategies are ineffective because they fail to identify as many as half of HIV-infected women (Barbacci et al., 1991). Belief that they are not at risk is the most common reason for patients' refusal of an HIV test, according to the committee's workshops and site visits. Many who deny risk do so because they are unaware of their partners' risk history.

Education programs also should address providers' confusion about HIV testing algorithms and interpretation of results. In low-prevalence areas, false positive results from initial screening with an ELISA (enzyme-linked immunosorbent assay) can account for at least two-thirds of all positive tests (if the prevalence of HIV in pregnant women is less than 5 per 10,000). By contrast, the rate of false positives in high-prevalence areas (200 per 10,000, for example) is about 5% (see Appendix K). Confirmatory testing with Western blot or immunofluorescence lowers false positives to almost zero. There are still problems with interpretation of indeterminate results, however, and providers need to know how to counsel women about the need for follow-up testing. Laboratories, under most circumstances, do not report initial positive results to patients until after confirmatory testing. Nevertheless, the committee was informed of several cases in which pregnant women were told of their positive initial ELISA test results, which turned out to be false positives, by providers who did not understand the need for confirmatory test results (Appendix G).

Education programs should also stress providers' potential malpractice liability for failing to offer an HIV test. As prenatal HIV testing increasingly becomes recognized as the standard of care, courts may rule that providers are negligent if they do not offer a test to a pregnant woman who later gives birth to an HIV-infected baby, or at least document the refusal of a test (King, 1991). As documented in Chapter 2, fear of malpractice has served as a powerful incentive for prenatal care providers to initiate other screening programs.

Improved Provider Practices

Information available to the committee through its workshops, site visits, and correspondence suggests a wide array of approaches to promote prenatal HIV testing by changing provider practices. Approaches include the preparation or dissemination of practice guidelines, such as those discussed in Chapter 6. There is also a variety of specific clinical policies that facilitate HIV testing, such as inclusion of HIV tests in the standard prenatal test panel and no longer requiring counseling as a prerequisite for HIV testing.

Clinical practice guidelines offer a means to facilitate HIV testing in the prenatal setting. Practice guidelines are "systematically developed statements to assist practitioners and patient decisions about appropriate health care for specific clinical circumstances" (IOM, 1990, 1992). Practice guidelines can be developed by federal or state health agencies, or by professional organizations, through a process of reviewing the relevant scientific and clinical literature and building consensus among pertinent professional and patient organizations. As described in Chapter 6, state and local health departments and a number of professional organizations have already prepared practice guidelines to implement the PHS counseling and testing guidelines (CDC, 1995b). Accepting this approach,

The committee recommends that professional organizations update their clinical practice guidelines to facilitate universal HIV testing, with patient notification, as a routine component of prenatal care.

In addition to their direct influence on clinical practices, guidelines of this sort issued by professional organizations have an important role to play in determining the standard of care used by the courts. The committee's recommendation for universal HIV testing with patient notification in the context of prenatal care is different from most existing practice guidelines, so professional organizations should consider rewriting their guidelines to be consistent with the committee's approach. Relevant state laws and regulations should also be reconsidered.

The development of clinical policies represents another approach to promoting prenatal HIV testing and appropriate care. Clinical policies are usually developed within a clinical department, practice, or health plan, and can be based on national standards. Clinical practice guidelines to implement the committee's recommendation for universal, routine testing with notification might, for example, include an HIV test on the checklist of clinical tests for which blood is drawn at the first prenatal visit, standing orders, and procedures to ensure that positive test results are delivered in a timely and appropriate way. Practice guidelines might also include clear identification of the essential components of post-test counseling for patients who test positive. Thus,

The committee recommends that all health care plans and providers develop, adopt, and evaluate clinical policies to facilitate universal prenatal HIV testing.

Institutional changes can lead to rapid increases in HIV test use. Kaiser Permanente of Northern California, for example, was able to increase test use throughout its service area from 50% to 63% in one year (from 1994 to 1995) by improving providers' ability to provide counseling and testing—for example, by ensuring access to educational materials and laboratory testing (Limata et al., 1997). In Southern California, prenatal HIV testing among pregnant Kaiser members rose from 55% to 85% between 1994 and 1997 (Pettiti, 1998). A provider survey conducted in Massachusetts found the adoption of an HIV clinical practice policy to be the single most important predictor of the occurrence of HIV prenatal testing (Allen et al., unpublished).

The availability of patient educational materials can also help to improve prenatal HIV testing rates, according to the committee's site visits and workshops. The need for clear and readily accessible patient educational materials is even greater under the committee's recommendation for routine prenatal testing with notification. As a result of its support for minimal pre-test counseling to reduce provider burden, the committee foresees greater emphasis on educational materials to inform patients about the test and its implications for the health of the mother and child. Educational efforts oriented to the public at large also should be undertaken to underscore the importance of HIV prenatal testing. The New Jersey Department of Health and Senior Services, for example, has developed a public education campaign that includes the use of posters, postcards, videos, and public service announcements (Appendix F). To encourage HIV prenatal testing among adolescents and immigrants, who are among the hard-to-reach populations (see below), educational materials and public service announcements should be tailored to individuals of different ages, cultures, and languages.

Outreach and counseling conducted by nurses, counselors, and other staff would increase the proportion of women tested by minimizing the burden of HIV counseling on physicians. Physicians at many of the sites visited by the Institute of Medicine (IOM) committee believed that counselors and nurses were more successful at counseling patients than they themselves. The Group Health Cooperative of Puget Sound, a large Kaiser-affiliated HMO (health maintenance organization) based in Seattle, Washington, recently took steps to improve HIV testing of pregnant women by (1) communicating with providers about the PHS recommendations, (2) integrating HIV education and counseling into prenatal classes usually given by registered nurses, (3) having test results available for review and discussion at the first visit with a prenatal care provider (midwife, obstetrician/gynecologist, or family practice physician), (4) making written support material for counseling and testing available to medical and nursing care providers, and (5) clearly defining appropriate steps for care of HIV-positive pregnant women (BlueSpruce, 1998).

Performance Measures and Contract Language

Health care plans and providers increasingly are held accountable for the services they provide through performance indicators such as measures of cost, quality of care, and patient satisfaction (IOM, 1996a). Performance measures for preventive services such as childhood immunizations and mammography screening are common. Another way to integrate public health goals and clinical practice is to develop contract language for managed care plans, especially those serving Medicaid populations. To take advantage of this approach,

The committee recommends that health care plans and providers adopt performance measures for a policy of universal HIV testing, with patient notification, as a routine component of prenatal care.

Performance measures are established by health care plans as a result of requirements for accreditation, participation in Medicaid or Medicare, and market demand. In the market-driven approach, health care plans voluntarily supply information relating to performance measures to enable purchasers to compare plans. If providers do not meet performance goals within the plan, the plan faces sanctions or consequences, such as loss of accreditation, loss of participation in Medicare or Medicaid, and/or loss of market share. With respect to HIV prenatal testing, few, if any, health care plans currently hold their providers accountable for a high rate of HIV prenatal testing. To implement this recommendation, groups that develop performance measures, such as the National Committee for Quality Assurance (NCQA), should develop and adopt specific performance indicators for prenatal testing.

The Group Health Cooperative has decided to measure "the proportion of pregnant women with chart documentation of informed consent or refusal for HIV antibody testing within three months of the initiation of pregnancy." The long-term goal, or "optimal performance," has been set at 95%. This is compared to approximately 50% in mid-1997, before the program described above was put into place. The Jefferson County (Alabama) health department has a reporting system that could be used to measure HIV testing rates in its prenatal clinics, but it does not link performance to specific rewards or sanctions (Appendix F).

Health plans can be held accountable for offering prenatal HIV tests or actually performing them. Estimating the proportion of women who are offered tests can be cumbersome because it relies on chart review, but some have suggested that this approach is preferable where testing is not mandatory, so that voluntary testing does not de facto become mandatory. It is usually easier to calculate the proportion of women who are actually tested because laboratory data frequently are computerized (Appendix D). Given the committee's emphasis on universal routine testing, the proportion of women in prenatal care actually tested would be an appropriate performance measure. Health care plans must, however, ensure patient confidentiality and guard against coercive testing when patients refuse to be tested.

Another approach to integrating public health goals and clinical practice is the development of contract language for managed care plans. In particular,

> **The committee recommends that health care purchasers adopt contract language supporting a policy of universal HIV testing, with patient notification, as a routine component of prenatal care.**

If universal HIV testing with patient notification is to become a routine component of prenatal care, contracts should not allow health insurers to deny benefits under "pre-existing conditions" or similar clauses based on the client's HIV status.

In 1997, as documented in Chapter 5, most women, and more than one-half of all Medicaid recipients were enrolled in some sort of managed care plan. The essence of managed care is that some entity is responsible for maintaining the health of every individual. This can be a major advantage when it comes to incentives to provide preventive services, such as prenatal care. Under fee-for-service systems, no one can be held responsible for pregnant women getting prenatal care. With managed care, the responsibility is clear, and plans can be held accountable for the services they provide, although few actually are. Thus the contracts that govern the care provided to patients in managed care systems can be powerful tools, and are especially important for increasing the number of women covered by Medicaid managed care.

Current Medicaid managed care contracts, however, are limited by what the states specify, and in most states, financing rather than public health agencies develop the contracts. Thus no one asks for contract provisions relating to perinatal transmission or other prevention issues (Wehr et al., 1998). Fewer than half the states that have Medicaid managed care contracts require HEDIS data, for instance. Managed care and insurance contracts typically do not mention specific conditions, but in 1996, 18 states mentioned HIV or AIDS in their contracts. Of those, ten are limited to a reference to counseling and testing as a covered service, usually only in the context of family planning services. Only one state, Florida, specifically assures access to the ACTG 076 protocol (Wehr et al., 1998).

A number of things could be specified in Medicaid managed care contracts. At a minimum, managed care organizations could be required to report what they tell their providers about prenatal testing and counseling and ZDV use. Managed care organizations could also be required to report on the proportion of women counseled and tested (or documented refusal), and the proportion of HIV-infected pregnant women who receive ZDV (whether there was a HEDIS question on this or not). Since many women qualify for Medicaid when they become pregnant, offering an HIV test could be a required part of the intake process (Wehr et al., 1998).

Improving Coordination of Care and Access to High-Quality HIV Treatment

Prenatal HIV testing can achieve its full value only if women who are found to be positive receive high-quality prenatal, intrapartum, and postnatal care for themselves and their children. In its workshop and site visits, however, the committee heard many unfortunate instances of inferior-quality HIV treatment and poor linkage to specialty care for women diagnosed with HIV. Thus,

The committee recommends efforts to improve coordination of care and access to high-quality HIV interventions and treatment for HIV-positive pregnant women.

This recommendation has two components. First, HIV testing in pregnancy should be seamlessly linked to specialty care for HIV-infected women identified in the prenatal setting. Without linkage, the committee's recommended policy of universal HIV testing, with patient notification, as a routine component of prenatal care would violate one of the fundamental criteria for public health screening, that is, there should be adequate facilities for diagnosis and resources for treatment for all who are found to have the condition, as well as agreement as to who will treat them.

As the committee's workshops and site visits have shown, providers' and patients' lack of knowledge of available resources have been barriers to HIV testing itself. If providers and patients do not know that resources are available for treatment, they will not believe that testing is valuable, nor will women who are tested benefit fully from it.

Second, optimal care for HIV-infected pregnant women and their babies is complex, and must be coordinated throughout the prenatal, intrapartum, and postnatal periods. Primary and prenatal care providers cannot all be experts on this care, especially in low-prevalence areas. They should, however, be able to refer patients for appropriate care in any area. A later section of this chapter discusses the resources and comprehensive infrastructure, including federal funding and a regional approach, needed to provide optimal care.

From the moment she is informed of her HIV-positive status, a pregnant woman must know that care is available, on a confidential basis, for herself and her unborn child. Information about, and referral to, care should be incorporated into post-test counseling. It also should be incorporated into pre-test counseling for women who initially refuse to be tested. Some women reject HIV testing out of misplaced fears that a positive result is a "death sentence." These women would be more inclined to accept testing with the knowledge that perinatal transmission often can be prevented and that HIV infection no longer signals an imminent death. Immediate linkage to care is also important for patients who are in a state of fear, shock, depression, or denial after the diagnosis. Some contemplate suicide or delay for months the decision to seek or accept treatment, according to the committee's site visits and workshops. This was especially true of adolescents and immigrants, as discussed below.

In many states, Medicaid will pay extra for an HIV test performed in a sexually transmitted disease (STD) clinic, but not for the same test performed as part of prenatal care because prenatal care is typically reimbursed as a package. During its site visits, the committee learned that some public prenatal clinics were taking advantage of this differential by requiring women in prenatal care to go to an STD clinic for HIV testing. Although in some cases the second clinic was "across the hall," it often required another visit, and more importantly, some women were reluctant to be seen in an STD clinic because of stigma. Systems issues such as this can have a major impact on use of testing, and must be addressed.

The ACTG 076 regimen requires initiation of ZDV therapy early in the prenatal period and continuing through the intrapartum and postpartum periods. As discussed in Chapter 4, optimal care increasingly involves complex antiretroviral therapy for most women as well as special obstetrical procedures. State-of-the-art specialty care for HIV-infected pregnant women is preferable to care provided by non-specialists. For these reasons, a coordinated system of service delivery and financing for both the mother and the child. Some pregnant patients, however, especially those in rural areas, must access HIV care in the primary care setting. In such cases, the primary care provider must be knowledgeable about HIV testing and treatment and in communication with HIV specialty care. Whatever the arrangement, patients must have a smooth transition from primary to specialty care.

Some of the highly coordinated programs visited by the committee not only furnish specialty care, but also ensure on-site access to medications, to clinical trials, and support services such as transportation and psychosocial services and assistance with applications for public programs that pay for their care, including medications (Appendixes E, F, and G). Ensuring continuity of funding for care for both women and children is also important, especially given the fragmentary nature of federal and state systems documented in Chapter 5.

Addressing Concerns about HIV Testing and Treatment

While lack of prenatal care and not being offered a test are the primary reasons why women are not being tested for HIV, some proportion of women refuse testing when offered. To enhance acceptance of routine HIV prenatal testing, therefore, providers should understand the constellation of reasons why some pregnant women refuse HIV testing. According to the committee's workshops and site visits, pregnant women reject testing because they deny risk; fear disclosure of test results will lead to abandonment, discrimination, and domestic violence; lack trust in the provider; and face religious, cultural, and linguistic barriers (see section on special populations, below). Thus,

The committee encourages the development of outreach and education programs to address pregnant women's concerns about HIV testing and treatment.

Public and private organizations can contribute to these programs, which could include making information available in prenatal care providers' offices and in the popular press.

Providers need to be sensitized to these attitudes to help them devise strategies or interventions designed to heighten acceptance of HIV testing. When a woman refuses to be tested, providers must continue to understand the reasons behind her refusal, and encourage testing while avoiding coercion. Providers' ability to persuade women to be tested is enhanced within a climate of trust in the prenatal care relationship and assurances of confidentiality. If testing becomes truly routine and integrated into prenatal care, some women's concerns may dissipate over time.

Once they agree to be tested, the overwhelming majority of patients who test positive accepts and complies with the ACTG 076 regimen. But this is not universally true. If they are to improve their acceptance and compliance, providers must understand the reasons that some women resist drug therapy. According to the committee's workshops and site visits, the major reasons for patients' resistance to antiretroviral therapy were concerns that it was a "poison" and might have long-term effects on the child; the side effects; the demanding regimen of administration, especially for babies; and fear that frequent drug administration would make it impossible to conceal their HIV status, in cases where disclosure is feared. Patients sometimes resort to removing prescription labels to evade disclosure.

RESOURCES AND INFRASTRUCTURE

When integrated into prenatal care, universal, routine HIV testing, with notification, is not costly, and could easily be covered by private insurance, Medicaid, and other prenatal care financing arrangements. Infected individuals are rare, so treatment costs are low when averaged over all women in a practice or health care plan. Indeed, analyses have shown that prenatal HIV testing and subsequent treatment of infected women and infants can be very cost-effective (Ecker, 1996; Gorsky et al., 1996; Mauskopf et al., 1996; Myers et al., 1998; see also Appendix K). In and of themselves, development and dissemination of policy goals will not achieve universal testing and optimal treatment. As the discussions in this chapter illustrate, a comprehensive infrastructure is needed. Maintaining this infrastructure requires federal funding, a regional approach, and ongoing surveillance program.

Federal Funding

The committee learned of many successful efforts to build the infrastructure in the New York metropolitan area, Alabama, and South Texas. Other similar examples were brought to the committee's attention at its workshops and in correspondence. The directors of these programs consistently said that federal funding for research and services was essential to maintain the necessary infrastructure, and, hence, the programs' success. The efforts called for in the earlier recommendations in this chapter will require similar or higher levels of investment. Beyond this, HIV does not respect state borders, so although the perinatal AIDS epidemic is concentrated in a few states, it is truly a national problem. Thus,

The committee recommends that federal funding for state and local efforts to prevent perinatal transmission, including both prenatal testing and care of HIV-infected women, be maintained.

The Administration and Congress should examine current budgets thoroughly for adequacy, particularly in light of the expanded programs recommended by the committee. Maintaining current program levels is the minimum requirement. The

Ryan White Comprehensive AIDS Resources Emergency (CARE) Act Amendments of 1996 (section 2625), for instance, authorized $10 million per year in grants to the states to carry out a series of outreach and other activities that would assist in making HIV counseling and testing available to pregnant women. The Congress, however, never appropriated funds for this purpose. Appropriating these funds now would go a long way towards building the infrastructure needed to lower perinatal transmission rates.

As discussed in Chapter 1, the Ryan White CARE Act Amendments of 1996 set up a decision process that could result in states' losing substantial amounts of AIDS funding unless they demonstrate substantial increases in prenatal HIV testing or a substantial decrease in HIV transmission rates, or institute mandatory newborn testing. In other words, under certain conditions, mandatory newborn testing would be required (to maintain federal funding) if current voluntary prenatal testing fails. The logic of this approach is unclear; newborn testing may confer benefits for HIV-infected newborns, but cannot prevent perinatal transmission. If the national goal is to prevent HIV transmission from mothers to children, the federal government should support, not undermine, prenatal testing and other state-based prevention efforts. The Ryan White CARE Act Amendments of 1996, paradoxically, could have the opposite effect.

Regional Approach

Health Resources and Services Administration (HRSA) currently funds a system of "HIV Programs for Children, Youth, Women, and Families" through Title IV of the Ryan White CARE Act. Many of these programs serve as de facto regional centers for specialized treatment of HIV-infected women and affected children and, to a lesser extent, coordination of prevention activities. Federal research funds in these and other centers also provide for both direct care and an infrastructure to support it. In FY 1998, HRSA funded 44 comprehensive direct service programs in 23 states, the District of Columbia, and Puerto Rico. Most are located in urban areas, but some serve rural areas (HRSA, 1998b). There is, however, no coordinated, regional approach. Thus,

The committee recommends that a regional system of perinatal HIV prevention and treatment centers be established.

This goal might be reached by expanding the mandate of existing centers, or by establishing new centers in areas not now covered.

The regional centers would assure optimal HIV care for all pregnant women and newborns, directly to those referred to the centers, and indirectly by working with primary care physicians who retain responsibility for the medical care of HIV-infected women. Moving beyond current practices, the regional centers would also help to develop and implement strategies to improve HIV testing in prenatal care, as discussed above.

As discussed above, optimal care for HIV-infected pregnant women and their babies is complex, and must be coordinated throughout the prenatal, intrapartum, and postnatal periods. Obstetric as well as prenatal care is necessary, as is care for the mother's own HIV disease. The committee's workshop and site visits have shown that substantial efforts to improve coordination of care and access to high-quality HIV treatment are still necessary, despite recent successes. To effectively identify HIV-infected women and prevent transmission, moreover, this infrastructure must include the education of prenatal care providers; the development and implementation of practice guidelines; the implementation of clinical policies, the development and adoption of performance measures and Medicaid managed care contract language for prenatal HIV testing; interventions to overcome pregnant women's concerns about HIV testing and treatment; interactions with HIV prevention programs and drug treatment programs; and efforts to increase utilization of prenatal care, as discussed in this chapter.

A Ryan White-funded program in Tampa, Florida, for example, provides nurse case managers for all pregnant women who are HIV-positive, whether they are being cared for by public or private providers. These case managers ease the baby's transition into a Title IV program, and provide supplementary services in conjunction with regular care providers. The program also works to improve compliance with Florida's law, which requires that all women in prenatal care be counseled and offered an HIV test. It is estimated that nearly all women who receive prenatal care in the public sector are tested, compared to 85% to 90% of the women in the private sector. To address this discrepancy, the program works with private sector physicians and group practices by sending nurses who visit offices, do chart audits, and make recommendations on how to improve testing rates. These nurses are viewed as individuals who can help the practices with HIV testing and who can link women and children with specialized HIV care when necessary, as well as "government auditors" (see Appendix H).

Defining the organization, funding, and operations of the recommended regional approach is beyond the scope of this report. Steps are needed, for instance, to ensure that regional centers do not allow private providers to "dump" patients and to not overly burden mothers with long distances to travel. To advance this plan, HRSA's Bureau of HIV/AIDS and its Maternal and Child Health Bureau, which together have authority and funding to deal with prenatal care and HIV treatment, should convene a national working group to implement this regional approach. The members of the working group should include representatives of Centers of Disease Control and Prevention (CDC) for their prevention authority, National Institutes of Health (NIH) because many of the existing centers receive significant research funding, and Health Care Financing Administration (HCFA) because of its oversight of Medicaid. State and local health authorities, representatives of managed care organizations, and representatives of the prenatal care providers should also be involved.

Surveillance

Surveillance systems are needed to support policy development and program evaluation regarding perinatal HIV transmission. Chapter 3 of this report illustrates how epidemiologic surveillance data can help to focus attention on critical dimensions of a public health problem. Such analyses are hampered, however, by the lack of national HIV prevalence data and the discontinuation, in 1994, of the Survey of Childbearing Women. Chapter 6 shows how data from provider and patient surveys, clinical and health plan records, and other sources such as birth certificates can be used to monitor the performance of providers and identify bottlenecks in prevention activities. Data of this sort, however, are not universally available, and often are defined differently from one population to another. Thus, in order to support the previous recommendation about performance measures, and to generally guide prevention efforts,

The committee recommends that federal, state, and local public health agencies maintain appropriate surveillance data on HIV-infected women and children as an essential component of national efforts to prevent perinatal transmission of HIV.

The universal testing approach that the committee recommends, as well as the call for health plan performance measures, should facilitate the development of appropriate public health surveillance systems.

The Ryan White CARE Act Amendments of 1996 could make it difficult to maintain the recommended surveillance system. The Act states that continued federal funding to the states could be contingent upon (see Chapter 1):

1. a 50% reduction (or a comparable measure for states with less than ten cases) in the rate of new AIDS cases resulting from perinatal transmission, comparing the most recent data to 1993 data; and
2. ensuring that at least 95% of women who have received at least two prenatal visits prior to 34 weeks of gestation have been tested for HIV.

The first of these measures is imprecise. Does the "rate of new AIDS cases" refer to the number per year, the proportion of all newborns with AIDS, the proportion of children born to HIV-infected mothers who have AIDS, or some other concept? Children born with HIV infection may not progress to AIDS for years, so monitoring new AIDS cases per se reflects prevention efforts far in the past. How should it be determined whether any specific case was the result of "perinatal transmission"? What should be the role of newborn HIV prevalence data in states with mandatory HIV reporting? Because of this imprecision, states would likely choose the most favorable statistic they have available to avoid the loss of federal funds. The law recognizes that in states with few cases of perinatal AIDS (less than ten) an alternative measure is needed because of the inherent statistical variation in rates based on small numbers, but fails to specify such a measure. In 1997, 39 states had fewer than ten perinatally transmitted AIDS cases (Chapter 3).

The second measure is overly precise. The restriction to "women who have received at least two prenatal visits prior to 34 weeks of gestation" seems to be based on the ACTG 076 protocol, but as Chapter 4 illustrates, women who start prenatal care late can also benefit from ZDV use. Since most health plans' data systems do not record prenatal care utilization in this much detail, the only way to compile these statistics would be to review individual medical charts, which is very costly. Birth certificates could be changed to include similar information, but currently only record prenatal care by trimester, and this information would have to be validated.

OTHER APPROACHES TO PREVENTING PERINATAL HIV TRANSMISSION

Although the committee's charge was focused on prenatal HIV testing and appropriate care, other ways to prevent perinatal transmission of HIV should be also considered. A detailed discussion of these interventions would be beyond the scope of this report, yet the committee believes that the following areas offer possibilities for preventing HIV infection in children, and should be included in a prevention package.

Primary Prevention of HIV Infection

Primary prevention of HIV refers to the avoidance of HIV infection in the general population before it occurs. Since perinatal transmission begins with infected mothers and their partners, primary prevention of HIV can contribute markedly to preventing perinatal transmission by lowering the number of HIV-infected women and their male partners. There are many established approaches to primary prevention of HIV: HIV/AIDS education, behavioral interventions, partner notification, treatment and prevention of sexually transmitted diseases, and community programs (IOM, 1994, 1995a, 1996b; NRC, 1989, 1990, 1991, 1995; CDC, 1997b, 1998b; NIH, 1997).

Beyond more general HIV prevention efforts, HIV prevention programs targeting drug users, as well as increasing drug treatment slots for HIV-infected pregnant women, appear to be especially vital. Injection drug use in women or their partners is the primary cause of perinatal AIDS, accounting for about 70%

of perinatal AIDS cases (Chapter 3). Drug treatment programs have higher HIV prevalence rates (2.9%) than at other testing sites, such as HIV counseling and testing sites, sexually transmitted disease clinics, and family planning programs (CDC, 1997d). Engaging drug abusers in drug treatment, needle exchange, and related programs is pivotal to primary prevention of HIV. Drug abuse treatment, and HIV prevention education given in the context of drug treatment, have been documented to reduce HIV risk behaviors, for example, drug use, risky injection practices, and number of sexual partners (IOM, 1995b, 1996b). Women found to be drug users in mandatory drug testing (see Chapter 2) need opportunities for treatment, not just identification and threats of removing their children. Similarly, needle exchange programs are effective in preventing HIV transmission (NRC, 1995). Targeted prevention programs also are essential in correctional settings, as discussed below.

Averting Unintended Pregnancy and Childbearing Among HIV-Infected Women

As a general proposition, pregnancies that are intended—consciously and clearly desired—at the time of conception are in the best interest of the mother and the child (IOM, 1995b). If a woman is infected with HIV, unintended pregnancy and childbearing clearly have special significance. For these reasons, preconception counseling represents an important opportunity to identify HIV-infected women who are considering pregnancy. Couples are increasingly being urged to plan their pregnancies (AAP and ACOG, 1997), and part of this planning process should be a visit to a health care provider to ensure that the woman enters pregnancy in optimal health. Such a preconception visit usually includes advice about nutrition, folic acid, weight, and tests for infectious and chronic diseases. Insofar as women and their partners avail themselves of this opportunity, preconception visits provide an early opportunity to obtain HIV testing for the woman and her partner. For those found to be HIV-positive, it provides a chance to consider avoiding pregnancy, and/or to be counseled about antiretroviral therapy during pregnancy.

Some women who know they are HIV-infected choose to become pregnant, especially now that the ACTG 076 regimen is available, but others become pregnant unintentionally. More women learn their HIV status in the course of their pregnancy. Nevertheless, improved knowledge of the consequences of unintended pregnancy (including HIV transmission) and the ways to avoid it as well as access to contraception can help to ensure that all pregnancies are intended (IOM, 1995b), and this would reduce, to some extent, the number of children born with HIV infection. The committee does not want to restrict reproductive choice (Faden et al., 1991), but notes that interventions for such women who choose to terminate unintended pregnancies can also be beneficial in reducing the number of children born with HIV infection. To be most effective, however, women must know their HIV status to be able to take action, and this requires testing. The more women know their HIV status early in pregnancy, the better able they will be to consider whether to continue a pregnancy as well as the benefits of antiretroviral therapy. After giving birth, HIV-infected women, like all women, should be counseled about contraception and given referrals for follow-up visits that support the woman's contraceptive choice. This is important for all women, but especially for women for whom the consequences of an unintended pregnancy are particularly great.

If such a program proves successful, it would be appropriate to implement comparable programs more broadly, but with clear provisions for women's right to refuse testing.

Increasing Utilization of Prenatal and Preconceptional Care

The purpose of prenatal care is to improve pregnancy outcomes, particularly for women at increased medical or social risk (IOM, 1988). Since the publication of the ACTG 076 results, the prenatal setting offers the additional opportunity for combating perinatal HIV transmission by HIV testing and by initiating effective treatment for women who test positive. Yet roughly 15% of HIV-infected pregnant women, many of whom are drug users, receive no prenatal care (Chapter 6). Therefore, increasing the proportion of women, especially drug users, who receive prenatal care should be a high priority.

The 1988 IOM report *Prenatal Care: Reaching Mothers, Reaching Infants* recommends activities to (1) remove financial barriers to care; (2) make certain that basic system capacity is adequate for women; (3) improve the policies and practices that shape prenatal services at the delivery site; and (4) increase public information and education about prenatal care. The improvements in prenatal care coverage documented in Chapter 6 show that progress is being made, but it is troubling that prenatal care utilization is especially limited among those women most likely to be infected with HIV.

Some recent policy changes at the federal and state level do not augur well for improving access to prenatal care, although their full impact is not yet known. The 1996 federal welfare reform legislation creates bureaucratic barriers to the receipt of Medicaid for low-income women, both those who receive cash benefits under the new state welfare programs and those who continue to be Medicaid-eligible when they find employment. The legislation also prohibits undocumented immigrants and certain categories of legal immigrants from receiving Medicaid, despite the fact that any child born to them in the United States automatically becomes a U.S. citizen.

With respect to drug abuse and pregnancy, several states have passed legislation mandating drug testing (prenatal or neonatal) and/or drug abuse treatment (see Chapter 2). Such legislation can have a chilling effect on the willingness of pregnant drug users to seek prenatal care, even in states where such laws have not been passed, according to the committee's site visits. Women also fear losing custody of their children if their drug use is discovered.

Enhanced HIV Prevention in Correctional Settings

Correctional settings—prisons and jails—offer a unique opportunity for prevention activities targeted at hard-to-reach women at risk for, or already infected with, HIV. The total number of incarcerated women was 74,730 in 1996, a threefold increase from 1985 (Bureau of Justice Statistics, 1997). The prevalence of HIV infection among incarcerated women is far higher than in the general community: 4% of female state prison inmates nationwide are known to be HIV-positive, with the proportion exceeding 10% in nine states. Women are more likely than men to be incarcerated for drug offenses. In Rhode Island, for instance, nearly half of incarcerated women are imprisoned for drug-related charges (Flanigan, 1998). Consequently, they generally serve shorter sentences and return to the community, where many will re-offend.

The proportion of pregnant women in correctional settings who are HIV-infected is not known, but can be inferred to be higher than that in the general community. The median age of incarcerated women (31 years) places them squarely in the reproductive period. Furthermore, 6.1% of women in state prisons in 1994 were pregnant upon admission. Women in correctional settings thus represent an important population for targeted prevention efforts. Despite the relatively high-prevalence of HIV and pregnancy, only 85% of pregnant women received a gynecological exam related to pregnancy upon admission, and only 69% received any prenatal care while incarcerated.

Many interventions could be introduced in correctional settings either for general primary prevention of HIV transmission or for prevention of perinatal transmission among HIV-infected pregnant women in particular. Interventions could focus on HIV testing and treatment, drug testing and treatment, prenatal care, and efforts to ensure continuity of care for HIV-positive patients who leave the correctional setting. Given the realities of the correctional system, however, utmost care must be taken so that interventions are seen to be in the best interest of those incarcerated. Interventions that take advantage of prisoners to protect others, especially if the interventions lack confidentiality and may put prisoners at risk for harm, can be counter productive.

The Rhode Island prison system provides a model comprehensive HIV testing and care program that is integrated with the community. The proportion of HIV-positive women in Rhode Island prisons at any given time is between 8% and 12% (Flanigan, 1998). As outlined to the committee at one of its workshops, Rhode Island mandates HIV testing for all individuals upon prison intake. For infected individuals, complete HIV care is available, and HIV patients are successfully linked to follow-up care in the community (Appendix D; see also Flanigan, 1998). The Rhode Island program has had a tremendous impact on HIV diagnosis statewide: 28% of HIV-infected women in the state were tested through the correctional system. An even higher percentage (39%) of HIV-infected injection drug-using women were identified through the correctional system.

Development of Rapid HIV Tests

Because reporting of conventional HIV tests takes about one to two weeks, an accurate rapid test, with results available in hours, might have applications in prenatal, labor, and delivery settings to prevent perinatal transmission in some groups of patients (Minkoff and O'Sullivan, 1998). Women and newborns identified with a rapid test late in pregnancy or intrapartum could receive the intrapartum or postpartum component of the ACTG 076 regimen, respectively. A truncated version of the ACTG 076 regimen appears to be effective in reducing perinatal transmission, although to a somewhat lesser extent than the full regimen (see Chapter 4).

While there is one commercially available Food and Drug Administration (FDA) approved rapid test, its rate of false positives is regarded as too high for use in most settings, though it may be beneficial in settings of high-prevalence (CDC, 1998g). The CDC is currently developing guidelines on the implementation and quality assurance of rapid HIV testing. New rapid tests are expected to become commercially available in the near future and, when used in conjunction with existing rapid tests, would have lower false positive rates.

In the prenatal setting, a rapid test might be especially valuable for women who are unlikely to return for test results. According to the committee's site visits and workshops, these women are more likely to be adolescents, drug users, undocumented immigrants, and/or homeless. In the labor and delivery setting, a rapid test might be valuable for women who have not been tested previously or have not received prenatal care. There is a higher prevalence of HIV infection in women who have not received prenatal care (Lindsay et al., 1991c; see also Chapter 6). The labor and delivery setting offers the last opportunity to interrupt HIV transmission via administration of intrapartum therapy and advice to avoid breast-feeding. Since this is not an ideal time to obtain consent to testing and to discuss the implications of a positive result, program design and implementation would need to address these issues.

Bellevue Hospital Center in New York City has applied for permission from the state department of health to launch a voluntary, rapid testing demonstration program (as an alternative to the mandatory newborn testing program). Under this program, all women in labor and delivery who previously have not been tested for HIV will be offered a test. Since women who do not agree to prenatal testing at this public hospital are considered to be a population with higher HIV prevalence, the positive predictive value of a test is higher than in other settings. When the test is positive, antiretroviral therapy is to be offered beginning immediately in the intrapartum period, even though the woman's status must be confirmed by more definitive tests.

A rapid test also may have broader application for HIV prevention in general, because many individuals fail to return for test results with conventional testing. In 1995, for example, 25% of individuals testing HIV-positive at publicly funded clinics did not return for their test results (CDC, 1997b). Sexually transmitted disease clinics and drug abuse treatment programs are among the sites that should introduce an accurate rapid testing program for the purpose of primary HIV prevention (CDC, 1998g).

POPULATION GROUPS THAT MAY FACE ADDITIONAL BARRIERS

The following section focuses on the issues involved with testing and coordinating care for HIV-positive pregnant women who are adolescents or immigrants. Another important special population is drug-using pregnant women, a topic covered later in this chapter. While there certainly are problems in the coordination of their care, the larger problem is drawing drug-using women into prenatal care in the first place. As documented in Chapter 6, drug users are substantially less likely than others to receive prenatal care. Women in prisons and jails are another population requiring special attention, and these issues have been taken up earlier in this chapter.

Adolescents

Adolescents are a critical, yet underrecognized, population that needs coordinated HIV services. An estimated 25% of HIV-infected adults nationwide acquired their infection as adolescents (Rosenberg et al., 1994). Among the barriers to accepting and complying with HIV treatment are the lack of linkages between testing and treatment programs; adolescents' perception of invincibility and difficulty understanding the abstract concepts of disease latency and probabilities of transmission. Adolescents may also be injection drug users, which makes them more likely to become HIV-infected, and more difficult to reach. In additon, some adolescents have chosen to leave their home or have been forced out. Apart from the multiplicity of problems created by homelessness, frequent changes of address or no home address jeopardize Medicaid eligibility.

A nationally recognized comprehensive treatment program for adolescents in New York City, the Adolescent AIDS Program of Montefiore Medical Center, has been successful in treating HIV-positive adolescents who are pregnant and reducing perinatal transmission of HIV. The program attributes its success in prevention of perinatal transmission to these features: labor-intensive outreach to adolescents and health care professionals to encourage testing with linkage to treatment; lack of financial barriers to testing and treatment through sliding fee scales and help with obtaining Medicaid and other public financing programs; accessibility to the program through subsidized transportation; a "one-stop shopping" approach enabling teenagers to receive counseling, testing, treatment, and medications for HIV at the same site—both during and after pregnancy (although obstetrical services are available through referral); and understanding the special needs and fears of adolescents.

Immigrants

Although they do not have higher HIV infection rates, many immigrant women face multiple barriers to the prevention of perinatal HIV transmission (Appendixes E, G, and H). The most formidable are cultural, financial, and legal, including potential loss of U.S. residency rights or citizenship. Many immigrants, particularly those who are undocumented, are reluctant to seek prenatal care because they distrust the health care system and fear being reported to the Immigration and Naturalization Service, which may lead to deportation. The foreignness of the language and the institutional atmosphere also lead to avoidance. Some minority groups equate hospitals with death. The cost of prenatal care is another obstacle. Many providers and programs provide free care or care at reduced cost, but federal law explicitly prohibits undocumented immigrants from receiving Medicaid.

Finally, the cost of treatment is yet another barrier. Few immigrants have private insurance or Medicaid, so the only avenues for uninsured women to pay for care is through programs such as health department clinics and community health centers that serve low-income, Medicaid-ineligible people. Children born to undocumented immigrants, however, are covered under Medicaid by virtue of being born in the United States, which confers U.S. citizenship. Nevertheless, in South Texas, undocumented mothers of children born in the United States do not seek care for their children because their use of Medicaid would interfere with other family members' residency or citizenship petitions in the future (Appendix G).

Even with the new program of federally funded state child health insurance programs (CHIPs, described in Chapter 5), a substantial fraction of low-income women and children will remain uninsured and HIV-infected children will be born ineligible for Medicaid. Continued support for public health clinics and neighborhood health centers and innovative insurance programs can help to provide prenatal and HIV testing care for these populations. The committee has seen examples of perinatal HIV centers that have been able to provide care for uninsured women, using combinations of private and governmental resources.

CONCLUSIONS

If the promise of the ACTG 076 findings—that perinatal transmission of HIV can largely be prevented—is to be fulfilled, the United States needs to adopt a goal that all pregnant women be tested for HIV, and those who are positive remain in care so that they can receive optimal treatment for themselves and their children. To meet this goal, **the United States should adopt a national policy of universal HIV testing, with patient notification, as a routine component of prenatal care.** Adopting this policy will require the establishment of, and resources for, a comprehensive infrastructure that includes education of prenatal care providers; the development and implementation of practice guidelines; the implementation of clinical policies, the development and adoption of performance measures and Medicaid managed care contract language for prenatal HIV testing; efforts to improve coordination of care and access to high-quality HIV treatment; interventions to overcome pregnant women's concerns about HIV testing and treatment; and efforts to increase utilization of prenatal care, as described above.

References

Acuff KL, Faden RR. A history of prenatal and newborn screening programs: lessons for the future. In: Faden RR, Feller F, and Powers M., eds. *AIDS, Women, and the Next Generation: Towards a Morally Acceptable Public Policy for HIV Testing of Pregnant Women and Newborns*. New York: Oxford University Press, 1991.

AIDS Policy Center for Children, Youth and Families. Fact sheet: Facts about access to HIV/AIDS drugs for children, youth, and families. April 1998.

AIDS Policy Center for Children, Youth and Families. Position statement on HIV testing. 1995.

Alderton D, CDC, HIV/AIDS Surveillance Branch, personal communication. April 8, 1998.

Allen, D, Gortmaker SL, Cotton DJ, Gardner JD. HIV counseling and testing by prenatal providers: impact of clinical policies on provider behavior. Unpublished.

American Academy of Pediatrics (AAP). Committee on Pediatric AIDS. Human milk, breastfeeding, and transmission of human immunodeficiency virus in the United States. *Pediatrics* 96:977–999, 1995a.

AAP. Provisional Committee on Pediatric AIDS. Perinatal human immunodeficiency virus test. *Pediatrics* 95:303–307, 1995b.

AAP and American College of Obstetricians and Gynecologists (ACOG*). Guidelines for Perinatal Care*. 4th Ed. Elk Grove Village, IL; Washington, DC: p. 75, 1997.

American Civil Liberties Union (ACLU). *HIV Surveillance and Name Reporting: A Public Health Case for Protecting Civil Liberties*. October 1997.

American College of Nurse Midwives. Division of Standards and Practices. Statement of HIV/AIDS. 1997.

American College of Obstetrics and Gynecology. Human immunodeficiency virus infections in pregnancy. *ACOG Educational Bulletin* 232, January 1997.

American Medical Association (AMA). Maternal HIV screening and treatment to reduce the risk of perinatal HIV transmission: An update report. Report 6 of the Council on Scientific Affairs (A-96). 1995.

AMA. Counseling and testing of pregnant women for HIV, Resolution 425. House of Delegates. 1996.

AMA. Counseling and testing of pregnant women for HIV [H-20.927]. *HOD Policy.* 1997.

Association of Maternal and Child Health Programs (AMCHP). Policy on HIV Counseling and Testing. 1995.

Association of Women's Health, Obstetric, and Neonatal Nurses (AWHONN). HIV Testing and Disclosure. 1995[www document] URL http://www.awhonn,org/resour/position/pshiv.html

Baba TW, Koch J, Mittler ES, Greene M, Wyand M, Penninck D, Ruprecht R. Mucosal infection of neonatal rhesus monkeys with cell-free SIV. *AIDS Res Hum Retrovirus* 10:351–357, 1994.

Barbacci MB, Repke JT, Chaisson RE. Routine prenatal screening for HIV infection. *Lancet* 337:709–711, 1991.

Barton JJ, O'Connor TM, Cannon MJ, Weldon-Linne CM. Prevalence of human immunodeficiency virus in a general prenatal population. *Am J Obstet Gynecol* 160:1316–1324, 1989.

Bayer R. Public health policy and the AIDS epidemic. An end to HIV exceptionalism? *N Engl J Med* 324(21):1500–1504, 1991.

Bell LJ. Survey of prenatal care providers' screening practices. *EPINotes: Disease Prevention and Epidemiology Newsletter* 19:1–2, 1997. South Carolina Department of Health and Environmental Control.

Biggar, RJ, Miotti PG, Taha TE, Mtimavalye L, Broadhead R, Justesen A, Yellin F, Liomba G, Miley W, Waters D, Chiphangwi JD, Goedert JJ. Perinatal intervention trial in Africa: effect of a birth canal cleansing intervention to prevent HIV transmission. *Lancet* 347:1647–1650, 1996.

Birkhead GS. New York AIDS Institute. Personal communication. 1998.

Birkhead GS, Warren BL, Charbonneau TT. Evidence of intermediate rates of perinatal HIV-1 transmission with partial 076 regimens: Results of observational study. Abstract presented at Fifth Conference on Retroviruses and Opportunistic Infections. Chicago, IL. February 1-5, 1998.

BlueSpruce J. Group Health Cooperative of Puget Sound. Personal communication, 1998.

Blum RW, Beuhring T, Wunderlich M, Resnick MD. Don't ask, they won't tell: The quality of adolescent health screening in five practice settings. *Am J Publ Health* 86:1768, 1996.

Borkowsky W, Krasinski K, Cao Y, Ho D, Pollack H, Moore T, Chen SH, Allen M, Tao PT. Correlation of perinatal transmission of human immunodeficiency virus type 1 with maternal viremia and lymphocyte phenotypes. *J Pediatr* 125:345–351, 1994.

Bremer JW, Lew JF, Cooper E, Hillyer GV, Pitt J, Handelsman E, Brambilla D, Moye J, Hoff R. Diagnosis of infection with human immunodeficiency virus type 1 by a DNA polymerase chain reaction assay among infants enrolled in the Women and Infants' Transmission Study. *J Pediatr* 129:198–207, 1996.

Bulterys M, Chao A, Dushimimana A, Saah A. HIV-1 seroconversion after 20 months of age in a cohort of breastfed children born to HIV-1 infected women in Rwanda. *AIDS* 9:93–94, 1995.

Bureau of Justice Statistics. *Correctional Populations in the United States, 1995.* 1997.

Byers Jr. RH, Caldwell MB, Davis S, Gwinn M, Lindegren ML. Projection of AIDS and HIV incidence among children born infected with HIV. *Stat Med* 17:169–181, 1998.

Cao Y, Krogstad P, Korber BT, Koup RA, Muldoon M, Macken C, Song JL, Jin Z, Zhao JQ, Clapp S, Chen IS, Ho DD, Ammann AJ. Maternal HIV-1 viral load and vertical transmission of infection: The Ariel Project for the prevention of HIV transmission from mother to infant. *Nat Med* 3:549–552, 1997.

Carusi D, Learman LA, Posner SF. Human immunodeficiency virus test refusal in pregnancy: A challenge to voluntary testing. *Obstet Gynecol* 91(4):540–545, 1998.

Centers for Disease Control and Prevention (CDC). Public Health Service guidelines for antibody testing to prevent HIV infection and AIDS. *MMWR* 36:509–515, 1987.

CDC Recommendations of the U.S. Public Health Service Task Force on the use of zidovudine to reduce perinatal transmission of human immunodeficiency virus. *MMWR* 43(RR-11), 1994.

CDC. 1995 revised guidelines for prophylaxis against *Pneumocystis carinii* pneumonia for children infected with or perinatally exposed to human immunodeficiency virus. *MMWR* 44(RR-4):1–10, 1995a.

CDC. U.S. Public Health Service recommendations for human immunodeficiency virus counseling and voluntary testing for pregnant women. *MMWR* 44(RR-7), 1995b.

CDC. AIDS among children—United States. *MMWR* 45(46):1–4, 1996a.

CDC. *HIV/AIDS Surveillance Report* 8(2), 1996b.

CDC. *AIDS Public Information Data Set: Data Through December 1996.* 1997a.

CDC. Fact sheet: Strategies for prevention of HIV in women. Atlanta: U.S. Department of Health and Human Services, 1997b.

CDC. *HIV/AIDS Surveillance Report* 9(2), 1997c.

CDC. HIV counseling and testing in publicly funded sites: 1995 summary report. Atlanta: U.S. Department of Health and Human Services, 1997d.

CDC. Update: Perinatally acquired HIV/AIDS, United States, 1997. *MMWR* 46(46):1085–1092, 1997e.

CDC. 1997 USPHS/IDSA guidelines for the prevention of opportunistic infections in persons infected with human immunodeficiency virus. *MMWR* 46(RR-12), 1997f.

CDC. Administration of zidovudine during late pregnancy and delivery to prevent perinatal HIV transmission—Thailand, 1996–1998. *MMWR* 47(8):151–154, 1998a.

CDC. Fact sheet: HIV prevention community planning: Successes and challenges. Atlanta: U.S. Department of Health and Human Services, 1998b.

CDC. Guidelines for the use of antiretroviral agents in pediatric HIV infection. *MMWR* 47(RR-4), 1998c.

CDC. Public Health Service Task Force's recommendations for the use of antiretroviral drugs in pregnant women infected with HIV-1 for maternal health and for reducing perinatal HIV-1 transmission in the United States. *MMWR* 47(RR-2):1–25, 1998d.

CDC. Report of the NIH panel to define principles of therapy of HIV infection and guidelines for the use of antiretroviral agents in HIV-infected adults and adolescents. *MMWR* 47(RR-05), 1998e.

CDC. Success in implementing PHS guidelines to reduce perinatal transmission of HIV—1993, 1995, and 1996. *MMWR* 47(33):688–691, 1998f.

CDC. Update: HIV counseling and testing using rapid tests—United States, 1998. *MMWR* 47(11):211–215, 1998g.

Chavkin W, Breitbart V, Elman D, Wise P. National survey of the states: Policies and practices regarding drug-using pregnant women. *Am J Publ Health* 88(1):117–119, 1998.

Ching S, Paul S, Goldman K. The diffusion of HIV counseling among New Jersey obstetricians and gynecologists: Factors influencing levels of implementation. New Jersey Graduate Program in Public Health, Fieldwork Project, May 1997.

Coates T, Stall R, Kegeles S, Lo B, Morin S, McKusick L. AIDS antibody testing: Will it stop the AIDS epidemic? Will it help people infected with HIV? *Am Psychol* 43:859–864, 1988.

Connor EM, Sperling RS, Gelber R, Kiselev P, Scott G, O'Sullivan MJ, VanDyke R, Bey M, Shearer W, Jacobson RL, Jimenez E, O'Neill E, Bazin B, Delfraissy JF, Culnane M, Coombs R, Elkins M, Moye J, Stratton P, Balsley J. Reduction of maternal–infant transmission of human immunodeficiency virus type 1 with zidovudine treatment. Pediatric AIDS Clinical Trials Group Protocol 076 Study Group. *N Engl J Med* 331(18):1173–1180, 1994.

Cozen W, Mascola L, Enguidanos R. Screening for HIV and hepatitis B virus in Los Angeles county prenatal clinics: A demonstration project. *J Acquir Immune Defic Syndr* 6:95–98, 1993.

Datta P, Embree JE, Kreiss JK, Ndinya-Achola JO, Braddick M, Temmerman M, Nagelkerke J, Maitha G, Holmes KK, Piot P, et al. Mother-to-child transmission of human immunodeficiency virus type 1: Report from the Nairobi study. *J Infect Dis* 170(5):1134–1140, 1994.

Davis K. Uninsured in an era of managed care. *Health Serv Res* 31:641–649, 1997.

Davis SF, Byers RH Jr., Lindegren ML, Caldwell MB, Karon JM, Gwinn M. Prevalence and incidence of vertically acquired HIV infection in the United States. *JAMA* 274(12):952–955, 1995.

Department of Health and Human Services. Fact sheet: Medicaid and acquired immune deficiency syndrome (AIDS) and human immunodeficiency virus (HIV) infection. March 1998. [www document] URL http://hiv.hcfa.gov/medicaid/obs11.htm

DHHS. *Volume 1. Natality. Vital Statistics of the United States.* Hyattsville, MD: National Center for Health Statistics, 1992.

Dickover RE, Garratty EM, Herman SA, Sim MS, Plaeger S, Boyer PJ, Keller M, Deveikis A, Stiehm ER, Bryson YJ. Identification of levels of maternal HIV-1 RNA associated with risk of perinatal transmission. Effect of maternal zidovudine treatment on viral load. *JAMA* 275(8):599–605, 1996.

D'Souza MP, Harden VA. Chemokines and HIV-1 second receptors. *Nat Med* 2:1293–1300, 1996.

Doyle A, Jefferys R, Kelly J. *State AIDS Drug Assistance Programs: A National Status Report on Access.* Menlo Park, CA: Henry J. Kaiser Family Foundation, 1997.

Duliege AM, Amos CI, Felton S, Biggar RJ, Goedert JJ. Birth order, delivery route, and concordance in the transmission of human immunodeficiency virus type 1 from mothers to twins. International registry of HIV-exposed twins. *J Pediatr* 126(4):625–632, 1995.

Dunn DT, Newell ML, Ades AE, Peckham C. Risk of human immunodeficiency virus type 1 transmission through breastfeeding. *Lancet* 340:585–588, 1992.

Dupont-Merck. Communication to Investigators, Efavirenz Information. 1998.

Ecker JL. The cost-effectiveness of human immunodeficiency virus screening in pregnancy. *Am J Obstet Gynecol* 174:716–721, 1996.

Ehrnst A, Lindgren S, Dictor M , Johansson B, Sonnenborg A, Czajkowski J, Sundin G, Bohlin AB. HIV in pregnant women and their offspring: Evidence for late transmission. *Lancet* 338:203–207, 1991.

Employee Benefits Research Institute (EBRI). Fact sheet: Characteristics of individuals with employment-based health insurance, 1987–1995. 1997. [www document] URL http://www.ebri.org/facts/ 0797fact.htm

EBRI. Issues of quality and consumer rights in the health care market. *EBRI Issue Brief* 196, April 1998.

Faden RR, Kass NE, Powers M. Warrants for screening programs: Public health, legal, and ethical frameworks. In: Faden RR, Feller G, Powers M, eds. *AIDS, Women, and the Next Generation: Towards a Morally Acceptable Public Policy for HIV Testing of Pregnant Women and Newborns.* New York: Oxford University Press, 1991.

Faden R, Chwalow AJ, Holtzman NA, Horn SD. A survey to evaluate parental consent as public policy for neonatal screening. *Am J Publ Health* 72(12):1347–1352, 1982.

Families USA Foundation. Field report: Balanced budget bill enacted. August 1997.

Fiscus SA, Adimora AA, Schoenbach VJ, Lim W, McKinney R, Rupar D, Kenny J, Woods C, Wilfert C. Perinatal HIV infection and the effect of zidovudine therapy on transmission in rural and urban counties. *JAMA* 275(19):1483–1488, 1996.

Fine A. *National Welfare Reform: Impact on Maternal and Child Health.* Washington, DC: Association of Maternal and Child Health Programs. 1997.

Flanigan T. The Miriam Hospital, Brown University. Personal communication, 1998.

Gamble V. A legacy of distrust: African Americans and medical research. *Am J Prev Med* 9:35–38, 1993.

Gamble, V. Under the Shadow of Tuskegee: African Americans and Health Care. *Am J Publ Health* 87:1773–1778, 1997.

Gorsky RD, Farnham PG, Straus WL, Caldwell B, Holtgrave DR, Simonds RJ, Rogers MF, Guinan ME. Preventing perinatal transmission of HIV: Costs and effectiveness of a recommended intervention. *Public Health Rep* 111(4):335–341, 1996.

Gostin LO, Ward JW, Baker AC. National HIV case reporting for the United States. A defining moment in the history of the epidemic. *N Engl J Med* 337:1162–1167, 1997.

Gostin LO, Webber D. The AIDS litigation project part II, HIV/AIDS in courts in the 1990s. *AIDS and Public Policy Journal* 13(2 Summer), 1998.

Gostin LO, Lazzarini Z, Ward J, Fleming P, Neslund V. State efforts to prevent perinatal HIV transmission: results of a national survey of state laws, regulations, policies, and guidelines. For Centers for Disease Control and Prevention. in Press.

Hale RW, Zinberg S. American College of Obstetrics and Gynecologists' position on HIV testing. *ACOG Clinical Review* 2(1):13, 1997.

Hamm RH, Donnell HD, Wilson E, Meredith K, Louise S. Prevention of perinatal HIV transmission: beliefs and practices of Missouri prenatal providers. *Missouri Epidemiologist* March–April:5–21, 1996.

Havens PL, Cuene BE, Hand JR, Gern JE, Sullivan BW, Chusin MJ. Effectiveness of intensive nurse case management in decreasing vertical transmission of human immunodeficiency virus infection in Wisconsin. *Pediatr Infect Dis J* 16(9):871–875, 1997.

Health Care Financing Administration (HCFA). Managed care trends. National Summary of Medicaid Managed Care Programs and Enrollment. June 30, 1997. [www document] URL http://www.hcfa.gov/medicaid/ome1997.htm

Health Resources and Services Administration (HRSA). Fact sheet: Title II Ryan White CARE Act. 1998a. [www document] URL http://www.hrsa.dhhs.gov/hab/OC/factshee/titii.htm

HRSA. Fact sheet. Title IV Ryan White CARE Act. 1998b.

Healton C, Howard J, Messeri P, Sorin MD, Abramson D, Bayer R. A balancing act: The tension between case-finding and primary prevention strategies in New York State's voluntary HIV counseling and testing program in women's health care settings. *Am J Prev Med* 12(1 Suppl):53–60, 1996.

Herczfeld, ND. A survey of prenatal care providers in Connecticut regarding their attitudes and practices pertaining to HIV/AIDS and pregnancy. Master of Public Health thesis, Yale University, Department of Epidemiology and Public Health, 1995.

Hill B, Nevada State Health Division, HIV/AID Programs Office. Personal communication, 1998.

Holtzman NA. Public participation in genetic policymaking: The Maryland commission in hereditary disorders in genetics and the law. In: Malinsky A, Annas GJ, eds. *Genetics and the Law*. New York: Plenum, 1984.

Husson RN, Lan Y, Kojima E, Venzon D, Mitsuya H, McIntosh K. Vertical transmission of human immunodeficiency virus type 1: Autologous neutralizing antibody, virus load, and virus phenotype. *J Pediatr* 126(6):865–871, 1995.

Institute of Medicine (IOM). *Reaching Mothers, Reaching Infants: Summary and Recommendations*. Washington, DC: National Academy Press, 1988.

IOM. *Clinical Practice Guidelines: Direction for a New Program*. Washington, DC: National Academy Press, 1990.

IOM. *HIV Screening of Pregnant Women and Newborns*. Washington, DC: National Academy Press, 1991.

IOM. *Clinical Practice Guidelines: From Development to Use*. Washington, DC: National Academy Press, 1992.

IOM. *AIDS and Behavior: An Integrated Approach*. Washington, DC: National Academy Press, 1994.

IOM. *Assessing the Social and Behavioral Science Base for HIV/AIDS Prevention and Intervention*. Washington, DC: National Academy Press, 1995a.

IOM. *The Best Intentions: Unintended Pregnancy and the Well-Being of Children and Families*. Washington, DC: National Academy Press, 1995b

IOM. *HIV and the Blood Supply: An Analysis of Crisis Decisionmaking*. Washington, DC: National Academy Press, 1995c.

IOM. *Measuring the Quality of Health Care—State of the Art*. Washington, DC: National Academy Press, 1996a.

IOM *Opportunities in Drug Abuse Research Committee on Opportunities in Drug Abuse Research*. Washington, DC: National Academy Press, 1996b.

IOM. *The Hidden Epidemic*. Washington, DC: National Academy Press, 1997.

Intercollegiate Working Party for Enhancing Voluntary Confidential HIV Testing in Pregnancy. Royal College of Paediatrics and Child Health. *Reducing Mother to Child Transmission of HIV Infection in the United Kingdom*. London, England: April 1998.

Irwin KL, Valdiserri RO, Holmberg SD. The acceptability of voluntary HIV antibody testing in the United States: A decade of lessons learned. *AIDS* 10:1707–1717, 1996.

Jones J. *Bad Blood: The Tuskegee Syphilis Experiment*. 2nd. ed.. New York: Free Press, 1993.

Jos PH, Marshall MF, Perlmutter M. The Charleston policy on cocaine use during pregnancy: A cautionary tale. *J Law Med Ethics* 23:120–128, 1995.

Kaiser Commission on the Future of Medicaid. Fact sheet: Medicaid and Managed Care. May, 1996.

Kaiser Commission on Medicaid and Uninsured. Unpublished estimates based on Current Population Survey, using ages 18–44 for women and under 18 for children. March 1996.

Kaiser Commission on Medicaid and Uninsured. *Uninsured in America: A Chart Book*. Menlo Park, CA: The Henry J. Kaiser Family Foundation, June 1998a.

Kaiser Commission on Medicaid and Uninsured. *Uninsured facts: The Uninsured and Their Access To Health Care*. Menlo Park, CA: The Henry J. Kaiser Family Foundation, July 1998b.

Kaiser Family Foundation. Abbot v. Bragdon: high court rules Americans with Disabilities Act protects patients with HIV. *Daily HIV/AIDS Report*. June 26, 1998a. [www document] URL http://report. kff.org/aidshiv/db2/1998/06/kh980626.1.html

Kaiser Family Foundation. Understanding the Impact of New Treatments on HIV Testing: Summary of a forum held on January 28–30, 1998. 1998b.

King P. Legal issues in voluntary screening for HIV infection in pregnant women. In: Faden RR, Feller F, Powers M., eds. *AIDS, Women, and the Next Generation: Towards a Morally Acceptable Public Policy for HIV Testing of Pregnant Women and Newborns*. New York: Oxford University Press, 1991.

Landesman SH, Kalish LA, Burns DN, Minkoff H, Fox HE, Zorrilla C, Garcia P, Fowler MG, Mofenson L, Tuomala R. Obstetrical factors and the transmission of human immunodeficiency virus type 1 from mother to child. The Women and Infants Transmission Study. *N Engl J Med* 334(25):1617–236, 1996.

Lewis K, Ellwood M, Czajka JL. Counting the Uninsured: A Review of the Literature. Occasional Paper No. 8. Washington, DC: The Urban Institute. 1998

Limata C, Schoen EJ, Cohen D, Black SB, Quesenberry Jr CP. Compliance with voluntary prenatal HIV testing in a large health maintenance organization (HMO). *J Acquir Immune Defic Syndr Hum Retrovirol* 15(2):126–130, 1997.

Lindegren ML. Prevalence of zidovudine use to reduce maternal–infant transmission, 1994–1995. Presentation at IOM Workshop on Perinatal Transmission of HIV, Washington, DC. April 1, 1998.

Lindegren ML, Byers RH, Fleming P, Thomas P, Wortley P, Gwinn M, Ward J. Status of the perinatal HIV epidemic in the United States: Success in perinatal prevention [abstract 23306]. Presented at the Twelfth World AIDS Conference, Geneva, Switzerland. June 28–July 3, 1998.

Lindsay MK. A protocol for routine voluntary antepartum human immunodeficiency virus antibody screening. *Am J Obstet Gynecol* 168(2):476–479, 1993.

Lindsay MK, Adefris W, Peterson HB, Williams H, Johnson J, Klein L. Determinants of acceptance of routine voluntary human immunodeficiency virus testing in an inner-city prenatal population. *Obstet Gynecol* 78(4):678–680, 1991a.

Lindsay MK, Feng TI, Peterson HB, Slade BA, Willis S, Klein L. Routine human immunodeficiency virus infection screening in unregistered and registered inner-city parturients. *Obstet Gynecol* 77(4):599–603, 1991b.

Lindsay MK., Peterson HB, Willis S, Slade BA, Gramling J, Williams H, Klein L. Incidence and prevalence of human immunodeficiency virus infection in a prenatal population undergoing routine voluntary human immunodeficiency virus screening, July 1987 to June 1990. *Am J Obstet Gynecol* 165(4, Pt 1):962–964, 1991c.

Lorenzi P, Masserei V, Laubereau B, Irion O, Kind C, Rudin C, Hirschel B, Kaiser L. Safety of combined anitretroviral therapies with or without protease inhibitors in pregnant HIV-infected women and their offspring [abstract No. 32453] Presented at the Twelfth World AIDS Conference. Geneva, Switzerland. June 28–July 3, 1998.

Lovvorn A, Quinn S. HIV testing of pregnant women: A policy analysis. *J Publ Health Policy* 18:401–432, 1997.

Louisiana Morbidity Report. Prevention of Perinatal HIV Transmission. 6(5):November–December, 1995.

Lurie P, Wolfe SM. Unethical trials of interventions to reduce perinatal transmission of the human immunodeficiency virus in developing countries. *N Engl J Med* 337:853–856, 1997.

Luzuriaga K, Bryson Y, Krogstad P, Robinson J, Stechenberg B, Lamson M, Cort S, Sullivan JL. Combination treatment with zidovudine, didanosine, and nevirapine in infants with human immunodeficiency virus type 1 infection. *N Engl J Med* 336(19):1343–1349, 1997.

Luzuriaga K, McQuilken P, Alimenti A, Somasundaran M, Hesselton R, Sullivan JL. Early viremia and immune responses in vertical human immunodeficiency virus type 1 infection. *J Inf Dis* 167:1008–1013, 1993.

Luzuriaga K, Sullivan JL. DNA polymerase chain reaction for the diagnosis of vertical HIV infection. *JAMA* 275(17):1360–1361, 1996.

Mandelbrot L, Le Cheandec J, Berrebi A, Bongain A, Benifla JL, Delfraissy JF, Blanche S, Mayaux MJ. Perinatal HIV-1 transmission: Interaction between zidovudine prophylaxis and mode of delivery in the French Perinatal Cohort. *JAMA* 280:55–60, 1998.

Mandelbrot L, Mayaux MJ, Bongain A, Berrebi A, Moudoub-Jeanpetit Y, Benifla JL, Ciraru-Vigneron N, Le Chenadec J, Blanche S, Delfraissy JF. Obstetric factors and mother-to-child transmission of human immunodeficiency virus type 1: The French perinatal cohorts. SEROGEST French Pediatric HIV Infection Study Group. *Am J Obstet Gynecol* 175(3 Pt 1):661–667, 1996.

Mason J, Preisinger J, Sperling R, Walther V, Berrier J, Evans V. Incorporating HIV education and counseling into routine prenatal care: A program model. *AIDS Educ Prev* 3(2):118–123, 1991.

Mauskopf JA, Paul JE, Wichman DS, White AD, Tilson HH. Economic impact of treatment of HIV-positive pregnant women and their newborns with zidovudine. Implications for HIV screening. *JAMA* 276(2):132–138, 1996.

Mayaux MJ, Teglas JP, Mandelbrot L, Berrebi A, Gallais H, Matheron S, Viraru-Vigneron N, Parnet-Mathieu F, Bongain A, Rouzioux C, Delfraissy JF, Blanche S. Acceptability and impact of zidovudine for prevention of mother-to-child human immunodeficiency virus-1 transmission in France. *J Pediatr* 131:857–862, 1997.

Michigan Department of Community Health. Improving the odds: Reducing perinatal HIV transmission: Report of the recommendations of the Maternal Child Health Advisory Committee, Subcommittee on Perinatal HIV Reduction. 1997.

Michigan Department of Community Health. Trends in perinatal HIV Transmission in Michigan. 1998.

Mills WA, Martin DL, Bertrand, Belongia EA. Physicians' practices and opinions regarding prenatal screening for human immunodeficiency virus and other sexually transmitted diseases. *Sex Trans Dis* 25(3):169–175, 1998.

Minkoff H, Burns SN, Landesman S, Youchah J, Goedert JJ, Nugent RP, Muenz LR, Willoughby AD. The relationship of the duration of ruptured membranes to vertical transmission of human immunodeficiency virus. *Am J Obstet Gynecol* 173(2):585–589, 1995.

Minkoff H, O'Sullivan MJ. The case for rapid HIV testing during labor. *JAMA* 279:1743–1744, 1998.

Mitchell B. Preliminary analyses of 1997 Texas birth certificate data, personal communication. Texas Department of Health, 1998.

Mofenson L. Session 11, Advances in HIV prevention: Prevention of perinatal HIV transmission. Presented at the Fifth Conference on Retroviruses and Opportunistic Infection. Chicago, IL. February 1–5, 1998.

Montana Department of Public Health and Human Services, Communicable Disease Control and Prevention Bureau, STD/HIV Section: DPHHS HIV Screening Survey Results. 1996

Myers ER, Thompson JW, Simpson K. Cost-effectiveness of mandatory compared with voluntary screening for human immunodeficiency virus in pregnancy. *Obstet Gynecol* 91(2):164–181, 1998.

National Academy of Sciences (NAS). *Genetic Screening: Programs, Principles, and Research.* Washington, DC: National Academy Press, 1975.

National Center for Health Statistics (NCHS). *Health. United States, 1996–1997 and Injury Chartbook.* Hyattsville, MD. 1997.

National Institutes of Health (NIH). Consensus statement. Newborn screening for sickle cell disease and other hemoglobinopathies. *JAMA* 258(9):1205–1209, 1987.

NIH. Interventions to prevent HIV risk behaviors. *NIH Consensus Statement* 15(2):1–41, 1997.

National Research Council (NRC). *AIDS: Sexual Behavior and Intravenous Drug Use.* Washington, DC: National Academy Press, 1989.

NRC. *AIDS: The Second Decade.* Washington, DC: National Academy Press, 1990.

NRC. *Evaluating AIDS Prevention Programs* (Expanded Edition). Washington, DC: National Academy Press, 1991.

NRC. *The Social Impact of AIDS in the United States.* Washington, DC: National Academy Press, 1993.

NRC. *Prevention HIV Transmission: The Role of Sterile Needles and Bleach.* Washington, DC: National Academy Press, 1995.

New York Department of Health, Maternal-Perinatal HIV Prevention and Care Program. Newborn HIV testing program update: Infants born February 1 to October 31, 1997. 1997.

New York Post. 13,000 Babies. January 5, 1938 p.1.

Newton ZB, Bell WC. HIV perinatal prevention project: Contact and survey of metro Atlanta obstetricians. *Georgia Obstetrical and Gynecological Society*, July 21, 1997.

Nyquist C. HIV testing of pregnant women in Colorado. Undated abstract.

Ohio Department of Health. Perinatal HIV counseling and testing survey. October 31, 1997.

Palasanthiran P, Ziegler JB, Stewart GJ, Stuckey M, Armstrong JA, Cooper DA, Penny R, Gold J. Breastfeeding during primary human immunodeficiency virus infection and risk of transmission from mother to infant. *J Infect Dis* 167:441–444, 1993.

Partika N. John A Burns School of Medicine, Department of Psychiatry, Kapiolani Medical Center for Women and Children, University of Hawaii at Manoa. Personal communication. 1998.

Partika N, Johnson J. Results of a survey of Hawaii ob/gyns and family practice physicians regarding perinatal transmission of HIV: During time period from July 1, 1996 to June 30, 1997. 1997.

Paul SM, Dimasi LG, Costa SJ, Beil J, Cross A, Morgan DH. Evaluation of ZDV administration to pregnant women and their children born in 1993 through 1996 in New Jersey [poster #23287] Presented at the Twelfth World AIDS Conference. Geneva, Switzerland. June 28-July 3, 1998a.

Paul SM, Cross H, Costa SJ, Pemberton G, Ching S, Dimasi L, Beil J, Palmer D, Pierce M, Caswell B, Morgan DH, Ziskin LZ. A comprehensive evaluation of implementation of the Public Health Service recommendations to prevent perinatal HIV transmission. Presentation at IOM Workshop. April 1, 1998b.

Pemberton G. Knowledge, attitude, beliefs and intentions surrounding AZT use: A study of pregnant women's perception. Master's thesis, New Jersey Graduate Program in Public Health, September 3, 1997.

Perez-Pena, R. Bill to track people infected with HIV gains in Albany. *New York Times.* June 19, 1998, P.A30.

Pettiti DB, Department of Research and Evaluation, Southern California Permanente Medical Group; Percentage of pregnant members of Southern California Kaiser Permanente tested for HIV by area, 1994–1997, Personal communication, April 30, 1998.

Phillips KA, Morrison KR, Sonnad SS, Bleecker T. HIV counseling and testing of pregnant women and women of childbearing age by primary care providers: Self-reported beliefs and practices. *Acquir Immune Defic Syndr Hum Retrovirol* 14:174–178, 1997.

Pilon. Alberta adds HIV test to prenatal screening. *Edmonton Sun.* August 6, 1998.

Pliner V, Weedon J, Thomas PA, Steketee RW, Abrams EJ, Lambert G, Greenberg B, Banji M, Thea DM, Matheson PB. Incubation period of HIV-1 in perinatally infected children, New York City perinatal HIV transmission collaborative study group. *AIDS* 12:759–766, 1998.

Popek EJ, Korber BT, Merritt L, Bardenguez A, Lee A, Hammill HA, Wiznia A, Viscarello R, Luzuriaga K, Van Dyke RB. Acute chorioamnionitis and duration of membrane rupture correlates with vertical transmission of HIV-1. Poster presented at the Fourth Conference on Retroviruses and Opportunistic Infections, Washington, DC, January 22–26, 1997.

Quinn S. Belief in AIDS as a form of genocide: Implications for HIV prevention programs for African Americans. *Journal of Health Education* 28:S6–S11, 1998.

RAND. Unpublished data from HIV Cost and Services Utilization Study. 1998.

Report of a Consensus Workshop. Maternal factors involved in mother-to-child transmission of HIV-1. *J AIDS* 5:1019–1029, 1992.

Rhame F, Maki D. The case for wider use of testing for HIV infection. *N Engl J Med* 320:1248–1254, 1989.

Riley CW. Perinatal HIV infection white paper. Virginia Department of Health, Division of STD/AIDS, January 1998.

Rodriguez EM, Mofenson LM, Chang BH. Association of maternal drug use during pregnancy with maternal culture positivity and perinatal human immunodeficiency virus transmission. *AIDS* 10:273–282, 1996.

Rogers MF. Epidemiology of HIV/AIDS in women and children in the USA. *Acta Paediatr* 421:15–16, 1997.

Rogers, MF, Caldwell MB, Gwinn ML, Simonds RJ. Epidemiology of pediatric human immunodeficiency virus infection in the United States. *Acta Paediatr* Suppl 400:5–7, 1994.

Rogers MF, Ou CY, Rayfield M, Thomas PA, Schoenbaum EE, Abrams E, Krasinski K , Selwyn PA, Moore J, Kaul A, et al. Use of the polymerase chain reaction for early detection of the proviral sequences of human immunodeficiency virus in infants born to seropositive mothers. New York City Collaborative Study of Maternal HIV Transmission and Montefiore Medical Center HIV Perinatal Transmission Study Group. *N Engl J Med* 320(25):1649–1654, 1989.

Rosenberg KD, Townes JM, Gonzales K, Modesitt SK, Fleming DW. HIV screening practices of Oregon prenatal care providers. Center for Disease Prevention and Epidemiology, Oregon Health Division. Undated abstract.

Rosenberg PS, Biggar RJ, Goedert JJ. Declining age at HIV infection in the United States. *New Engl J Med* 167:1096–1099, 1994.

Royce RA., Walter EB, Eckman A, Bennett B. Public health efforts to prevent vertical HIV transmission in North Carolina. Presentation at IOM Workshop on Perinatal Transmission of HIV, Washington, DC, April 1, 1998.

Rubin T. Health Care Finances Administration (HCFA): Impact of the PHS voluntary testing recommendations: Results from providers and patient survey and state data systems. Presentation at the IOM Workshop on Perinatal Transmission of HIV, Washington, DC, April 1, 1998.

Ruff AJ, Coberly J, Halsey NA, Boulos R, Desormeaux J, Burnley A, Joseph DH, McBrien M, Quinn T, Losikoff P, et al. Prevalence of HIV-1 DNA and p24 antigen in breast milk and correlation with maternal factors. *J Acquir Immune Defic Syndr* 7:68–73, 1994.

Sage AC, Mahon B, Colfort Jr. JM. HIV counseling and testing practices of prenatal care providers in California. Unpublished.

Scarlatti, G, Hodara V, Rossi P, Muggiasca L, Bucceri A, Albert J, Fenyo EM. Transmission of human immunodeficiency virus type 1 (HIV-1) from mother to child correlates with viral phenotype. *Virology* 197(2):624–629, 1993.

Schoen EJ. Northern California Kaiser Permanente Health Plan. Personal communication, 1998.

Scott R. Sickle-cell anemia,high prevalence and low priority. *N Engl J Med* 282:164–165, 1970.

Segal AI. Physician attitudes toward human immunodeficiency virus testing in pregnancy. *Am J Obstet Gynecol* 174(6):1750–1756, 1996.

Semba RD, Miotti P, Chiphangwi JD, Saah AJ, Canner JK, Dallabetta GA, Hoover DR. Maternal vitamin A deficiency and mother-to-child transmission of HIV-1. *Lancet* 343:1593–1597, 1994.

Shakarishvili A, Schulte J, Levine W, Kreitner S, Caldwell B, St. Louis M. Lack of timely prenatal care among women infected with HIV: Implications for prevention of perinatal HIV transmission in the United States. Abstract presented at the Eleventh International Conference on AIDS, Vancouver, BC, July 7–12, 1996. [www document] URL http://sis.nlm.nih.gov/aidsabs.htm

Siegel K, Gorey E. HIV-infected women: Barriers to AZT use. *Soc Sci Med* 45(1):15–22, 1997.

Silverman NS, Rohner DM, Turner BJ. Attitudes toward health-care, HIV infection, and perinatal transmission interventions in a cohort of inner-city, pregnant women. *Am J Perinatol* 14(6):341–346, 1997.

Simonds RJ, Rogers M. Impact of the PHS voluntary testing recommendations. Results from CDC's surveillance and enhanced surveillance systems. Presentation at IOM Workshop on Perinatal Transmission of HIV, Washington DC, April 1, 1998.

Simpson JL, Nadler HL. Maternal serum alpha-fetoprotein screening in 1987. *Obstet Gynecol* 69:134–134, 1987.

Simpson W, Hart G, Johnston FD, Goldberg DJ, Boyd FM. Comparison of opt-in and opt-out HIV testing in antenatal care: uptake and acceptability in Edinburgh, Scotland [abstract #43120]. Abstract presented at the Twelfth World AIDS Conference, Geneva, Switzerland. June 28-July 3, 1998.

Sperling RS, Shapiro DE, Coombs RW, Todd LA, Herman SA, McSherry GD, O'Sullivan MJ, Van Dyke RB, Jimenez E, Rouzioux C, Flynn PM, Sullivan JL. Maternal viral load, zidovudine treatment, and the risk of transmission of human immunodeficiency virus type 1 from mother to infant. Pediatric AIDS Clinical Trials Group Protocol 076 Study Group. *N Engl J Med* 335(22):1621–1629, 1996.

Sprecher S, Soumenkoff G, Puissant F, Degueldre MD. Vertical transmission of HIV in 15 week fetus. *Lancet* 2:288–289, 1986.

Stoddard T, Reiman W. AIDS and the rights of the individual: Toward a more sophisticated understanding of discrimination. *Milbank Q* 68 (Suppl 1):143–174, 1990.

Study EC. Natural history of vertically acquired human immunodeficiency virus-1 infection. *Pediatrics* 94:815–819, 1994.

Thea DM, Steketee RW, Pliner V, Bornschlegel K, Brown T, Orloff S, Matheson PB, Abrams EJ, Bamji M, Lambert G, Schoenbaum EA, Thomas PA, Heagarty M, Kalish ML. The effect of maternal viral load on the risk of perinatal transmission of HIV-1. New York City Perinatal HIV Transmission Collaborative Study Group. *AIDS* 11(4):437–444, 1997.

Thomas S, Quinn S. Presidential apology for the Study at Tuskegee (1997*). 1998 Medical and Health Annual.* Chicago, IL: Encyclopedia Britannica, 280–281, 1997.

Turner BJ, Markson L, Hauck W, Cocroft J, Fanning T. Prenatal care of HIV-infected women: Analysis of a large New York State cohort. *J Acquir Immune Defic Syndr Hum Retrovirol* 9(4):371–378, 1995.

Turner BJ, McKee-Nelsen L, Fanning TR, Hauck WW. Prevention of vertical HIV transmission with zidovudine: Projected impact of HIV testing and prenatal care. *AIDS Care* 9(5):577–588, 1997.

U.S. Public Health Service (USPHS). Syphilis in Mother and Child. Supplement 7 to Venereal Disease Information (Washington, DC: Government Printing Office, 1940), 1.

Urban Institute. Counting the Uninsured: A Review of the Literature. Occasional Paper No. 8. 1998.

Ventura SJ, Peters KD, Martin JA, Maurer JD. Births and deaths: United States, 1996. *Monthly Vital Statistics Report* 46(1S2):12. Hyattsville, MD: National Center for Health Statistics. 1997.

Ventura SJ, Martin JA, Curtin SC, Mathews TJ. Report of final natality statistics, 1996. *Monthly Vital Statistics* 4(11):43. Hyattsville, MD: National Center for Health Statistics. 1998.

Walter EB, Elliott AJ, Regan AN, Drucker RP, Clements DA, Wilfert CM. Maternal acceptance of voluntary human immunodeficiency virus antibody testing during the newborn period with the Guthrie card. *Pediatr Infect Dis J* 14:376–381, 1995.

Walter EB, Lampe MA, Livingston E, Royce RA. How do North Carolina prenatal care providers counsel and test pregnant women for HIV? Survey measures knowledge of HIV testing benefits. *NC Med J* 59:105–109, 1998.

Webber MP, Schoenbaum EE, Bonuck KA. Correlates of voluntary human immunodeficiency virus antibody testing reported by postpartum women. *JAMWA* 52(2):89–92, 1997.

Wehr E, Fagan M, Blake S, Rosenbaum S. *HIV/AIDS Related Provisions of Medicaid Managed Care Contracts.* Menlo Park, CA: Henry J. Kaiser Family Foundation. 1998.

Weil A. The new children's health insurance program. Should states expand Medicaid? New Federalism: Issues and Options for the States. Series A (A13), Washington, DC: Urban Institute. 1997

Weiser B, Nachman S, Tropper P, Viscosi KH, Grimson R, Baxter G, Fang G, Reyelt C, Hutcheon N, Burger H. Quantitation of human immunodeficiency virus type 1 during pregnancy: Relationship of viral titer to mother-to-child transmission and stability of viral load. *Proc Natl Acad Sci USA* 91(17):8037–8041, 1994.

Weisman C. Women's use of health care. In Falik MM, Collins KS, eds. *Women's Health: The Commonwealth Survey.* 25–32. Johns Hopkins University Press, 1996.

Wilson JMG, Jungner F. Principles and practice of screening for disease. Public Health Paper 34. Geneva: WHO, 1968.

Wisconsin AIDS/HIV Program. HIV antibody testing among pregnant women in Wisconsin, 1996. April 1997.

Wiznia AA, Crane M, Lambert G, Sansary J, Harris A, Solomon L. Zidovudine use to reduce perinatal HIV type 1 transmission in an urban medical center. *JAMA* 275(19):1504–1506, 1996.

World Health Organization (WHO). HIV and infant feeding. July 17, 1998. [www document] URL http:// www.unaids.org/unaids/document/epidemio/infant.html

Wortley PM, Fleming PL. AIDS in women in the United States. *JAMA* 278(11):911–916, 1997.

Ziegler JB, Johnson RO, Cooper DA, Gold J. Postnatal transmission of AIDS-associated retrovirus from mother to infant. *Lancet* 1:896–898, 1985.

APPENDIXES

APPENDIX

A

Committee and Staff Biographies

Marie C. McCormick, M.D., Sc.D. (*Chair*), graduated from Emmanuel College (B.A. in chemistry) and from the Johns Hopkins Medical School (M.D.) and the John Hopkins School of Hygiene and Public Health (Sc.D.). She completed her training in pediatrics at the Johns Hopkins Hospital. She has served on the faculty of the University of Illinois Abraham Lincoln Medical School, the Johns Hopkins Medical School and School of Hygiene and Public Health, and the University of Pennsylvania. She joined Harvard initially as an associate professor of pediatrics at the Harvard Medical School, and later became the Sumner and Ester Feldberg Professor and Chair of the Department of Maternal and Child Health, Harvard School of Public Health, and professor of pediatrics at the Harvard Medical School. Since completing her training, she has pursued two overlapping research interests: the effect of health services on perinatal and infant outcomes at birth, with a particular focus on elucidating the factors influencing the outcomes of very premature infants, and the evaluation of programs for children and their families. She has written on the health outcomes of infants born at risk, the services that may influence such outcomes, and the broader effect of child health and developmental programs. She was elected to the Institute of Medicine (IOM) of the National Academy of Sciences in 1997 and has been a member of the Board on Health Promotion and Disease Prevention since 1993. She chaired the earlier IOM Committee on Perinatal and Newborn Screenings for HIV Infection (1990–1991).

Ezra C. Davidson, Jr., M.D. (*Vice-Chair*), is associate dean, primary care, and professor (past chairman 1971–1996) of the Department of Obstetrics and Gynecology, the Charles R. Drew University of Medicine and Science. He currently holds professorships in obstetrics and gynecology at the University of California, Los Angeles and Dartmouth Schools of Medicine. He was chief-of-service, Department of Obstetrics and Gynecology at King/Drew Medical Center in Los Angeles (1971–1996). He was a Robert Wood Johnson Health Policy Fellow at the IOM (1979–1980), during which time he served as a health adviser to Senator Bill Bradley of New Jersey. He has served on a number of IOM–National Academy of Sciences (NAS) study committees on issues of national health policy and has worked with government and private organizations in this regard. He has served the American College of Obstetricians and Gynecologists as President (1990–1991) and national secretary for six years. His other major organizational responsibilities have included chair of the Board of Trustees of the National Medical Association and president of the Association of Professors of Gynecology and Obstetrics. He has chaired the Secretary's Advisory Committee on Infant Mortality (U.S. Department Health and Human Services) and the Advisory Committee for Reproductive Health Drugs of the Food and Drug Administration (FDA). He serves on the National Institutes of Health (NIH) Advisory Committee to the Director and the Advisory Committee on Clinical Research. He is a member of the Council on Graduate Medical Education (COGME) and the California Wellness Foundation's Board of Directors. He has been elected to the National Black College Alumni Hall of Fame, Fellowship ad eundem, Royal College of Obstetricians and Gynaecologists, and the IOM.

Fred Battaglia, M.D., graduated from Cornell University (B.A.) and Yale University School of Medicine. After service as a medical intern at Johns Hopkins Hospital, he spent two years doing research in the Department of Biochemistry in Cambridge, England, and the Department of Physiology at Yale University School of Medicine. His served his residency at Johns Hopkins University after which he completed a fellowship in the Laboratory of Perinatal Physiology in San Juan, Puerto Rico. He has been a professor of pediatrics and obstetrics-gynecology at the University of Colorado School of Medicine since 1969 and served as the chairman of the Department of Pediatrics from 1974 to 1988. He was elected to the Institute of Medicine in 1986. He has served on advisory committees to the March of Dimes; the Joseph P. Kennedy, Jr., Foundation; the National Institutes of Health, and several foundations. He is a member of several editorial boards.

Ronald S. Brookmeyer, Ph.D., is professor in the Department of Biostatistics at the Johns Hopkins University School of Hygiene and Public Health. He has a Ph.D. in statistics from the University of Wisconsin. He has authored more than 90 scientific articles and books in biostatistics, epidemiologic methods, and AIDS and is coauthor of the book entitled *AIDS Epidemiology: A Quantitative Ap-*

proach. His research has included statistical methods in epidemiologic studies of AIDS. He was one of the developers of the back-calculation method that is widely used for estimating and projecting the size of the epidemic. In 1992, he was awarded the Spiegelman gold medal by the American Public Health Association for contributions to health statistics. His National Research Council (NRC) committee service includes the Committee on National Statistics, the Committee on Statistical Issues in AIDS Research, and the Panels on Needle Exchange Programs and Social Security Disability Research. He has also served on the Clinical Research Committee for the AIDS Research Advisory Committee of the National Institute of Allergy and Infectious Diseases (NIAID) He was on the editorial board of *Statistics in Medicine* from 1985 to 1994 and has served on the regional advisory board of the Biometrics Society and as chair of the Biometrics Section of the American Statistical Association. He is a fellow of both the American Statistical Association and the American Association for the Advancement of Science.

Deborah Cotton, M.D., M.P.H., is professor of medicine and public health, Boston University School of Medicine, and director, Office of Clinical Research, Boston University Medical Center. She also serves as assistant provost of the Boston University Medical Campus. Dr. Cotton received her A.B. cum laude from Brandeis University, M.D. cum laude from Boston University, and M.P.H. from the Johns Hopkins University. A specialist in infectious diseases, Dr. Cotton's research concerns the clinical epidemiology of AIDS. Dr. Cotton is a nationally recognized authority on AIDS in women. She is co-editor of the recently published textbook *The Medical Management of AIDS in Women* with Heather Watts, M.D., and a member of the editorial board of the *Journal of Women's Health*. Dr. Cotton served as a member and then chairman of the FDA's Antiviral Advisory Committee, from 1989 to 1994, and chaired the meeting of the committee at which approval of zidovudine to prevent perinatal transmission of HIV was recommended. Dr. Cotton currently serves on the Advisory Council of the NIH Office of AIDS Research and is a member of the IOM Board on Health Sciences.

Susan Cu-Uvin, M.D., is assistant professor of obstetrics and gynecology (research) at Brown University. She provides primary care and obstetric-gynecologic care to HIV-infected women at the Immunology Center, the Miriam Hospital, Providence, Rhode Island. Her research activities focus on HIV shedding in the genital tract of women and its relevance to heterosexual and mother-to-infant transmission. Dr. Cu-Uvin graduated from the University of the Philippines College of Medicine and finished a residency in obstetrics and gynecology. She completed a three-year fellowship in HIV/AIDS at The Miriam Hospital, Brown University, and became an attending physician in immunology and geographic medicine.

Nancy Kass, Sc.D., is associate professor and director of the Program in Law, Ethics, and Health, Johns Hopkins School of Public Health, and senior faculty in the Bioethics Institute, Johns Hopkins University. She also is a fellow of the Kennedy Institute of Ethics, Georgetown University. She received her B.A. from Stanford University, completed doctoral training in health policy from the Johns Hopkins School of Public Health, and was awarded a National Research Service Award to complete a postdoctoral fellowship in bioethics at the Kennedy Institute of Ethics, Georgetown University. Dr. Kass conducts empirical work in bioethics and health policy. Her publications are primarily in the fields of HIV/AIDS policy, genetics policy, and research ethics. She is coeditor (with Ruth Faden) of *HIV, AIDS and Childbearing: Public Policy, Private Lives* (Oxford University Press, 1996). She served as consultant to the President's Advisory Committee on Human Radiation Experiments from 1994 to 1995 and currently is vice-chair of the Johns Hopkins School of Public Health Institutional Review Board.

Patricia King, J.D., is the Carmack Waterhouse Professor of Law, Medicine, Ethics, and Public Policy at the Georgetown University Law Center. She is a senior research fellow with the Kennedy Institute of Ethics. She is a member of the Institute of Medicine Council. She has served on several NRC and IOM committees, including the Commission on Behavioral and Social Sciences and Education (1992–1995), the IOM Committee to Study the Social and Ethical Impact of Biomedicine (1992–1994), the IOM Committee on Assessing Genetic Risks (1991–1993), and the IOM Board on Health and Science Policy (1989–1994). King has served as deputy assistant attorney general, Civil Division, of the U.S. Department of Justice; and as deputy director of the Office of Civil Rights, U.S. Department of Health, Education, and Welfare. She has a J.D. from Harvard Law School and a B.A. from Wheaton College.

Lorraine V. Klerman, Dr.P.H., is Professor of the Department of Maternal and Child Health, School of Public Health, University of Alabama at Birmingham. She also holds appointments in the Department of Pediatrics, the Civitan International Research Center, and the Lister Hill Policy Center. She is a health services researcher with particular interest in health delivery systems for economically deprived women and children. She is the author of *Alive and Well? A Research and Policy Review of Health Programs for Poor Young Children,* and numerous journal articles and book chapters on poverty, adolescent pregnancy, school absence, and related subjects. She is a graduate of Cornell University and the Harvard School of Public Health. In 1996, she received the American Public Health Association's Martha May Eliot Award for exceptional health services to mothers and children.

Katherine Luzuriaga, M.D., graduated from the Massachusetts Institute of Technology (S.B. in applied biology and M.S. in nutritional biochemistry) and the

Tufts University School of Medicine (M.D.). After a research fellowship in infectious diseases at the University of Massachusetts Medical School, Dr. Luzuriaga joined the faculty there and is currently associate professor of pediatrics. Dr. Luzuriaga's research activities have focused on understanding the viral and immunopathogenesis of early vertical HIV-1 infection. She has also been active in the development of antiretroviral therapies for children through the Pediatric AIDS Clinical Trials Group. Dr. Luzuriaga is a 1997 recipient of the Elizabeth Glaser Scientist Award from the Pediatric AIDS Foundation.

Ellen J. Mangione, M.D., M.P.H., is director of the Disease Control and Environmental Epidemiology Division of the Colorado Department of Public Health and Environment. She received a B.A. from Smith College; has an M.D. from the College of Physicians and Surgeons, Columbia University; and has an M.P.H. from the University of California, Berkeley. She completed her training in internal medicine at the Boston University Medical Center and a fellowship in infectious diseases at the University of Colorado Health Sciences Center (UCHSC). She is a graduate of the Epidemic Intelligence Service and the Preventive Medicine Residency of the Centers for Disease Control and Prevention (CDC), Public Health Service. She is board-certified in internal medicine, public health, and general preventive medicine, as well as infectious diseases. She is an assistant clinical professor in the Infectious Disease Division and the Department of Preventive Medicine and Biometrics, UCHSC. Dr. Mangione has been a consultant to the Office of Technology Assessment and is a member of an Environmental Protection Agency Science Advisory Committee. She has been involved in disease control projects in Liberia, Burkina Faso, and North Yemen. In addition to a strong interest in environmental epidemiology and international health, she has responsibility for statewide disease control activities in Colorado, including tuberculosis, immunization, and STD/HIV control and surveillance programs.

Douglas Morgan, M.P.A.,* is assistant commissioner, Division of AIDS Prevention and Control, New Jersey Department of Health and Senior Services. He received his undergraduate degree, a B.A. in chemistry, from Rutgers, the State University, Newark, New Jersey, and his masters in public administration from New York University. From 1989 to 1990, he was executive director of the Minority Health Institute, University of Medicine and Dentistry of New Jersey. He was formerly assistant secretary for medical care programs with the Maryland Department of Health and Mental Hygiene. He is a member and former chair of the National Alliance of State and Territorial Directors. He serves on the U.S. CDC's Advisory Committee for HIV/STD Prevention and the Columbia School of Public Health's Advisory Committee for the Public Health Community Schol-

---

*Resigned from the committee on April 20, 1998.

ars Program. On April 1998, he accepted a position with the Division of Service Systems, HIV/AIDS Bureau, Health Resources and Services Administration.

Stephen B. Thomas, Ph.D., graduated from the Ohio State University (B.S. in health education), Illinois State University (M.S. in community health), and Southern Illinois University (Ph.D., in community health). Currently he is a tenured associate professor of community health in the Department of Behavioral Sciences and Health Education, and director of the Institute for Minority Health Research at the Rollins School of Public Health of Emory University in Atlanta. From 1986 to 1993, he was on the faculty of the Department of Health Education at the University of Maryland in College Park. His research is focused on community-based interventions to prevent AIDS, substance abuse, and violence among racial and ethnic minority populations. He has written extensively on the social construction of AIDS in the African-American community. He represented Emory University at the White House for the Presidential Apology to Survivors of the Syphilis Study at Tuskegee. He has served as evaluation consultant to the Southern Christian Leadership Conference, the Walter Reed Army Institute of Research, the Baltimore County Public School System, the United Methodist Church Office of the Resident Bishop, Kaiser Permanente, and numerous community-based organizations serving minority populations. He has given testimony before the Presidential Commission on HIV and Senator Paul Coverdale's Commission on Drug Interdiction. He has served as a legislative intern for Senator Paul Simon. He was a consultant to the IOM-NAS Study Committee on Preventing HIV Transmission: The Role of Sterile Needles and Bleach. He currently serves on the editorial boards of *Health Education and Behavior* and the *Journal of Health Education*. At Emory University he is on the Board of Directors for the Center for Ethics in Public Policy and the Professions. Dr. Thomas believes that we must become more skilled in the use of community-based social change strategies as a primary means to advance health promotion and disease prevention programs that are scientifically sound, ethnically acceptable, and culturally competent.

Sten H. Vermund, M.D., Ph.D., is professor of epidemiology, medicine, and pediatrics at the University of Alabama at Birmingham. He also serves as Director, of the Division of Geographic Medicine. His training is from Stanford University (human biology), Albert Einstein College of Medicine (medicine), Columbia University (pediatrics and epidemiology), and the London School of Hygiene and Tropical Medicine (tropical public health). From 1988–1994, he served as the chief of the Vaccine Trials and Epidemiology Branch in the Division of AIDS at NIAID where he helped launch initiatives in perinatal transmission prevention, women's health, and prevention clinical trials. His current research activities include the natural history of HIV among adolescents; STD control and HIV prevention in high-risk but low-HIV-prevalence areas of Asia,

Central America, and the Caribbean; HIV prevention studies in Zambia; clinical epidemiology of HIV in Alabama; molecular epidemiology of *Pneumocystis carinii;* and several non-AIDS infectious disease epidemiology projects including the study of bacterial vaginosis and early preterm birth. Dr. Vermund serves on the Prevention Research Advisory Committee for the Office of AIDS Research at NIH, on the Centers and Programs Scientific Review Committee of the National Institute on Drug Abuse, and as a scientific adviser to the Pediatric AIDS Foundation, the Catalonia Ministry of Health AIDS Research Institute, the Center for Urban Epidemiologic Studies of the New York Academy of Medicine, and the Columbia University Center for AIDS Research.

Liaison to the Board on Health Promotion and Disease Prevention

Robert Fullilove, Ed.D., is currently the associate dean for community and minority affairs at Columbia University's School of Public Health. He is also an associate professor of clinical public health and codirector of the Community Research Group at the New York State Psychiatric Institute. Prior to joining the Faculty of Medicine at Columbia, Dr. Fullilove was the assistant director of multicultural inquiry at the University of California, San Francisco, and the Bayview Hunters Point Foundation, which was headed by his wife, Dr. Mindy Fullilove. The Fulliloves have made numerous presentations on HIV disease among people of color and have published extensively. Their research encompasses a wide range of topics including crack cocaine use and sexually transmitted disease in the AIDS era; trauma-related disorders and their impact on sexual risk taking; and science, mathematics, and medical education for African Americans and other students of color. Dr. Robert Fullilove received his B.A. from Colgate University (1966), his M.S. from Syracuse University (1972), and his Ed.D. from Columbia University (1984). Since 1995, he has served on the IOM's Board of Health Promotion and Disease Prevention. Since 1997, he has served as a member-nominee to the CDC's Advisory Committee on HIV and STD Prevention. He is also a widely exhibited painter and a self-described "francophile."

Staff

Michael A. Stoto, Ph.D., is a senior staff officer of the Institute of Medicine, and was formerly the director of the Division of Health Promotion and Disease Prevention. Dr. Stoto directed the IOM's effort in support of the U.S. Public Health Service's *Healthy People 2000* project and has worked on IOM projects addressing a number of issues in public health, health statistics, health promotion and disease prevention, vaccine safety and policy, environmental health, and AIDS. Dr. Stoto led the staff responsible for the reports *Veterans and Agent Orange:*

Health Effects of Herbicides Used in Vietnam; HIV and the Blood Supply: An Analysis of Crisis Decisionmaking; Healthy Communities: New Directions for the Future of Public Health; and *Improving Health in the Community: A Role for Performance Monitoring.* Dr. Stoto received an A.B. in statistics from Princeton University and a Ph.D. in statistics and demography from Harvard University, and was formerly an associate professor of public policy at Harvard's John F. Kennedy School of Government. He is an adjunct associate professor of biostatistics at the Harvard School of Public Health and, at the completion of the perinatal transmission project, will become professor and chair of the Department of Epidemiology and Biostatisics at the George Washington University School of Public Health and Health Services.

Donna A. Almario, B.A., is the project and research assistant on the perinatal transmission of HIV study. Ms. Almario joined the Division of Health Promotion and Disease Prevention in October 1997. Prior to joining the Institute of Medicine, she worked as a research assistant studying breast cancer at Georgetown University Medical Center's Lombardi Cancer Center. Ms. Almario graduated from Vassar College with a biopsychology degree in May 1996.

APPENDIX

B

Context of Services for Women and Children Affected by HIV/AIDS

Barbara Aliza

The development of new opportunities to substantially reduce the risk of perinatal HIV transmission and more effectively treat those already infected not only has significant implications for improving maternal, fetal, and infant health, but places new demands on the health care system with respect to how services are funded and delivered. The introduction of new, more potent drugs, more effective therapeutic regimens, new tools for monitoring and assessment, and knowledge of how and when perinatal HIV transmission takes place has brought intensified efforts in both the public and private sector to reach out to all women of reproductive age with information, counseling, testing, and treatment services. At the same time that the need to simplify access to these services has become critical to maximizing prevention and treatment opportunities, the organization and funding of needed services has grown even more complex.

This appendix identifies the range of services available on the community level to women and children affected with HIV disease in order to provide a framework for understanding the opportunities for treatment and prevention. After describing the population of women and children affected by HIV and discussing what we know about where women and children go for care, the appendix profiles a variety of providers offering services to this population. It then discusses the major sources of funding for HIV-related services and the implications of a number of policy issues, including welfare reform, changes in Medicaid, public and private sector managed care, the Health Insurance Portability and Accountability Act, and the Americans with Disabilities Act.

SOURCE OF CARE FOR WOMEN, CHILDREN, AND ADOLESCENTS

Women's access to the health care system varies by income, ethnicity, and education (Wyn et al., 1996). How and where women seek health care reflects both the structure and the organization of the health care system, as well as women's awareness or knowledge of health care practices and their satisfaction with health care professionals (Falik, 1996). The majority of women and children in the United States receive care in a private provider's office. The more affluent and educated a woman is, the more likely she is to use two providers—an obstetrician–gynecologist and an internist or family care practitioner (Weisman, 1996). Most adolescents receive health care at community teen clinics, school-based clinics, community family practices, private family practices, and private pediatric practices (Blum et al., 1996).

The poor or nearly poor, the population most affected by HIV infection, is more likely to use publicly funded providers or programs (public and nonprofit hospitals, community health centers, family planning clinics, and public health clinics (Lyons et al., 1996). Most children, youth, and families affected by AIDS depend on these "safety net" programs for their care. While more than 61% of women in care for HIV (Rand, 1998) and 90% of children (under 18) with AIDS (DHHS, 1998) receive care paid for through the Medicaid Program, the rapid growth of public managed care programs for those on Medicaid is moving service delivery into the managed care setting.

The significant developments in prevention and treatment for women and children and the efforts to promote the application of these developments have taken place in the context of a health care system that is undergoing a revolution in structure and funding. Significant changes in Medicaid and welfare programs, the growing presence of managed care in both the public and private sector, the growing number of uninsured, and the recently introduced Children's Health Insurance Program are having a significant impact on our health care system, affecting not only the availability of quality services, but also access to services.

The lack of a unified set of goals or policies that guides how health care services in the United States are organized challenges our ability to respond optimally to an epidemic as complex and challenging as HIV/AIDS. An array of federal, state, and local laws, regulations, policies, institutions, and funding mechanisms not only shapes the services in any given locality (Hess, 1994) but determines who has access to those services. The current mix of public and private services and funding streams not only varies significantly from state to state and community to community, but is undergoing rapid change and is financially vulnerable. In addition to a growing number of uninsured and a reduction in public funding of health care services, the rapid growth of managed care is competing for clients in both the public and the private sector and reduces the ability of public programs, and private sector programs using public funds, to subsidize care through Medicaid reimbursement (Davis, 1997).

TABLE B.1   Community-Level Health Care Providers

Private Providers	Public and Nonprofit Providers
Obstetricians/gynecologists	State and local public health clinics
Pediatricians	Public and nonprofit hospitals
Family practice practitioners	Community health centers
Nurse midwives	Family planning clinics
Nurse practitioners	WIC clinics
Managed care organizations	STD clinics
AIDS service organizations	Healthy Start sites
Home testing/counseling	School-based health centers
	Prisons
	Drug treatment facilities
	State HIV testing/counseling centers

NOTE: STD = sexually transmitted disease; WIC = Special Supplemental Nutrition Program for Women, Infants, and Children.

Women and children with, or at risk for HIV/AIDS must rely on a broad array of preventive, diagnostic, treatment, and support services to maximize their health and quality of life. The current mix of service delivery structures available on the community level can be organized into two somewhat arbitrary categories: *public and nonprofit providers* and *private providers*, neither of which is purely private or exclusively public. Some private providers receive differing amounts of public funding for their patients, and many public and nonprofit providers use a combination of public and private providers to deliver services. This section describes community-level providers listed in Table B.1.

Public and Nonprofit Providers

State and Local Public Health Services and Clinics

Local Health Departments[1] These administrative and service units of local and/or state governments employ at least one full time person and carry some responsibility for the health of an area smaller than the state. The estimated total local health department (LHD) expenditure is $8 billion. Most of the nearly 3,000 LHDs are located in 47 states and fall under the authority of local government and health boards rather than state public health infrastructure. As the locus of public health and prevention services in a community, the majority of LHDs play an important role in providing or assuring maternal and child health services and

---

[1]Data in this section from the *National Profile of Local Health Departments,* Washington, D.C., 1993 and 1995.

TABLE B.2 Percentage of Local Health Departments Providing
Specific Services

Services	Percentage	Services	Percentage
WIC services	78	HIV/AIDS treatment	33
Prenatal care	64	Well-child clinics	79
Obstetrical care	33	EPSDT services	72
STD testing and counseling	71	Child sick care	39
Family planning	68	Children with special needs services	65
STD treatment	66	School health services	60
HIV counseling and testing	68		

NOTE: EPSDT = Medicaid's Early Periodic Screening, Diagnostic, and Treatment Program; STD = sexually transmitted disease; WIC = Special Supplemental Nutrition Program for Women, Infants, and Children.

many provide services that target communicable diseases such as HIV, tuberculosis, and sexually transmitted diseases (STDs).

Population served: By definition, the population served by an LHD includes all persons within the unit's jurisdiction. The provision of personal health services varies considerably from community to community; 68% offer such services to all persons in their jurisdiction, while 32% limit those services to a target population.

Services provided: Services offered directly or by contract include such population-based services as health education and risk reduction, community outreach and education, and communicable disease screening. Services relevant to maternal and child health are listed in Table B.2.

Funding: Local health departments access a variety of funding sources, including, for example, state funds (including maternal and child health program funds), local community funds, Medicaid, federal government program grants, patient fees, and private foundations.

State Title V Maternal and Child Health and Children with Special Health Care Needs Clinics and Service: These clinics and services are operated directly by the State Title V Maternal and Child Health (MCH) Program, which is funded by the Title V Maternal and Child Health Services Block Grant (Title V of the Social Security Act). Although some state Title V MCH programs directly run clinical services in a community or on a regional basis, most support care indirectly through grants and contracts to local health departments and community-based providers and facilities. For this reason the program is an important source of funding for services for women and children and is detailed in the discussion of funding sources.

Public and Nonprofit Hospitals

Public Hospitals. There are more than 100 public hospitals and health systems in large metropolitan areas, mostly under the authority of state or local governments or agencies. The exact number of public hospitals in smaller towns and communities is unknown. Public hospitals are referred to as "safety net providers" and are major referral centers, teaching hospitals, and providers of care for low-income populations and populations who are poor and uninsured.

Population served: More than 90% of patients served are either Medicaid recipients, Medicare beneficiaries, or the uninsured. Although public hospitals traditionally serve many patients that other hospitals will not serve, they have experienced a reduction in obstetrical patient volume in recent years, owing in great part to competition from public and private sector managed care.

Services provided: These include preventive and primary care, specialized health services, emergency and trauma care, high-risk pregnancy services, HIV/AIDS care and neonatal intensive care. Many of the public hospitals have created a network of primary care clinics through the community and sometimes provide mobile health units and outpatient hospital units.

Funding: Funding sources include Medicaid, state and local subsidies, private insurance, and foundations.

Nonprofit Hospitals. In many communities without public hospitals, nonprofit hospitals, especially university-affiliated facilities, serve the poor, providing the same safety net as public hospitals. In 1996, there were over 3,000 nonprofit hospitals across the country with more than 2.6 million births.[2] These facilities often provide the same range of health care services to women and children, including those affected by HIV/AIDS, and experience many of the same pressures as public hospitals related to adequate reimbursement by public and private third party payers and the burden of uncompensated care. Nonprofit hospitals are under the authority of community boards and are open to all residents of a community.

Funding: Funding sources often include Medicaid, state and local grants, private insurance, and grants from foundations.

Community Health Centers[3]

These public and private nonprofit community-based organizations directly or indirectly, through contracts and cooperative agreements, provide primary

---

[2]Data from the American Hospital Association (1998).

[3]Data provided in this section come from the *Analyses from the 1996 Uniform Data System* conducted by MDS Associates, Inc. and Stickgold and Associates. Principal authors were Deborah Lewis-Idema and Beverly Wiaczek.

health and related services to residents of a defined geographic area, specifically a medically underserved area. Located in 55 states and territories, there are more than 685 federally qualified community-based organizations receiving federal money that serve more than 10 million people a year with a network of 5,500 primary care providers. Under the authority of the Federal Bureau of Primary Health Care and community boards, these organizations fund 3,032 service delivery sites, including freestanding health clinics (1,889), shelters (298), schools (195), social service centers (123), health departments (106), mobile vans (80), substance abuse treatment facilities (71), HIV/AIDS clinics (41), mental health clinics (38), migrant camps (37), hospitals (37), and public housing (36). There are more than 100 clinics that meet the statutory requirements for a health center but do not receive federal funds. These clinics qualify for the same cost-based reimbursement from Medicaid and are referred to as federally qualified health center (FQHC) "look-alikes." There are an additional 200 nonprofit community-based clinics that do not receive federal money and have not applied for "look-alike" status.

Population served: Although this varies from community to community, the target populations are the medically underserved, the poor, and disadvantaged, including minorities, women of childbearing age, infants, persons with HIV infection, substance abusers and/or homeless individuals and their families. Women of childbearing age constitute almost one-third of the population served; children account for 42%. In 1966, 10% of females (age 13–44) served were known to be pregnant with less than 1% known to be HIV-positive; 65% were below the federal poverty level and 20% fell between 100% and 200% of poverty.

Services provided: These also vary according to the needs of the community. The most common services are those that target mothers and children, including the provision of such enabling services as case management, education, outreach, interpretation, transportation, child care, and discharge planning. Obstetrical and gynecological care is provided by 90% of grantees; 75% provide perinatal services and less than 50% provide labor and delivery services. Less than 1% of patient encounters included HIV testing, although 85% of grantees report providing this service.

Funding: Sources of funding for community, migrant, and homeless health centers include, in order of frequency, the Bureau of Primary Health Care, Medicaid, the Ryan White CARE Act, state and local grants, private insurance, Medicare, patient fees, and foundation grants and contracts.

Family Planning Clinics[4]

Under the authority of the Office of Population Affairs (OPA), Department of Health and Human Services (DHHS), this national network of clinics is funded

---

[4]Data from the National Family Planning and Reproductive Health Association (1998).

by Title X of the Public Health Service Act through grants to approximately 80 public and private nonprofit grantees for the provision of family planning information and services. In 1994 the health department was the sole grantee in 27 states and seven territories and a primary grantee in another ten states (Kaesar et al., 1996). Clinic sites include state and local health departments, hospitals, university health centers, Planned Parenthood affiliates, independent clinics, and other public and nonprofit agencies. Title X clinics are community-based, located in every state and in three-fourths of U.S. counties. They serve as an important entry point into care and, for some, the only source of service.

Population served: Among those served are approximately 4 million women of reproductive age. The majority of clients are young, have never borne a child (Kaeser et al., 1996), have incomes below 150% of the federal poverty level (FPL), are uninsured, and do not qualify for Medicaid.

Services provided: These include community education and outreach, contraceptive information and services, pregnancy testing, gynecological examinations, basic lab tests, and other screening services for STDs and HIV, high blood pressure, anemia, and breast and cervical cancer.

Title X clinics operate under uniform federal regulations and guidelines that "often serve as the blueprint for state family planning programs." A 1987 directive from the federal OPA, requires clinics to "offer, at a minimum, education on HIV infection and AIDS, counseling on risks and infection prevention, and referral services." They may also provide risk assessment, counseling, and tests. The directive further notes that if testing is done, it should be targeted. It emphasizes the importance of "offering effective methods of family planning to sexually active HIV-infected women who run a high risk of perinatal transmission in pregnancy and who run a significant risk of transmitting HIV to other sexual partners." Guidelines for Title X grantees are currently under development, in collaboration with the Centers for Disease Control and Prevention (CDC).

Funding: Sources of funding for family planning clinics may include Title X funds, state funds (including state maternal and child health program funds), Medicaid, private insurance, and patient fees. There is no charge for patients under 100% of the FPL and a sliding scale fee for patients up to 250% FPL.

Special Supplemental Nutrition Program for Women, Infants, and Children[5]

Supplemental foods, nutrition education, and health care referrals provided to low-income pregnant, postpartum, and breast-feeding women, and to infants and children up to their fifth birthday. Administered on the federal level by the

---

[5]Data in this section were provided in the fact sheet, WIC: Building a Better future for America's Children, National Association of WIC Directors and from the WIC Program Office, Food and Nutrition Service, U.S. Department of Agriculture (1997).

Food and Nutrition Service, U.S. Department of Agriculture (USDA), funds are provided directly to state health agencies which, in turn, distribute them to local agencies. Special Supplemental Nutrition Program for Women, Infants, and Children (WIC) programs are located in every state, most Indian Reservations and in all U.S. territories. There are 1900 local agencies and approximately 10,000 clinic sites. Local agencies often have multiple satellite sites throughout the community.

Population served: Eligibility is based on nutritional risk and an income less than or equal to 185% of FPL. This includes 7.4 million to 7.5 million infants, children, and women, of whom approximately 1.7 million were pregnant or post-partum women. Approximately 20% of all pregnant women in the United States are in WIC, 40% of whom enroll within the first trimester of pregnancy. Two-thirds of participants live at or below the poverty line and one-third do not participate in other federal assistance programs.

Services provided: These include a food package determined by the participants' specific needs and designed to provide high levels of protein, iron, calcium, and vitamins A and C. For women who cannot or should not breast-feed, iron-fortified infant formula is available for their infants. WIC also provides nutrition education and counseling, and referrals for pre- and postnatal health care (such as HIV testing), drug abuse education, and promotion of immunizations.

The USDA is expecting to issue formal (written) directives on working with HIV-positive women sometime this year, in addition to a policy document issued by the USDA and DHHS in November 1997 on the contraindications to breast-feeding. The National Association of WIC Directors (NAWD) is also in the final stages of drafting a policy paper on working with HIV-positive women and is expecting to finalize it in the fall of 1998. New York and New Jersey have established specific guidelines related to HIV for WIC programs in their state that have been used as models in a recent conference for WIC programs. Both the guidelines developed by USDA and NAWD will suggest that WIC agencies advise women to know their HIV status, and if HIV-positive, not to breast-feed.

Sexually Transmitted Disease Clinics

Funded in partnership between CDC's Division of Sexually Transmitted Disease (STD) Prevention and state and local health agencies, more than 3,000 clinics provide dedicated services to prevent and treat STDs. Although some are located at family planning clinics and hospitals, most are located in state and local public health departments. These clinics are the primary source of HIV testing in public facilities. Authority is shared by CDC and state and local health agencies.

Population served: This includes both men and women, although men use these clinics in far greater numbers than women. The population is most often poor, uninsured, and experiencing symptoms.

Services provided: Among these are pre- and post-test counseling for HIV and safe sex, testing and treatment for a variety of STDs, partner notification, and education and training for community providers.

Healthy Start Sites

Funded by the Maternal and Child Health Bureau in the Department of Health and Human Services, this national demonstration program was founded in 1991 to reduce infant mortality and low birthweight, especially in high-risk populations. The program was founded on the principle that strategies developed by the community were needed to address the causes of these problems. Located in 60 selected communities, the program focuses on (1) increasing community awareness (2) coordinating services between public and private agencies, and (3) building partnerships.

There are no available data on the numbers of women served who have been counseled and/or tested for HIV or who are HIV-positive. Although some individual sites may have developed policies related to HIV counseling, testing, and risk reduction, there is no formal guidance from the federal agency related to HIV perinatal transmission, except for the Public Health Service (PHS) guidelines.

School-Based Health Centers[6]

Found in more than 900 schools across the country, school-based health centers provide a comprehensive range of physical and mental health services to children and adolescents. Although they vary from community to community, all centers are located in schools and operated by health professionals, usually a multidisciplinary core team of primary care professionals—often a nurse practitioner or physician assistant, possibly a part-time pediatrician or family practitioner, and a social worker. Centers focus on assuring that patients are linked to a continuum of care, as needed, often establishing a network with community providers.

Population served: School-age children are served, although individual schools may limit or target specific age groups. Usually about half the students in a school use the services, especially those with limited access to care.

Services provided: These include a range of preventive and primary care, counseling, and linkage to a continuum of care in the community. There is no available information on what percentage of these health centers provides HIV counseling and/or linkage to testing and treatment services, but these centers are often the first and may be the only contact with medical services for adolescents.

---

[6]Data provided by "School-Based Health Centers. Making the Grade." Washington, D.C., George Washington University, 1998.

Data for 1993 indicate that 16% of services are for reproductive health and 23% are for preventive health.

Funding: Funding sources may include the state maternal and child health program, other state funding, local funds, foundations, and reimbursement from public and private insurance.

Prisons[7]

A range of health care services is available through the prison system to the 1.725 million persons in prisons and jails throughout the country at any one time. Approximately 5% to 7% of prisoners are women (120,000). AIDS incidence among state and federal prisoners is 20 times the rate in the population at large. Ninety-two percent of female prisoners are of childbearing age (under 45) and a greater percentage of female prisoners are HIV-positive. Access to health care services and testing, counseling, and therapeutic regimens for HIV varies significantly from jurisdiction to jurisdiction. The fact that roughly 700,000 women are released from prisons each year highlights both the importance and the difficulty in establishing and maintaining good access to needed HIV services.

Services provided: Services provided in the city and county jail systems and the state and federal prison systems are difficult to characterize because of their variability. While many prisons directly provide health care services by their own staff, the practice of contracting with outside agencies is rapidly increasing. Contracts generally are arranged with university medical schools and correctional health care companies, the latter on a capitated basis. The policy for HIV testing of pregnant females is the same as for other inmates in most systems. Seven state systems and the federal prison system have mandatory or routine testing of incoming pregnant women, but provide voluntary or on-request testing for other inmates. There are no data about routine counseling of pregnant inmates regarding testing. A survey conducted by ABT Associates, Inc. revealed that 90% or more of prisons report the availability of prenatal care, ZDV therapy and combination therapies. Information on how accessible these services are to inmates is not available, nor is there any information about follow-up and referral once a prisoner is identified and/or treated and then released.

Drug Treatment Facilities[8]

Funded primarily through the Federal Substance Abuse, Prevention, and Treatment Block Grant, totaling $1.3 billion, and state and local funds, this public

---

[7]Much of the data in this section was obtained in an interview with Theodore Hammett, ABT Associates, Boston, MA, April 9, 1998.

[8]1995 funding sources obtained from state Resources and Services Related to Alcohol and Other Drug Problems: Fiscal Year 1995, National Association of State Alcohol and Drug Abuse Directors, Inc.

system of drug treatment facilities consists of approximately 10,000 treatment sites. Funds are distributed to 60 entities, including all states, the District of Columbia, Puerto Rico, the Virgin Islands, and the Pacific Trust, for the purpose of planning, carrying out, or evaluating related activities. States distribute the funds through a county or regional intermediary, which in turn distributes the funds to treatment facilities. The state is almost always a purchaser of care and sometimes a manager, but rarely provides the service directly, especially within a community.

Population served: 28% to 30% of those served are women. States are required to set aside a minimum of 5% of the funds for treatment of pregnant women and women with children. Pregnant women are also given priority enrollment in all treatment services, and states are required to maintain spending for treatment at the FY 1994 levels. All states with ten or more AIDS cases per 100,000 population must carry out one or more projects that make early intervention services for HIV infection available on-site.

Services provided: States are required to provide primary care, prenatal care, and child care to the women served under the 5% set-aside. Most grantees contract with primary care providers for such care. There is no requirement to do HIV testing and counseling, although many conduct risk assessments for tuberculosis (TB) and HIV as part of their protocol. In addition to the regular block grant activities, there are 54 demonstration projects specifically targeting pregnant and postpartum women, and in these projects, pre- and post-test counseling are required. Most of these projects are ending this fiscal year and the remaining 18 end in FY 1999.

The Substance Abuse and Mental Health Services Administration (SAMHSA) has disseminated guidance regarding screening and assessment issues for projects focusing on specific populations. The Center for Substance Abuse Treatment (CSAT) has disseminated guidance related to HIV counseling and testing through a protocol developed for treatment providers and primary care providers (Series 11), a protocol for screening for infectious disease for patients in treatment (Series 6), and for a protocol improving treatment for drug-exposed infants (Series 5). The movement of Medicaid recipients into managed care has resulted in a reduction of coverage for substance abuse treatment services. There has also been an increase in cases of criminal prosecution for pregnant women who are substance abusing and in mandatory testing, reporting, and treatment (Chavkin et al., 1998).

Funding: Additional funding comes from Medicaid, other federal programs (Ryan White CARE Act and the Department of Justice), and private insurance.

State Testing/Counseling Centers

Administered by state AIDS directors, approximately 10,000 testing and counseling centers (including anonymous testing sites) throughout the country receive the bulk of their funding from the CDC through a cooperative agreement with the state. In states with a high incidence of HIV, additional money is more likely to be provided. Thirty percent of the sites are dedicated, mostly anonymous, and are frequently linked to medical facilities; 30% are located in STD clinics, and the remainder are a mix of provider sites, including community health centers, hospitals, prisons, family planning clinics, drug treatment centers, and, occasionally, private providers.

Private Providers

The following providers are important sources of primary care and obstetrical care for women.

Obstetricians/Gynecologists

More than 37,000 physicians in the United States specialize in obstetrics and gynecology, 28,000 of whom are actively involved in providing obstetrical care. Obstetrician-gynecologists are often used by women for both specialty care related to reproductive health and primary care (Weisman et al., 1996). Ninety percent of obstetricians-gynecologists are affiliated with the American College of Obstetricians and Gynecologists (ACOG), a professional association.

ACOG has disseminated the PHS guidelines for counseling and antibody testing to prevent HIV infection and AIDS, as well as specific information to its members related to prevention of perinatal HIV transmission, including (1) an educational bulletin in January 1997 that discussed clinical, legal, and ethical issues and recommended that all pregnant women be counseled and encouraged to be tested by the provider; (2) ethical guidance for patient testing (October 1995); and (3) a Committee on Ethics "opinion" related to physician's responsibilities. ACOG has also produced patient education materials for providers, specifically recommending counseling and testing.[9]

Pediatricians

There are approximately 53,000 members of the American Academy of Pediatrics (AAP), an estimated 75% to 80% of board-certified pediatricians (not all of whom practice in the United States). Pediatricians are concerned with the physical and psychosocial growth, development, and health of the individual child beginning prior to birth throughout infancy, childhood, adolescence, and early adulthood. Surveys of academy membership indicate that 90% to 95% provide direct patient care and 75% provide health supervision or primary care for at least some of their practice time. Thirty-five percent of children visiting a

---

[9]Data and information provided by ACOG, April 10, 1998.

pediatrician in a typical week are 2 or under, while only 17% of the cases are adolescents (ages 12–21.) No data are available to indicate what percentage of pediatricians are conducting HIV counseling and testing or what percentage of the cases seen are HIV-positive.[10]

The AAP has issued several statements to its members that follow the lead of the PHS guidelines: (1) The *Role of Pediatricians in Prevention and Intervention* (1993); (2) *Perinatal Human Immunodeficiency Virus Testing* (1996); (3) *Evaluation and Medical Treatment of the HIV-Exposed Infant* (1997); and (4) a joint statement with ACOG on testing for HIV (1997).

Family Practice Practitioners[11]

There are more than 84,000 practicing family physicians, family practice residents, and medical students with an interest in family practice. Family physicians (FPs) and general practitioners (GPs) are responsible for more outpatient medical visits than any other specialty and place a high priority on preventive health services. More than 30% provide obstetrical care in their practice and more than 90% provide pediatric care. The National Ambulatory Medical Care Survey of 1993 revealed that 0.12% of all office visit conditions in family practice were for HIV; counseling in HIV transmission was given in 0.54% of visits by GPs-FPs; HIV testing was included in 0.13% of visits.

The American Academy of Family Physicians has adopted as its policy the section "Guidelines for Counseling and Testing for HIV Antibody" from the CDC's (1987) PHS guidelines. The academy recommends universal HIV counseling and voluntary testing for all pregnant women and supports the enactment of state laws providing for reporting HIV.

Nurse Midwives[12]

There are more than 5,000 nurse midwives in clinical practice in the country and more than half are employed in a hospital or physician practice. Nurse-midwifery practice is legal in all 50 states and the District of Columbia. Certified nurse midwives (CNMs) are educated in nursing and midwifery and provide primary care to women of childbearing age, including prenatal, labor, and delivery care, postpartum care; gynecological exams; newborn care; assistance with family planning decisions; preconception care; menopausal management; and counseling in health maintenance and disease prevention.

Nurse midwives attended more than 205,000 births in the United States in

---

[10]Data provided by the AAP.

[11]Information provided by the American Academy of Family Physicians.

[12]Information in this section provided by the American College of Nurse Midwives, Washington, DC.

1994, more than 5% of all the nation's births. Ninety percent of visits to CNMs are for preventive and primary care; 20% for care outside the maternity cycle. Seventy percent of women seen by a CNM are "considered vulnerable by virtue of their age, socioeconomic status, education, ethnicity, or location of residence."

The American College of Nurse Midwives first issued a statement on HIV/ AIDS in 1991 with revisions in 1996 and 1997. The statement calls for all women to be counseled on HIV risk behaviors and risk reduction strategies and, following counseling, to be offered HIV testing with informed consent.

Nurse Practitioner[13]

There are approximately 50,000 nurse practitioners in the United States. A nurse practitioner is a registered nurse who has advanced education and clinical training in a health care specialty area, including women's health, neonatal/ perinatal health, family practice, and pediatrics. Practice settings include private offices, community health centers, public health clinics, hospital clinics, and family planning clinics. Approximately 67% of nurse practitioners practice in a private setting and 33% work in a public setting. Many of their patients have incomes below the federal poverty level.

The American Academy of Nurse Practitioners published the PHS guidelines in its journal and disseminated a joint letter with CDC calling members' attention to the guidelines.

Managed Care Organizations

These organizations provide health services through a single point of entry and formal enrollment and manage patient care to assure an emphasis on preventive and primary care and a reduction in inappropriate utilization and costs (Aliza et al., 1996). A variety of managed care arrangements now play a major role in providing health care, including full risk plans (health maintenance organizations [HMOs] or health insurance organizations [HIOs]), limited risk prepaid health plans (PHPs) and fee for service primary care case management (PCCM). Managed care organizations (MCOs) either employ or contract with providers for patient care services. The number of persons enrolled in such plans is growing rapidly in both the public and the private sector, but especially among women, children, and youth enrolled in Medicaid, the predominant payer for the population affected by HIV. In 1996, 13.3 million Medicaid beneficiaries were enrolled in some form of managed care, a fourfold increase since 1991; 90% of HIV-positive mothers are covered by Medicaid (Kaiser Family Foundation, 1998).

---

[13]Information in this section provided by the American Academy of Nurse Practitioners, Washington, DC.

All states, except Alaska, are pursuing some type of managed care initiative. Enrollment of Medicaid recipients averages almost 50% across states, and ranges from less than 10% to 100%. The Balanced Budget Act of 1997 allows state Medicaid programs to: (1) convert to managed care without obtaining waivers; (2) require enrollment for most beneficiaries; and (3) permit MCOs easier entry into the Medicaid managed care market. Managed care contracts, like traditional insurance contracts, do not typically identify specific conditions. In 1996, 18 states referenced counseling and testing as a covered service, usually only in the context of family planning services, and one state (Florida), assured access to the AIDS Clinical Trials Group protocol number 076 (ACTG 076) (Wehr et al., 1998).

AIDS Service Organizations[14]

AIDS service organizations (ASOs) can be loosely defined as nonprofit community-based organizations offering a range of services to the affected population. Because of the range of services offered and funding received by these organizations, not only is it difficult to define them, but there is no precise count of the number of organizations. Most ASOs are located in cities receiving funds from the Ryan White Title I Emergency Relief Grant Program for Eligible Metropolitan Areas—areas with a high incidence of HIV/AIDS—although there are also many in smaller cities and towns throughout the country.

Population served: This generally includes the affected population as a whole, although some organizations may focus their efforts on a particular segment of the population (homosexual men, minorities, women).

Services provided: These range from referral to counseling and testing, and education, to the full range of comprehensive clinical and support services offered by a handful of organizations in major metropolitan areas. Approximately 90 ASOs receive funding directly from the CDC to provide health education/risk reduction services defined as outreach, risk reduction counseling, prevention case management, and community-level intervention to change perceptions of risk.

Home Testing/Counseling [15]

The first home collection HIV test was approved in 1996 and was available from two manufacturers until June 1997. There is currently only one manufacturer, Home Access Health Corporation, that provides testing kits. The kits costs $40–$50 and allow users to remain anonymous; results are obtained by telephone

---

[14]Information provided by the AIDS Action Council, Washington, DC.

[15]Data from Home Access Health Corporation (1996). *Home Access: HIV Counseling and Testing Report.* Home Access Health Corporation 1(1) September 1997.

BOX B.1
Data Reported by Home HIV Testing Kit Manufacturers

- Tests submitted from 50 states, D.C., Puerto Rico, and the Virgin Islands;
- 97% of users called for results, compared to 44% in STD clinics and 83% in voluntary counseling and testing clinics (CDC, 1997)
- Prevalence rate of 0.9% was three times the general U.S. prevalence of 0.3%, but less than that of individuals tested at publicly funded test sites (1.6%);
- 5% of samples were unsuitable;
- Women comprised of 37% of home testing kit users, with 17% testing positive;
- Home kits are being used by many individuals who have not been previously tested;
- Many of those testing positive expected their tests to be negative;
- 65% of HIV-positive clients received referrals for services;
- 23% refused referrals citing an existing source of care, and 5% hung up upon receive a positive result; 10% called back for additional counseling; and 8% asked the counselor to discuss the results with their partner.

---

using a code number. The home user collects blood spots at home and sends the specimens by mail for laboratory testing. Users are required to telephone for recorded pre-test counseling and are offered the opportunity to speak with a trained counselor. Positive results are provided by a counselor and negative results are received through a recorded message, with the option to speak to a counselor.

Supporters of home testing expected that it would increase access to testing and encourage individuals who might not be tested otherwise. Manufacturers agreed to report data to the CDC. For home test data, see Box B.1.

SOURCES OF FUNDING FOR HIV/AIDS SERVICES FOR WOMEN, CHILDREN, AND ADOLESCENTS

The number of Americans who do not have health insurance coverage has continued to grow. Nearly 41 million persons under age 65 were without public or private health insurance in 1996 (Kaiser Commission on Medicaid and the Uninsured, 1998). Approximately 19% of women of child-bearing age (18–34 years) and 10% of children under 18 are not insured (Kaiser Commission on Medicaid and Uninsured, 1998). There are a number of reasons for this growth in the uninsured, not the least of which is the cost of coverage for the employer, the employee, and the individual purchaser. The fact that an individual or family does not have health insurance significantly influences their access to health care services and, therefore, the ability to access important preventive health services such as counseling and testing for HIV. The uninsured are less likely to see a doctor and three to four times more likely to report having problems accessing the health care they need. They are also more likely to delay or go without medical care, even if the lapse in coverage was only temporary. The uninsured are twice as likely as those with private insurance to be hospitalized for avoidable complications (Kaiser Family Foundation, 1998).

Maximizing prevention of HIV/AIDS and its transmission requires a broad array of services at the community level—outreach, education, counseling, testing, access to treatment and medications, and support services. Many services at the community level receive funding and/or support from multiple federal, state, and both public and private local sources, including philanthropy.

Private Insurance

Most women of childbearing age (70%) and children (66%) have their health care paid for through private insurance.[16] Private insurance is usually obtained directly through employment or as a dependent of an employed person. Private health insurance on an individual basis is much more expensive, and the percentage has declined steadily over the past decade (EBRI, 1997). In 1996 only 15% of women in care with an asymptomatic HIV diagnosis (CD4 count of 500 or above) had private insurance; 60% had public insurance (Medicaid and Medicare); and 25% had no insurance (Rand, 1998). The number with private insurance declined as the disease progressed to AIDS (CD4 count below 200), while the number with public insurance increased to 70% (Rand, 1998).

With developments in HIV prevention and treatment options and the promulgation of PHS guidelines by the CDC in 1994, local, state, and federal agencies have made multiple efforts, especially in states and communities with a high incidence of HIV infection, to inform providers and the public and to promote counseling and testing of pregnant women wherever services are offered. Federal monies flow into the community either directly through grants to public and private providers or indirectly, through state agencies, which in turn allocate funds in a manner specific to their mandate.

Federal funds consist of project or program dollars that support administrative and/or clinical and support services (e.g., Ryan White Comprehensive AIDS Resources Emergency (CARE) Act, Title V MCH, Community Health Centers), and reimbursement dollars for specific services (Medicaid) and pharmaceuticals (ADAP). State funding consists of matching fund contributions required by a specific program (e.g., Title V MCH services), shared funding (e.g., CDC programs) or supplemental funds used to expand service support. Community providers also often receive grants from foundations and local governments to pro-

---

[16]Unpublished estimates from the Kaiser commission on Medicaid and Uninsured. Based on the March 1996 *Current Population Survey,* using ages 18-44 for women and under 18 for children.

vide services, and some engage in fund-raising from the individuals and businesses in their community.

The following discussion presents a brief description of the major sources of federal funding reaching the community. A number of smaller funding sources are scattered throughout federal agencies in the form of grants to the providers discussed in the previous section or in the form of demonstration grants.

Medicaid

Medicaid (Title XIX of the Social Security Act), the second largest publicly financed health care program, provided health and long-term care coverage to approximately 36.8 million Americans in 1996—the elderly, the disabled, women, and children (DHHS, 1998). Over 61.5% of women in care for HIV are insured by Medicaid (Rand, 1998). Medicaid also pays for the care of about 90% of children with AIDS (DHHS, 1998). Medicaid is the largest single payer of direct medical services for people with AIDS, totaling approximately $3.5 billion in FY 1998 (DHHS, 1998).

Medicaid is an entitlement that guarantees eligible individuals access to a minimum level of benefits, established by the federal government, regardless of where they live, but individuals must meet state income and resource criteria and fall within specific categories. States have the option, however, of adding eligibles and services to their Medicaid program from a federally established list and still receiving a federal match. Thirty-four states offer a "medically needy" option that permits those with too much income to otherwise qualify by offsetting their excess income with medical or remedial expenses. Medicaid covers only 62% of the poor, and since the 1996 legislation, coverage for legal immigrants, children with disabilities, and individuals with substance abuse and alcoholism has been either eliminated or restricted (AIDS Action Council, 1998b). In most states, persons eligible for SSI disability benefits are automatically eligible for Medicaid.

States share the cost of the program with the federal government, paying between 20% and 50% of the cost. The full range of Medicaid services identified in a state plan must be provided to persons with HIV disease. Some states offer optional services, such as targeted case management, preventive services, and hospice care. Medicaid currently covers all Food and Drug Administration (FDA) approved prescribed drugs, including those used for prophylactic treatment of AIDS-related opportunistic infections, and drugs for treatment of HIV disease and prevention of perinatal HIV transmission. Although states are required to cover these drugs for people on Medicaid and can participate in Medicaid's drug rebate contract, many states have imposed limitations by restricting the number of prescriptions a patient can purchase in a month, the number and terms of refills, a requirement for prior authorization, and a determination of "medical necessity." Medicaid has issued a directive to states requiring that those which include drugs and cover the HIV population in managed care, and to ensure that those drugs are available in managed care formularies. Medicaid covers the provision of ZDV to HIV-positive pregnant women and their infants to prevent the transmission of HIV. Medicaid's Early and Periodic Screening, Diagnostic, and Treatment (EPSDT) Program provides services to children and adolescents (under 21) that are "medically reasonable and necessary," whether they are identified in the plan or not.

The dramatic growth in Medicaid's use of managed care over the last decade has moved many of those with HIV into the managed care setting and placed increased demands on states to monitor and assure access to the full range of quality services needed for management of HIV within managed care organizations (see the discussion of Medicaid issues in the section Important Issues Affecting Services).

Social Security

Social Security has two programs that can offer benefits to eligible persons with HIV/AIDS. For persons who work, Social Security Disability Insurance (SSDI) provides monthly benefits to persons disabled by a medical condition that is expected to last at least a year or end in death and is serious enough to prevent them from doing substantial work. The amount of the monthly benefit depends upon how much was earned while working. After 24 months on SSDI, the recipient becomes eligible for Medicare, which helps pay for hospital and hospice care, lab tests, home health care, and other medical services.

Supplemental Security Income (SSI) is intended for those who have not worked enough to qualify for Social Security or whose benefits are low and resources limited. Children with disabilities who live in low-income families may qualify for the SSI Disabled Children's Program (SSIDCP). In most states, eligibility for SSI makes one eligible for Medicaid coverage.

Child Health Insurance Program

Recently enacted, Child Health Insurance Program (Title XXI-Social Security Act) (CHIP) is intended to enable states to expand health insurance coverage to low-income children up to age 19. About $40 billion in federal funds will be provided over the next 10 years with a requirement for matching state funds. States may expand the Medicaid program and/or create or expand a separate state health insurance program. States must submit a state plan (17 states had filed plans as of February 1998) that includes standards and methods for establishing and continuing eligibility and for finding and enrolling eligible children. Eligibility is limited to children whose families have incomes at or below 200% of the poverty level or 50% above the state's current Medicaid eligibility limit and who are not eligible for Medicaid or covered by other health insurance. States may choose how to determine family income.

States that choose to expand their Medicaid program must provide the same benefits under CHIP. States that do not expand Medicaid can either choose popular benefit packages or develop equivalent ones. In response to the information that 11 million infants, children, and adolescents were uninsured last year, 3 million of whom were estimated to be eligible for Medicaid, CHIP requires and supports outreach to Medicaid-eligible children.

There are important implementation issues that will affect eligibility and services for the HIV-infected population. If a state chooses to expand Medicaid with CHIP funds, the comprehensive Medicaid benefit package would be available to children and become an entitlement. Choosing a separate health insurance program that uses commercial plan packages may not meet the multiple special needs of a child with HIV/AIDS and the benefits can be capped by the state's allocation. A separate plan would also allow for premiums and cost sharing, while a Medicaid expansion would preclude passing on costs to families in the form of cost sharing. Some state Medicaid plans, however, have received waivers for cost sharing. No matter which plan a state chooses, it has considerable flexibility in determining family incomes and which groups of children to cover.

Health Resources and Services Administration[17]

Health Resources and Services Administration (HRSA) is located within the DHHS and contains four bureaus, three of which directly support services that benefit individuals and families affected by HIV/AIDS—the HIV/AIDS Bureau, the Bureau of Primary Health Care, and the Bureau of Maternal and Child Health. The following are the major HRSA programs supporting service delivery on the community level.

Ryan White Programs (Titles I, II, III, IV, and Part F)

The Ryan White CARE Act, administered by the HIV/AIDS Bureau, funds the delivery of HIV/AIDS care, services, and training. The purpose of the act was to improve the quality and availability of care for people with HIV/AIDS and their families. Total appropriations for the CARE Act for FY 1998 were $1.15 billion. Amendments to the Ryan White CARE Act in 1996 intensified the focus on prevention of perinatal HIV transmission and provided additional funding to states adopting the new CDC guidelines for offsetting costs related to such activities as outreach, voluntary testing for HIV, and mandatory testing of newborns.

Title I: HIV Emergency Relief Grant Program for Eligible Metropolitan Areas. Formula and supplemental grants to Eligible Metropolitan Areas (EMAs)

---

[17]Information on Ryan White titles from HRSA (1997a,b). Data provided by the HIV/AIDS Bureau.

disproportionately affected by the HIV epidemic. Grants are awarded to the chief elected official of the city or county that administers the health agency providing services to the greatest number of people living with HIV in the EMA. An HIV health services planning council representative of providers and people living with AIDS sets priorities for the allocation of funds. Services may include outpatient health care, support services, and inpatient case management. Providers may be public or nonprofit entities. There are 49 EMAs in 19 states, Puerto Rico, and the District of Columbia.

At a minimum, the city must allocate a percentage of grant funds for providing services to women, infants, and children, including treatment measures to prevent perinatal transmission of HIV, equal to the percentage of women, infants, and children with AIDS in the total AIDS population. HRSA FY 1995 data indicate that overall, 34% of those served by Title I grantees were women and children.

Title II: HIV Care Grants to States. Formula grants are given to states and territories for health care and support services. Grants are awarded to the state agency designated by the governor, usually the health department. Services may include home- and community-based health care and support services, continuation of health insurance coverage, and pharmaceutical treatments through the AIDS Drug Assistance Program (ADAP). HRSA data indicate that in 1995, 25% of those served by Title II grantees were women and children.

ADAP provides funds to states to make protease inhibitors and other therapies available to uninsured and underinsured individuals with HIV. These funds are available in all 50 states, the District of Columbia, Puerto Rico, the Virgin Islands, and Guam. Administered by state AIDS directors, each state sets its own financial and medical eligibility criteria, and determines the type and number of drugs covered and their purchase and distribution. In 1996, 83,000 persons with HIV disease were served; $52 million in supplemental funds were appropriated in 1996 to supplement the $53 million committed by states from their Title II awards. The total national ADAP budget for FY 1997 was $385 million, a 221% increase from FY 1996, with the majority of funds coming from federal sources, including the $167 million designated for ADAP (Doyle et al., 1997).

ADAP is the second largest source of payment for HIV/AIDS drugs and is a "last resort" payment program that varies significantly from state to state as to who has access. Fifteen states have waiting lists for ADAP enrollment and/or for access to protease inhibitors (AIDS Policy Center for Children, Youth, and Families, 1998). The demand for ADAP funds has increased dramatically as the number of persons with HIV has grown and new therapeutic regimens have been developed. In 1997, four state programs did not cover protease inhibitors and two states covered only one. Five states did not cover any of the prophylactic drugs strongly recommended in the 1997 guidelines, and only two states had the full complement recommended. (CDC, 1997; Doyle et al., 1997).

Title III: HIV Early Intervention Services. Grants are awarded for early intervention services for low-income, medically underserved people in existing primary care systems. To date, 166 facilities in 34 states, Puerto Rico, and the District of Columbia have been awarded funds. Nearly half of the funds have been given to community and migrant health centers; the other half have been distributed to homeless programs, local health departments, family planning programs, diagnostic and treatment centers for hemophilia, federally qualified health centers, and private nonprofits. In FY 1995, 39% of the programs targeted services to women and children.

Title IV: Coordinated HIV Services and Access to Research for Children, Youth, Women, and Families. Grants are awarded to (1) promote the development and operation of systems of primary health care, social services, and outreach that benefit children, youth, women, and families in a comprehensive, community-based, family-centered system of care; (2) emphasize prevention within systems to reduce the spread of HIV infection; and (3) link comprehensive systems of care with HIV/AIDS clinical research trials and other research activities, thereby increasing access to care. There are currently 65 projects funding 350 care sites in 27 states, Puerto Rico, and the District of Columbia, serving mostly poor, minority families with limited access to transportation and housing. Data from 1996 indicate that 11,200 adolescents were served, 14% of whom were pregnant. Approximately 100,000 adolescent and adult women were served through Title IV prevention, outreach, and education efforts.

In collaboration with the Special Projects of National Significance (SPNS) program, Title IV funds the Women's Initiative for HIV Care and Reduction of Perinatal HIV Transmission. Three-year cooperative agreements have been awarded to ten sites in ten states to develop models of care that enhance outreach and HIV counseling and testing services for women of childbearing age, especially during pregnancy. The program also offers perinatal ZDV prophylaxis and ongoing care for mothers with HIV and their children. Program goals include (1) facilitation of early identification through outreach, counseling, and voluntary testing; (2) facilitation of access to and utilization of a comprehensive system of care that includes ZDV prophylaxis to reduce perinatal HIV transmission; (3) promotion of consumer education; (4) training of providers; and (5) evaluation of the efficacy of strategies and models.

Title V (formerly Part F). SPNS funding supports the development of models of HIV/AIDS care designed to address hard to reach populations and to be replicable. In 1996 there were 62 grantees focusing on a variety of issues—including, for example, managed care, infrastructure development, training, reduction of barriers for rural residents, women, adolescents, and children, integration of mental health and primary care services, and services for correctional populations.

Three of the grantees were women centered programs. The SPNS program has collaborated with the SAMHSA and the National Institute of Mental Health, to co-fund eleven mental health services demonstration projects for people living with HIV/AIDS.

The HIV/AIDS Dental Reimbursement Programs assist dental schools and post-doctoral dental programs with uncompensated costs incurred in providing oral health treatment to HIV-positive patients.

The AIDS Education and Training Centers is a national network of 15 centers that conduct education and training programs for health care providers who want to learn more about the counseling, diagnosis, treatment and management of care for individuals with or at risk for HIV/AIDS. These centers work with community-based HIV/AIDS organizations, health professions schools, hospitals, health departments, community health centers, medical societies, and other organizations.

Maternal and Child Health Services Block Grant

Administered by the Maternal and Child Health Bureau (MCH), the Title V (Social Security Act) MCH Services Block Grant enables state health agencies to establish a state-level program consisting of both the MCH and Children with Special Health Care Needs (CSHCN) programs to form the locus of responsibility in each state for health-related services to mothers and children. The State Title V MCH program is a federal–state partnership in which states are allowed considerable discretion in determining how to use federal funds to meet the unique needs of their respective jurisdictions. Although activities vary from state to state and depend upon how the state is organized, MCH and CSHCN programs engage in such core public health activities as assessment, policy development, and assurance. Assurance activities include, but are not limited to direct and indirect support of clinical and support services for women and children, including those affected by HIV/AIDS. While some states directly provide services in the community or on a regional level, the bulk of support for service delivery is provided indirectly through grants and contracts with community-based providers, including local health departments, community health centers, hospitals, university medical centers, school-based and school-linked health clinics and programs, public and private community agencies, and private providers. Total Title V appropriations for FY 1998 were $683 million, with $564.9 million allocated to states on a formula basis in the form of a block grant.

States must match federal funds $3 for every $4 and must dedicate 30% of block grant funding to preventive and primary care for children, and 30% for children with special health care needs. Most of the remaining funds are used for pregnant women and infants. Title V programs serve more than 17 million women of reproductive age, infants, children, and youth. Roughly one-third of all pregnant women in the United States receive Title V-supported prenatal care. A 1995 survey of Title V programs (Brown and Aliza, 1995), indicated that children with HIV/AIDS are eligible for preventive and primary care services in all Title V MCH, programs and for CSHCN services, including case management, in 90% of the programs reporting. A high degree of collaboration related to HIV/AIDS was noted with family planning programs, state AIDS offices, STD programs, local health agencies, and Ryan White activities, particularly the Title IV program for women, children, youth, and families.

In November 1995, the Association of Maternal and Child Health Programs developed and distributed to all state Title V MCH and CSHCN programs, a document entitled *Opportunities for Reducing Transmission of HIV to Infants: Guidelines for State Title V Program Leadership* (Kagan and Aliza, 1995).

Federal Health Center Programs

Administered by the Bureau of Primary Health Care, the four federal health center programs (Section 330 of the Public Health Service Act) consist of the migrant health centers program, health care for the homeless, health services for residents of public housing, and the community health center program. These programs, formerly authorized under Sections 329, 330, 340, and 340A, have been consolidated under one section, Section 330, and are an important source of funding for services in specific geographical areas designated as underserved. The total appropriation for FY 1998 is $826 million.

Services required of health centers includes primary care services, diagnostic laboratory and radiologic services, preventive health services (prenatal and perinatal services, screening for breast and cervical cancer, well child services, immunizations, screening for communicable diseases, elevated blood lead levels and cholesterol, pediatric eye, ear, and dental screenings, family planning services, preventive dental services), emergency medical services, and pharmaceutical services. Health centers also are required to provide referrals to providers, including substance abuse and mental health services, patient case management services, support services, and education of patients and the general population.

Centers for Disease Control and Prevention Programs

The CDC is an agency of the DHHS. Its purpose is to promote health and quality of life by preventing and controlling disease, injury, and disability. The CDC encompasses eleven centers, institutes, and offices. The National Center for HIV, STD, and TB Prevention is the major locus for HIV prevention activities. The Center for Chronic Disease Prevention and Health Promotion also plays a role in HIV prevention and the Division of Adolescent and School Health supports counseling related to HIV/AIDS in the school health setting.

Division of HIV/AIDS Prevention[18]

Located in the National Center for HIV, STD, and TB Prevention, the division has 65 cooperative agreements (CAs), totaling $250 million, with all states, territories, the District of Columbia, and Puerto Rico, and with six cities (New York City, Houston, Chicago, San Francisco, Los Angeles, and Philadelphia). These projects fund 10,000 counseling and testing sites. Part I of the CA provides funds for counseling, testing, referral, and partner notification; Part II supports health education and risk reduction, including street and community outreach, risk reduction counseling, prevention case management and linkage to other services, and community-level intervention to change perceptions of risk. The CAs require a community planning process whereby health departments, affected communities, providers, and scientists get together to plan the health department's application to the CDC.

In addition to cooperative agreements with states, the CDC offers competitive funding grants and demonstration grants. Examples of these vehicles are: (1) 20–40 grants to minority organizations within communities to provide services to meet unmet needs related to HIV/AIDS; and (2) 5–6 demonstration project grants to health departments that emphasize prevention and linkage to care with a particular focus on reducing perinatal transmission.

Division of STD Prevention[19]

Located in the National Center for HIV, STD, and TB Prevention, this division has 65 funded projects totaling $80 million dollars, with all states, territories, the District of Columbia, Puerto Rico, and with six cities (New York City, Chicago, Los Angeles, Philadelphia, San Francisco, and Baltimore). These projects fund 3,000 STD clinics, most of which are located in state and local public health departments. Other sites include some family planning clinics and hospitals. These clinics are the primary source of HIV testing in public facilities, although the population using these clinics is primarily male, poor, uninsured, and experiencing symptoms of an STD. Every patient using clinic services gets pre- and post-test counseling for HIV and education concerning safe sex practices. Be cause of the demand for services, most of the effort in providing follow-up involved those who test positive; 82% of those who test positive are brought back for follow-up.

There are three sources of funding for STD clinics: (1) CDC funds can be used for management, consultation, technical assistance, some staff, and travel;

---

[18]Information provided by the Division of HIV/AIDS Prevention, CDC.
[19]Information provided by the Division of STD Prevention, CDC.

(2) state funds can be used for medical supplies, laboratory services, disease intervention, and some staff; and (3) local funds usually provide the facilities and primary staff for the clinic.

Division of Adolescent and School Health

In addition to monitoring the incidence and prevalence of risks among youth, this division supports every state and territorial education agency and 18 local education agencies that serve cities with the highest number of reported AIDS cases. Division of Adolescent and School Health's (DASHs) efforts in this area focus on assisting these agencies to develop and implement HIV-related school policies and student curricula and training teachers to carry out prevention efforts.

Substance Abuse and Mental Health Services Administration Programs

An agency under the Department of Health and Human Services, Substance Abuse and Mental Health Services Administration (SAMHSA) has three centers that provide substance abuse and mental health services, with a FY 1997 budget of approximately $1.4 billion. The three centers include: the Center for Mental Health Services (CMHS), the Center for Substance Abuse Prevention (CSAP), and the Center for Substance Abuse Treatment (CSAT). There are two offices within the agency that coordinate services related to women and AIDS—the Office for Women's Services and the Office on AIDS. CSAT administers the block grant program supporting the 10,000 substance abuse treatment facilities throughout the country that receive federal funds, and is responsible for residential and treatment programs for pregnant and postpartum women; demonstration projects that target special populations, including those with HIV; and programs that address the needs of people under the criminal justice system. CSAP has a number of projects focused on women that are ending this year. No new targeted programs are planned.

The Prevention and Treatment of Substance Abuse Block Grant Program is funded at $1.3 billion and is intended to address substance abuse in states and cities. It requires that 35% of funds be spent on alcohol prevention and treatment; 35% on drug prevention and treatment; 20% on supporting primary prevention; and 10% for pregnant and postpartum women and women with dependent children.

State AIDS Programs

State agency staff have programmatic responsibility for administering HIV/ AIDS health care, prevention, education, and supportive service programs funded by the state and federal governments. All 50 states, the District of Columbia, Puerto Rico, the U.S. Virgin Islands, and the U.S. Pacific Islands have AIDS programs at the state or territorial level. The bulk of funding for HIV/AIDS services administered through state AIDS directors comes from the CDC. CDC prevention dollars are provided for testing, counseling, and outreach; Ryan White Title II dollars are provided with the requirement that community planning groups determine how funds are to be distributed; and state funds are provided at state discretion. State AIDS programs fund testing and counseling services, education, and outreach services in existing community-based service settings through grants and contracts; some testing and counseling centers are run directly by the state.

National Institutes of Health Research Programs[20]

One of eight health agencies of the PHS, DHHS, the National Institutes of Health (NIH) is comprised of 24 separate institutes, centers, and divisions. In addition to supporting intramural research, NIH uses 81% of its funding to support the research of non-federal scientists in 1,700 research settings throughout the country and abroad, including universities, medical schools, hospitals, and research institutions.

Extramural research grants related to HIV are provided to institutions across the country to conduct peer-reviewed research. These research efforts offer women and children affected by HIV, who meet the protocol criteria, important opportunities to access care through participation in research protocols. One of the Ryan White Title IV program mandates is to assist women and children with HIV in accessing research protocols. The three major clinical trial networks are the Pediatric AIDS Clinical Trials Group (PACTG), the AIDS Clinical Trials Groups (ACTG), and the Terry Beirn Community Programs for Clinical Research on AIDS (CPCRA). ACTG research focuses translating basic research discoveries into clinical research, while the PACTG evaluates interventions to prevent perinatal transmission and to improve the quality of life of HIV-infected infants, children, and adolescents. The CPCRA enrolls adults to studies in primary care settings. The two institutes noted below work closely together and provide the bulk of NIH-supported ACTG research for women and children.

National Institute of Child Health and Human Development

In FY 1997, the National Institute of Child Health and Human Development (NICHD) budget dedicated almost $23 million to pediatric ACTG research in an independent network of 30 to 40 clinical centers located in 15 states, the District of Columbia, and Puerto Rico. A subset of eleven centers specifically conducts

---

[20]Information provided by the National Institute of Child Health and Human Development, National Institute of Allergy and Infectious Diseases, and the Office of AIDS Research, National Institutes of Health.

research that includes obstetric and newborn patients in addition to pediatric patients. Research funds support individual clinic budgets for staff and patients and care-related services, including enhancement of recruitment and retention of patients. Pregnant women access clinical trials research through the PACTG arm; there are limited opportunities to access treatment unrelated to pregnancy (e.g., cervical dysplasia). Grantees are almost all university, hospital-based clinics and some community-based providers. There is currently a new collaboration with the Ryan White Title IV grantees to establish linkages to research sites related to nutrition research.

National Institute of Allergy and Infectious Diseases

National Institute of Allergy and Infectious Diseases (NIAID) is the institute that expends the majority of NIH funding for extramural PACTG research. In FY 1997, NIAID dedicated $32 million to PACTG research (32% of which was targeted specifically to women), and $69.6 million to adult ACTG research (approximately 22.5% of which was specifically targeted to women). NIAID has 21 clinical sites (or main units) with multiple subunits, located in 14 states, the District of Columbia, and Puerto Rico. Research dollars are provided in the form of long term cooperative agreements, and grants and are expended for a core of fixed costs related to staffing based on the number of patients in a given period. NIAID conducts the CPCRA described above.

AUTHORITY FOR POLICY DECISIONS AND OVERSIGHT

A description of the agencies and bodies that may exercise general or specific authority over some or all of the services provided by providers profiled on the community level accurately reflects the complexity of our health care system. An individual provider may have one or many agencies and/or government and community bodies that have oversight responsibilities and guide policies for service delivery. Providers in the private practice setting are responsible to their licensing boards and the policies and oversight of the organizations with whom they contract to deliver services. Public providers tend to use multiple funding streams and so must respond to the authority of each of the funders, as well as state and local governing bodies.

By law and custom, responsibility in health affairs is shared by federal, state, and local authorities. As a result, there is often an effort on the part of federal and state entities to avoid from issuing too many regulations or offering what might be perceived by their respective constituents as "excessive" guidance. Many of these authorities "recommend" rather than "require." The degree to which responsibility or authority is shared among these authorities has fluctuated. The locus of responsibility for decisions about public benefits has clearly shifted over this decade. Recent welfare legislation embodies this fundamental change in how and where decisions are made about public benefits. Decisions on who should get what benefits and for how long has devolved from the federal to the state level and, in many states, to the local level to varying degrees. The variability that has always existed from community to community in the organization, structure, and funding of health care services has increased accordingly, creating important challenges to mounting an effective effort to reduce HIV perinatal transmission.

IMPORTANT ISSUES AFFECTING SERVICES

There are a number of important issues that significantly affect the structure, funding, and the delivery of services to women, children, and youth affected by HIV. Although some of these issues have been briefly touched on in the sections that describes the health care system and funding mechanisms, they can be examined as part of the larger picture of significant public policy and health care system changes that have taken place during this decade.

Welfare Reform

Welfare reform legislation is probably the most sweeping of the changes that have important implications for the health of women and children affected by HIV. The Personal Responsibility Work Opportunity Reconciliation Act (PRWORA), referred to as welfare reform, passed in 1996 and included changes not only to welfare but to the SSI program, food stamps, Medicaid, and immigrant eligibility for means-tested benefits. The welfare program, which almost exclusively served women and children, was replaced by the Temporary Assistance to Needy Families (TANF) block grant program, effectively ending the Aid for Families with Dependent Children (AFDC) entitlement to a guarantee of cash assistance to all eligible individuals. Briefly,

- recipients may receive benefits for no more than five years over a lifetime and must adhere to work requirements; states may apply even stricter limits.
- TANF recipients who would have qualified under former AFDC rules are guaranteed Medicaid and pregnant women retain Medicaid eligibility during pregnancy, even if they lose their eligibility for TANF benefits.
- although states have the option of serving "current" qualified legal immigrants (those residing in the United States on August 22, 1996), the definition of "qualified immigrants" has been narrowed as has their access to certain benefits; disabled and elderly immigrants who fall in this category and were receiving SSI and derivative Medicaid benefits on the above date may maintain those benefits;
- new immigrants (those entering the country after passage of the bill) will not be eligible for "federal means-tested public benefits" such as food stamps, TANF, or Medicaid, for their first five years in the United States, but may be

served in community health centers and state MCH programs and receive public health assistance (not Medicaid) for immunizations and testing and treatment of the symptoms of communicable disease;

• undocumented immigrants are barred from federal public benefits, and from state and local programs, and their presence must be reported to the Immigration and Naturalization Service (INS); and

• cash assistance is not available to individuals convicted of drug felonies, even if they are seeking drug treatment (Children's Defense Fund, 1997; San Francisco AIDS Foundation, 1997).

The impact of these changes on access to care and, therefore, primary and secondary prevention opportunities for reducing perinatal transmission is significant and complex. Most women with or at risk for HIV have low incomes, are uninsured, and/or often rely on government programs to support their access to health care. Women with HIV disease may become impoverished because the disease itself prevents them from working or because of the expenses associated with it. Women's traditional linkage with the Medicaid program often came with their enrollment in AFDC (the former welfare program). With reduced access to welfare due to changes in eligibility and the imposition of time limits and sanctions, women may not be aware of their potential eligibility for Medicaid or how to access the program. Although many states have attempted to ease access to Medicaid for those applying for TANF benefits by creating a single application for TANF and Medicaid, access has been made more complicated for those not eligible or interested in TANF benefits because separate routes to Medicaid have not been effectively established in many jurisdictions. With access to both welfare and health care services restricted to certain categories of legal immigrants and unavailable for the undocumented, opportunities for prevention and treatment are more limited. Many undocumented women are fearful of accessing care because of INS reporting requirements. Women seeking drug treatment may not have the financial support they need because of the prohibition on benefits for those with a prior conviction.

While there are still opportunities for many women to access health services, the PRWORA is new and so sweeping that there is still much confusion on the part of potential recipients and those administering the new law. States are just beginning to develop the capacity and systems needed to appropriately inform and educate staff and reach out to potential recipients with information and mechanisms for linkage to appropriate services.

Medicaid

Some important policy changes affect this program's relationship to HIV prevention and treatment services for women and children. As previously noted, Medicaid plays a critical role in providing health care for low-income people living with HIV/AIDS, with more than 61.5% of women in care for HIV (Rand, 1998) and 90% of children with AIDS (DHHS, 1998) relying on this program for health care coverage. The costs associated with Medicaid have been rising and there have been several efforts to change the entitlement status of the program, impose per capita caps, and change the structure of payments to providers. While the program remains an entitlement, passage of the Balanced Budget Act of 1997 resulted in several important changes:

• Medicaid has experienced funding cuts in two important areas that affect HIV services. In response to abuses by states, the disproportionate share hospital (DSH) payments, which compensate hospitals serving a large volume of uninsured and Medicaid patients, have been curbed and reporting requirements imposed. The DSH program is important to health care access for people with HIV and AIDS by supporting such safety net providers as outpatient HIV clinics at public and nonprofit hospitals across the nation. The second cut in Medicaid comes from repeal of the Boren Amendment, which established a standard for reimbursement to hospitals and nursing homes. States must now provide public notice of their rates and how they were calculated.

• States now have the authority to mandate that beneficiaries enroll in managed care plans without application to the federal government; plans can consist of only Medicaid beneficiaries, and states can impose cost sharing charges allowed under fee for service plans. These changes may well affect the ability of persons with HIV to access services needed for their care (see comments in following section, below.)

• States now have the option to extend Medicaid coverage for 12 months for all children, whether or not they continue to meet income eligibility tests. This provision is expected to expand coverage by up to one million children.

• States have the option of creating a Medicaid "buy-in" for persons whose income is under 250% of poverty and who would be eligible for SSI, if their income were not too high. This has important implications for increasing access to Medicaid for women with HIV (Families USA Foundation, 1997).

Managed Care

Enrollment in managed care arrangements has increased dramatically in this decade. The percentage of employees enrolled in managed care plans increased from 48% in 1992 to 855 in 1997 (Employee Benefit Research Institute, 1998). Almost 50% of Medicaid recipients were enrolled in managed care in 1997, with two states reporting 100% enrollment and five states reporting more than 80% enrollment (HCFA, 1997). The movement into managed care represents a fundamental change in the way health care services are delivered in both the public and the private sector, raising issues of access to care and quality of care.

• Through public sector managed care arrangements, women, children, and youth are the population moving most quickly into managed care. This population as a whole and those with or at risk for HIV/AIDS have unique and complex needs requiring a broad array of multidisciplinary medical and support services. Many of the managed care organizations (MCOs) may not have the experience or expertise necessary to work with low-income populations or populations with the complex medical and social needs of those with HIV. They also may not have experience working with multiple public and private providers to assure access to specific services.

Some of the problems encountered by persons with HIV enrolled in MCOs include reduced access to specialty care providers, including HIV specialists; reduced access to specific drug formularies and specific services; clinical decisions with the appearance of cost as the dominant factor; limitations placed on the information providers can provide; and insufficient time to meet with providers. Relationships need to be built with the type of providers that adolescents seek out—teen clinics, school health clinics, community family practice sites, and family planning clinics. More time is needed to gain experience providing HIV specialty services and to build systems that can monitor and evaluate the quality of care in the managed care setting and provide oversight. One strategy that some states have chosen is to carve out specific services or populations, such as those with disabilities, so as to ensure a focus on the multiple and special needs of the population.

• Medicaid managed care arrangements compete for public providers and private community-based providers serving the uninsured and publicly insured. Before the advent of managed care, these providers were frequently the only providers for the poor or nearly poor patient. Reimbursement from Medicaid for eligible populations gave these providers the ability to cross-subsidize the uninsured or underinsured patient (Davis, 1997). Medicaid competition is threatening the ability to support services to those without adequate insurance coverage. In addition, "many public hospitals and . . . providers of care to the poor with a mission to render care to the uninsured are being sold to private, for-profit organizations without a comparable mission to provide uncompensated care" (Wehr et al., 1998).

The movement towards managed care has important implications for all those served, particularly for those who have a high level of need. Work is in progress on the national level to establish a patient's bill of rights for managed care settings and to establish oversight mechanisms that include monitoring and evaluation.

Health Insurance Portability and Accountability

The Health Insurance Portability and Accountability Act (HIPAA), passed in 1996, attempts to address a number of issues for people with pre-existing conditions, including those with HIV/AIDS. The law prohibits group health plans, insurers, and managed care organizations from denying coverage because of pre-existing conditions if the person had been insured for an uninterrupted 12 month period prior to the application. In addition, the law

- limits to 12 months the time a person can be subject to a pre-existing medical condition exclusion if they had no previous health care coverage;
- guarantees the availability of individual health insurance policies for those who leave jobs and maintain previous coverage;
- prohibits denial of coverage in group plans to persons in poor health; and
- requires insurers to sell plans to small employers and guarantees renewal for both small group and individual coverage.

The law did not specify what benefits a health plan must include and did not guarantee that health insurance coverage would provide adequate care or be affordable. In addition, there are a number of issues involving AIDS and private insurance coverage that remain unresolved at this time. These include questions about whether health plans can exclude from coverage individuals who have received a diagnosis of HIV infection before coverage; whether an employer can restructure a health plan to reduce benefits for a specific type of illness after a claim has been filed; and whether specific services will be considered "medically necessary" and, therefore covered under insurance plans.

Americans with Disabilities Act

The Americans with Disabilities Act (ADA) of 1990 protects against discrimination in the workplace, housing, and public accommodations for people with disabilities, including people living with HIV/AIDS. On June 25, 1998 the decision by the U.S. Supreme Court has important implications for anti-discrimination protections for individuals with asymptomatic HIV disease in employment, insurance, and services offered by business and government (AIDS Action Council, 1998a). The ruling determined that "HIV infection satisfies the statutory and regulatory definition of physical impairment during every stage of the disease." This means that persons with asymptomatic HIV cannot be excluded under the ADA and should have access to non-discriminatory and high quality health care. The decision also determined that reproduction was a major life activity for the purposes of the ADA and that HIV infection limits the ability to reproduce.

CONCLUSION

The current revolution that is taking place in our health care system, as well as the complexities in its structure and funding, both challenge our efforts to institute effective policies for reducing perinatal HIV transmission and provide new opportunities. While multiple efforts have been made to inform providers and promote strategies for reducing perinatal transmission, more needs to be done. There is a need for a broader dissemination of more explicit guidance, the development of incentives for prevention efforts, and identification and maximization of opportunities for intervention.

REFERENCES

AIDS Action Council. *Bragdon v. Abbott: an HIV Civil Rights Case.* 1998a.

AIDS Action Council. *Medicaid and HIV/AIDS.* 1998b.

Aliza B, Brown T, Fine A, Lynch L. *Partnerships for Healthier Families: Principles for Assuring the Health of Women, Infants, Children, and Youth Under Managed Care Arrangements.* Association of Maternal and Child Health Programs. November 1996.

Blum RW, Beuhring T, Wunderlich M, Resnick MD. Do not ask, they won't tell: The quality of adolescent health screening in five practice settings. *American Journal of Public Health* 86:12, 1768, 1996.

Brown T, Aliza B. *A Changing Epidemic: How State Title V Programs Are Addressing the Spread of HIV/AIDS in Women, Children, and Youth.* The Association of Maternal and Child Health Programs, 1995.

CDC. 1997 USPHS/IDSA guidelines for the prevention of opportunistic infections in persons infected with human immunodeficiency virus. *MMWR* 46(RR-12), 1997.

Chavkin W, Breitbart V, Elman D, Wise P. National survey of the states: policies and practices regarding drug using pregnant women. *American Journal of Public Health* 88(1):117–119, 1998.

Children's Defense Fund. *Health Provisions in the Welfare Law* (April 25, 1997).

Davis K. Uninsured in an era of managed care. *Health Services Research* 31:641–649, 1997.

Department of Health and Human Services. Fact sheet: Medicaid and acquired immune deficiency syndrome (AIDS) and human immunodeficiency virus (HIV) infection. March 1998. [available on-line: http://hiv.hcfa.gov/medicaid/obs11.htm]

Doyle A, Jefferys R, Kelly J. *State AIDS Drug Assistance Programs: A National Status Report on Access.* Menlo Park, CA: Henry J. Kaiser Family Foundation, 1997

Employee Benefits Research Institute (EBRI). Fact sheet: Characteristics of individuals with employment-based health insurance, 1987–1995. 1997. [www document] URL http://www.ebri.org/facts/0797fact.htm.

EBRI. Issues of quality and consumer rights in the health care market. *EBRI Issue Brief* 196, April 1998.

Falik M. Introduction: Listening to women's voices, learning from women's experiences. In Falik MM, Collins KS, eds. *Women's Health: The Commonwealth Survey.* Baltimore, Md.: Johns Hopkins University Press; 4, 1996.

Families USA Foundation. Field report: balanced budget bill enacted. August 1997

George Washington University. *School-Based Health Centers. Making the Grade.* Washington, D.C.: George Washington University, 1998.

Health Care Financing Administration (HCFA). Managed care trends. National Summary of Medicaid Managed Care Programs and Enrollment. June 30, 1997. [available on-line http://www.hcfa.gov/medicaid/ome1997.htm]

HRSA (Health Resources and Services Administration). *HIV/AIDS Bureau (December 1997)* .

HRSA. *HIV/AIDS Programs (August 1997).*

Hess C. The organization of maternal and child health services. In *Maternal and Child Health Practices.* eds., H Wallace, R Nelson, and P Sweeney. Third Party Publishing Co. 4th Edition, 1994.

Home Access Health Corporation. *Home Access: HIV Counseling and Testing Report.* 1997

Kaeser L, Gold R, and Richards C. *Title X at 25.* Washington, DC.: The Alan Guttmacher Institute, 1996.

Kagan J and Aliza B. *Opportunities for Reducing Transmission to HIV to Infants: Guidelines for State Title V Program Leadership.* 1995.

Kaiser Commission on the Future of Medicaid. *Fact Sheet: Medicaid's Role for Persons with HIV/AIDS,* 1996.

Kaiser Commission on Medicaid and Uninsured. *Uninsured in America: A Chart Book.* Menlo Park, CA: The Henry J. Kaiser Family Foundation, June 1998.

Kaiser Family Foundation. *Fact Sheet: Medicaid and Managed Care,* 1998.

Kaiser Family Foundation. *Uninsured in America: Key Facts About Gaps in Health Insurance Coverage Today.* 1998.

Lyons B, Salganicoff A, Rowland D. Poverty, access, and health care, and the Medicaid's critical role for women. In Falik MM, Collins KS, eds. *Women's Health: The Commonwealth Survey.* Baltimore, Md.: Johns Hopkins University Press, 1996.

National Association of WIC Directors. *WIC: Building a Better Future for American's Children.* Washington, D.C.: WIC Program Office, Food and Nutrition Service, USDA, 1997.

RAND. Unpublished data from HIV Cost and Services Utilization Study. 1998.

San Francisco AIDS Foundation. *Renewing the Commitment: A New Era for HIVAIDS Care, Treatment and Services.* 1997.

Wehr E, Fagan M, Blake S, Rosenbaum S. *HIV/AIDS Related Provisions of Medicaid Managed Care Contracts.* Menlo Park, CA: Henry J. Kaiser Family Foundation. 1998.

Weisman, C. Women's use of health care. In Falik MM, Collins KS, eds. *Women's Health: The Commonwealth Survey.* Baltimore, Md.: Johns Hopkins University Press, 1996.

Wyn R, Brown ER, Yu H. Women's use of preventive health services." In *Women's Health: The Commonwealth Survey.* eds. MM Falik and K Scott Collins. Baltimore, Md.: Johns Hopkins University Press, 1996, 50.

Workshop I Summary

Miriam Davis

The Institute of Medicine (IOM) Committee on Perinatal Transmission of HIV held a workshop on February 11, 1998, to explore the rationale for, and response to, the 1995 Public Health Service (PHS) guidelines for universal counseling and voluntary testing of pregnant women for HIV (CDC, 1995). This summary covers workshop topics on the origin of the PHS guidelines; the positions of medical organizations; state policies and laws to implement the PHS guidelines; and the history and implementation of a mandatory newborn testing law in New York State. Workshop speakers and participants represented a broad spectrum of public health organizations at the federal, state, and local level. Health care providers and patients also participated.

THE ORIGIN OF THE PUBLIC HEALTH SERVICE GUIDELINES

The development of the 1995 PHS guidelines was triggered by the results of the AIDS Clinical Trials Group protocol number 76 (ACTG 076) demonstrating a two-thirds reduction in perinatal transmission with zidovudine (ZDV) (Connor et al., 1994). Prior to 1995, PHS guidelines recommended counseling and testing only of high-risk women or of women from high-prevalence geographic areas. When initial guidelines on counseling and testing were issued in 1989, HIV-positive pregnant women were advised merely to consider avoiding pregnancy until more was known and to avoid breast-feeding. At that time, effective means of treatment and prevention had yet to be developed, according to Dr. Martha Rogers of the PHS, one of the principal authors of both the old and the new guidelines.

Over the next decade, the policy climate changed dramatically with medical and scientific advances in early treatment of HIV and prevention of perinatal transmission. In 1994, the PHS formally inaugurated policy development to revise its earlier guidelines. After seeking broad input, especially from HIV-positive women and their advocates, the PHS proposed new guidelines in the *Federal Register*. The guidelines were revised in accordance with comments received during a 45-day comment period and were issued in final form on July 7, 1995. The guidelines proposed universal counseling and voluntary testing, in lieu of a more targeted approach to either high-risk women or high-prevalence states. The rationale for universal counseling was that many HIV-infected pregnant women and newborns in low-risk groups and low-prevalence states still were not being tested and treated. The universal approach was seen by the PHS, according to Dr. Rogers, as a means of stimulating the development of a counseling, testing, and treatment infrastructure in low-prevalence states and regions.

The PHS adoption of voluntary, as opposed to mandatory, testing was recommended for the following reasons: the policy had widespread support, particularly from patients for whom adherence to a demanding drug regimen is essential for prevention of transmission; mandatory testing was thought to be a deterrent to prenatal care; the risks of testing positive (e.g., discrimination and domestic violence) would outweigh the benefits in some cases; and experience had indicated that a high rate of acceptance was achievable since more than 90% of women accept testing when offered in several reported studies. Although the guidelines did not explicitly specify how patient consent to testing was to occur, Dr. Rogers pointed out that two types of patient consent are consistent with the intent of the PHS guidelines: the "right of refusal" (in which women are tested routinely unless they expressly refuse) and the "recommended with consent" (in which testing is recommended by the health care provider but performed only after explicit consent).

POSITIONS OF MEDICAL ORGANIZATIONS

Four professional organizations shared with the IOM committee their respective positions on HIV counseling and testing of pregnant women. The American Medical Association was the only one of the four to endorse mandatory testing of pregnant women and newborns. The other three organizations were in accord with the PHS in supporting universal counseling and voluntary testing of pregnant women. None of the organizations is actively monitoring the impact of its policies on member attitudes and practices.

American Medical Association

The American Medical Association (AMA) supports mandatory testing of all pregnant women and newborns. This policy, according to Dr. John Henning of the AMA Department of STD and HIV, was adopted in June 1996 after contentious debate by the AMA House of Delegates, its policy setting body. The formal policy states, "The American Medical Association supports the position that there should be mandatory HIV testing of all pregnant women and newborns, with counseling and recommendations for appropriate treatment." Dr. Henning observed that the debate centered upon medical benefits to the infant versus protecting the rights of the patient (i.e., the pregnant woman).

Because the voting was very close and not all of the 550 delegates were present for the vote, the delegates reconsidered the policy at the next meeting in December 1996. They began by considering a resolution to rescind mandatory testing, but, again after heated debate, the recision resolution was successfully reversed to reaffirm the need for mandatory testing. The AMA's position on mandatory testing is an outgrowth of its earlier policy that testing should be voluntary, unless the benefits of newborn testing are demonstrated sufficiently to warrant mandatory testing.

Participants reacted to the AMA position by questioning the effectiveness of mandatory testing and the procedural impact of the AMA position. Workshop participants expressed surprise with mandatory testing in light of its possible deterrence to prenatal care; experience suggesting that women overwhelmingly agree to be tested voluntarily; and the possibility of harm to women from their partner if they proceed with testing. Dr. Henning said that the overriding impetus for the passage of the policy was the life of the newborn. In later discussion, the terms of the AMA's debate, which pit the life of the newborn against the rights of the mother, was criticized as a false dichotomy by Mr. Tim Westmoreland, a representative of the Elizabeth Glaser Pediatric AIDS Foundation. Instead, the debate over mandatory versus voluntary testing should be cast, in his view, as "what doesn't work" versus "what works." In response to other questions, Dr. Henning cited the AMA's position as a policy, not a law or mandate, for physician behavior; consequently, AMA members are not monitored for their compliance. The policy remains in force unless further action is taken by the House of Delegates.

American College of Obstetricians and Gynecologists

The American College of Obstetricians and Gynecologists (ACOG) endorses voluntary, as opposed to mandatory, HIV testing of pregnant women. Its position, passed in August 1995 and reaffirmed in 1996, advocates (1) routine counseling of all pregnant women as part of prenatal care; (2) voluntary testing with consent; and (3) documentation of refusal of testing in the patient's chart. Dr. Michael Greene, an ACOG representative, also noted that ACOG recommends that pre-test counseling should include information about high-risk behaviors, vertical transmission, availability and effectiveness of therapy, and the potential social and psychological implications of testing positive. ACOG also recommends, on a voluntary basis, contacting sexual partners of HIV-positive patients, as well as sharing test information with health care professionals, including pediatricians. ACOG policies are developed by one of its standing committees, which then forwards its recommendations to the ACOG executive committee for a vote to establish policy. ACOG members provide an estimated 85% of all obstetrical care in the United States; the remainder is provided mostly by midwives and family practitioners.

Discussion of the ACOG position focused on why some obstetricians appear to be failing to routinely counsel pregnant women. While ACOG does not monitor obstetrician practices in relation to its policies, Dr. Greene speculated about the possible reasons: obstetricians view counseling as time- and resource-consuming and as engendering unnecessary patient anxiety among many patients at low risk. They also may not have developed channels of referral to specialty care for those testing positive. One participant pointed out that screening for alpha-fetoprotein testing for birth defects provides a model, embraced by practicing obstetricians, of pre- and post-test counseling and linkages to genetic counseling and specialty care.

American Academy of Pediatrics

The American Academy of Pediatrics (AAP) favors universal counseling and voluntary testing of pregnant women. It also recommends testing of all newborns whose mothers either are HIV-positive or have unknown HIV status. The AAP's recommendations include the following key points: (1) Routine HIV education and routine testing, with consent, should be performed for all pregnant women. Consent can take the form of the right of refusal in order to facilitate rapid incorporation of HIV testing into routine practice. (2) All testing programs should evaluate the percentage of women who refuse testing. In cases of poor acceptance rates, programs should analyze why and make changes. (3) Newborn testing should be performed, with maternal consent, when the mother's HIV status is unknown. If the newborn tests positive, the mother should be notified and receive referral for her testing and treatment. (4) Results of maternal testing should be provided to the pediatric health care provider. (5) Comprehensive HIV-related medical services should be available to all infected mothers, infants, and other family members (AAP, 1995). These recommendations were developed by a standing committee, the Committee on Pediatric AIDS. The AAP committee's recommendations were forwarded to the executive committee of the AAP and were approved for publication.

During the discussion, Dr. Gwendolyn Scott was asked why the AAP favored voluntary testing and what evidence it considered about the deterrent effects of mandatory testing for women seeking health care. She replied that personal experience, rather than hard data, was pivotal in persuading the AAP committee to embrace voluntary testing. The committee viewed voluntary testing as critical to ensuring a pregnant woman's compliance with the complex course of treatment needed for herself, her child, and possibly her older children.

National Medical Association

The National Medical Association (NMA) position on HIV testing of pregnant women, presented by Dr. Rani Lewis, asserts that (1) all health care professionals should offer counseling and voluntary HIV testing to all pregnant women on a confidential basis; (2) health care professionals should offer ZDV therapy to pregnant women and newborns without attempting to coerce treatment; (3) amniocentesis, fetal scalp electrode placement, or measures that lead to prolonged rupture of the fetal membranes should be avoided, as should breast-feeding; and (4) confidentiality, while extremely important, should not extend to withholding test information from other health care workers, such as pediatricians, for whom the information has medical significance. Dr. Lewis also observed that women who refuse testing are most likely to refuse treatment for themselves and their children. Some low-income and minority women view testing as threatening because, in their eyes, the diagnosis and the hospital experience in general are equated with death. She expressed concern that mandatory testing would leave women who refuse treatment for their children vulnerable to allegations of child abuse. She also noted that the NMA is very concerned about heightening discrimination against a population that already experiences a disproportionate share of discrimination. In view of the public health emphasis on testing, she stressed the importance of providing equal emphasis on funding for counseling and treatment. The NMA position was developed by its AIDS Task Force and adopted by its Executive Committee. The NMA is a 175-year-old organization for physicians of color and physicians who primarily care for patients of color.

Most of the discussion centered on NMA's support for disclosure of test results to other health care professionals, despite the importance of confidentiality. Some participants claimed that disclosure would act as a deterrent to testing, to which Dr. Lewis responded that NMA accepted the fact that some women would be deterred, but felt that disclosure to the pediatrician was paramount.

Response to the Positions of Medical Organizations

Mr. Tim Westmoreland, the Washington representative of the Elizabeth Glaser Pediatric AIDS Foundation, served as the respondent to the panel of medical organizations. His foundation favors counseling and voluntary testing of all pregnant women. He pointed out that mandatory testing not only discourages women from testing, but also ushers in the possibility of mandatory treatment. He described mandatory testing of newborns as a bad opening to what necessarily will become a complicated relationship between the physician and the family. The test itself is the simplest part of the newborn's HIV diagnosis and treatment.

If the mother declines the test and is overruled by a mandatory policy, the initiation of a good doctor/patient interaction over the long and complex regimen of drugs and monitoring will be difficult. Yet without such a treatment regimen, the test itself is pointless unless the state is prepared to take every child away from parental custody. In addition, he made several legal, financing, and policy observations. He stated that none of the positions of the medical organizations carries the force of law, except for the PHS guidelines, which are required of recipients of certain federal funds under Title II of the Ryan White Comprehensive AIDS Resources Emergency (CARE) Act. He noted that the PHS guidelines, by virtue of establishing a standard of care, also may have legal consequences: physicians, even those in private practice and thus not technically covered by the guidelines, who fail to offer counseling and testing may be subject to malpractice under certain circumstances. He expressed his concern over the inadequacy of counseling, testing, and treatment practices and evaluation in Medicaid managed care plans, whose enrollment is burgeoning. He also expressed concern that discrimination against asymptomatic HIV-infected people may surge if the Supreme Court decides this term that the Americans with Disabilities Act does not extend protections to HIV-infected, yet asymptomatic, individuals until they progress to AIDS. Finally, he observed that support for mandatory testing provides a false sense of accomplishment for policy makers, because it may absolve them of responsibility to address the more complicated issues of financing research, treatment, and other forms of patient care.

STATE LAWS AND POLICIES ON HIV TESTING OF PREGNANT WOMEN AND NEWBORNS

Preliminary results were summarized from a survey of state laws and policies to implement the PHS guidelines or prevent perinatal transmission through other measures. The results, presented by Zita Lazzarini of the Harvard School of Public Health, were available from 43 states and 2 territories, with at least 7 others expected (Gostin et al., in press).

The survey found that most states have moved quickly to implement the PHS guidelines. Eighty-seven percent had policies on counseling and testing of pregnant women, the vast majority of which require voluntary testing with informed consent. Several states have routine testing with the right of refusal. No states require mandatory testing of pregnant women. Several states indicated that approximately 90% to 95% of pregnant women are willing to be tested when testing is offered, but not all pregnant women (50% to 75%) were actually offered testing. Seventy-seven percent of states had policies on treatment, none mandatory, and 44% had policies on testing of newborns. New York is the only state that mandates newborn testing. In general, states responded mostly with policies rather than laws or regulations, and policies were mostly voluntary. In light of state actions, the authors concluded that policy makers should consider ongoing evaluation data from the states before changing existing state efforts.

Response to State Survey

One overarching sentiment expressed by participants was the need to monitor and evaluate states' implementation of their laws, regulations, and policies. State surveillance efforts were seen as crucial in examining the full impact of policies in reducing transmission rates. In addition, monitoring of individual service sites, especially those under Medicaid managed care, was deemed to be important. Given the dynamic financing environment, participants expressed concerns about testing without consent, undertreatment, or denial of treatment to patients in managed care. A Health Care Financing Administration (HCFA) representative observed that implementation of the PHS guidelines to reduce perinatal transmission requires coordination at many levels and between providers and payers. State laws that require providers to offer HIV counseling and testing to pregnant women may be more effective if there are laws or requirements to report on compliance. A state's Medicaid agency can require Medicaid-contracting managed care organizations (MCOs) to report on rates of HIV counseling and testing of pregnant women. Quality assurance measures related not only to counseling and testing, but to actual delivery of all components of treatment to reduce perinatal transmission (antepartum, intrapartum, postpartum), can be developed and tracked. National Committee for Quality Assurance (NCQA), Joint Commission for Accreditation of Healthcare Organizations (JCAHO), and other organizations may be able to help in developing measures. AIDS Education and Training Centers (AETCs) can train providers. These organizations are in a position to offer incentives to encourage counseling, testing, treatment, and record keeping. They also can sanction organizations that fail to do so. Some participants suggested the utility of a program-by-program scorecard of performance, indicating the percentage of pregnant women who are offered counseling and pursue testing, and the percentage who fill ZDV prescriptions (as recorded by the pharmacy) for themselves and their children. One participant commented that the provider infrastructure is in place, but the incentives are not.

Some of the participants were disappointed by states' disproportionate emphasis on counseling and testing, rather than on treating. They saw treatment of the mother as essential for her health, as well as for her ability to care for, and administer treatment to, the newborn. An HIV-infected woman at the workshop criticized the inequity of state and federal policies that seemed to focus so much attention on the mother and seemingly insufficient attention on the father, who, in her case, had infected seven other women besides herself. She expressed her frustration that policies not only failed to protect these women, but also made them feel solely responsible for the plight of their infants.

After the workshop, it was reported that all states have certified, as required by the Ryan White CARE Act Amendments of 1996, that they have appropriate partner notification activities in place for known HIV-infected individuals.

HISTORY AND IMPLEMENTATION OF NEW YORK'S NEWBORN TESTING LEGISLATION

New York has the highest pediatric AIDS caseload in the nation. The State of New York passed legislation in June 1996 mandating that all newborns be tested for HIV. The sponsor of the legislation, Assemblywoman Nettie Mayersohn, described its origins. From 1987 to the mid-1990s, Centers for Disease Control and Prevention (CDC) had established a surveillance system for monitoring the spread of HIV among heterosexual women and infants. This system included anonymous testing of all newborns in New York and other states. Even after CDC terminated the program, New York continued the surveillance system with its own funds until 1997, when the program was converted from monitoring/ surveillance function to a programmative function involving mandatory newborn testing. Prior to the legislation, about 1,500 to 1,800 newborns had tested positive each year, out of approximately 185,000 births. Neither the mother nor the health professionals knew of the mother's infection. According to Ms. Mayersohn, the HIV-positive newborns were being discharged without referral for treatment that could have prolonged or saved their lives. Ms. Mayersohn saw the situation as "criminal to deny the most innocent and the most helpless victims of the epidemic the care to which they are entitled." She successfully advocated for mandatory newborn testing, but she did not support mandatory testing of pregnant women.

Dr. Guthrie Birkhead of the New York AIDS Institute described implementation of the New York legislation. All women in the state are required to be informed in the labor and delivery setting of the imminent HIV testing of the newborn. When the woman's HIV status is unknown, full-fledged pre-test counseling is required. Newborn test results are returned to the hospital by two to three weeks after birth. If the women are identified then, there is sufficient time to begin newborns on *Pneumocystis carinii* pneumonia (PCP) prophylaxis at four to six weeks of age, but insufficient time to advise women against breast-feeding. New York has established a referral network of AIDS centers where newborns and mothers can be treated. Of the more than 185,000 newborns tested over a nine-month period from February 1997 to October 1997, 60 HIV-positive infants were born to mothers who were unaware of their infection. Before the legislation was implemented in 1997, New York State instituted, by regulation, a consented testing program. This earlier program had two components: (1) voluntary notification to mothers of their newborn test results, and (2) mandatory prenatal counseling (with recommended HIV testing) in all state-regulated facilities (e.g., hospitals, clinics, and staff model HMOs, but not in private offices of physicians). While the subsequent mandatory newborn testing legislation superseded the first component of the program, it did not affect the mandatory prenatal counseling component for state-regulated facilities. Since the vast majority of HIV-positive women receive prenatal care in these facilities, many pregnant women still are required to receive counseling about perinatal transmission.

Reaction to the New York Legislation

Reaction to the New York legislation was offered by several designated respondents as well as by workshop participants. Most disagreed with the New York legislation and were skeptical about the effectiveness of mandatory newborn testing in reducing perinatal transmission.

Dr. Amitai Etzioni, a professor at George Washington University, was the only respondent to offer qualified support for mandatory newborn testing (Etzioni, 1998). He framed the question of mandatory versus voluntary newborn testing as one that weighs the potential harm to the mother, in terms of her privacy and autonomy, against the interests of the child. He preferred voluntary testing, performed in the prenatal setting and with consent, to mandatory newborn testing. But he did not feel that voluntary testing alone would completely eliminate the problem of perinatal transmission because a small proportion of women would not agree to be tested. He emphasized that privacy is not an absolute legal right and there are circumstances in which legislation is justified to violate privacy concerns. He viewed mandatory newborn testing as appropriate because the interests of the newborn should take priority; however, at the same time, he argued for policies to improve counseling when test results are released, to increase voluntary prenatal testing, to increase penalties against unauthorized disclosure of test results, and to increase penalties for discrimination against those who test positive. He likened New York's conversion from the anonymous to the mandatory program to a clinical trial that is halted because early signs of success make it unethical to continue the study in a blinded fashion.

Dr. Alan Fleischman, with the New York Academy of Medicine, articulated his fervent opposition to the New York legislation. He disagreed with the premise that mandatory testing prevents HIV transmission for two fundamental reasons: (1) test results are not available in sufficient time for the mother to avoid HIV transmission through breast-feeding, and (2) mandatory testing discourages women from obtaining prenatal care from a health care system they see as punitive.

Dr. Fleischman argued instead that mandatory testing may *increase* the likelihood of HIV transmission. He suggested that the specter of mandatory testing of newborns discourages obstetricians from counseling women in pregnancy, when prevention would be far more effective, because of the assurance that the newborn eventually will be tested. Likewise, pediatricians may also be discouraged from advising women against breast-feeding when the newborn's HIV status is unknown.

Dr. Fleischman also presented results from his national surveys of neonatologists' attitudes towards HIV-infected babies. The surveys revealed neonatologists, the physicians who care for critically ill newborns, to be a somewhat unexpected source of discrimination against HIV-positive newborns. Surveys conducted in 1991 and 1996 probed neonatologists' attitudes about lifesaving procedures for HIV-infected infants through a series of hypothetical vignettes about how they would treat these infants' non-HIV-related conditions, such as surgery for intestinal blockage and correction of a heart defect. Results from the 1991 survey found neonatologists' recommendations for lifesaving procedures to vary with HIV status: neonatologists were less likely to recommend lifesaving procedures for infants who were HIV-infected or whose mothers were HIV-infected (with infants' status unknown) than for infants with no known HIV risk (Levin et al., 1995). Neonatologists in the survey also placed very low value on the quality of life for at-risk or HIV-infected infants, a valuation that was consistent with their willingness to withhold treatment recommendations. The results from the 1996 survey were virtually identical, despite widespread knowledge of progress with ZDV for HIV prevention and treatment. Results did not vary by location or region. Neonatologists held the same attitudes about withholding treatment for HIV-infected or at-risk infants in 1996 as they did in 1991. In the discussion, a number of participants expressed shock of the results and the implications of withholding treatment from HIV-exposed infants who later proved to be HIV-negative. One participant speculated that neonatologists' attitudes might have been colored by their own fear of performing invasive procedures on infants with HIV. The participant recommended revising the survey to include vignettes with non-invasive procedures to test whether fear shaped neonatologists' attitudes.

Theresa McGovern of the HIV Law Project, an organization that provides advocacy and legal services for low-income women in New York City, stated that her organization favors voluntary testing during pregnancy. It joined other organizations in a lawsuit to block implementation of mandatory newborn testing. Their opposition was predicated upon the law's ineffectiveness, flawed implementation, and its premise that women would not be receptive to testing during pregnancy. Ms. McGovern referred to studies showing that women overwhelmingly accept testing. In her experience, women were not being offered the test. She stated, "Frankly, I was angry at the notion of [how] after years of provider failure to recognize and treat this disease in women and children, legislation would be passed as if the women were negligent." She echoed concerns about the receipt of test results being too late to prevent transmission through breast-feeding. She was distressed about the quality of pre-test counseling at the time of delivery, and about women not receiving appropriate care and treatment once they had been identified through the program as HIV-positive.

One of the women whom Ms. McGovern represents, a 25-year-old woman who is also the mother of a six-month-old daughter, relayed her own experiences with the mandatory newborn testing program in New York. Having received no prenatal counseling about HIV, she learned that she and her daughter were HIV-positive two weeks after her daughter's birth and after she had begun breast-feeding. She said, "This diagnosis caused me a great deal of pain and anguish. I considered suicide, I considered killing my baby and myself because I was just so upset that I was HIV-positive, my baby was HIV-positive, what was I going to do with this baby, we both were going to die, who was going to raise her if she wasn't positive and I was the only one positive. . . . My daughter has had two positive PCR (polymerase chain reaction) tests since birth. I am destroyed that I breast-fed and that I continued to expose my daughter to HIV through breast milk. . . . I am deeply disturbed and angry about the lack of information that I was given during my pregnancy. I know that if I had been well informed I would have made choices that were best for myself and my child."

Some participants questioned the cost-effectiveness of the New York legislation and asked how funds might better be spent on improving rates of voluntary testing among pregnant women. Dr. Birkhead noted that the incremental cost of newborn HIV testing is relatively low (about one dollar for each screening test) because HIV is only one of a panel of tests run on newborn blood samples collected for other purposes. The PCR follow-up test is more expensive ($50 to $100 each), but is only performed on about 1,000 out of 185,000 samples. These are the collective costs of identifying approximately 60 infants statewide whose mothers' HIV-positive status was unknown before delivery. Dr. Etzioni argued that programs to educate providers and pregnant women were likely to be more expensive than New York's newborn testing program, but the costs alone should not determine whether the approach is voluntary or mandatory.

Much of the discussion surrounded the importance of voluntary testing of pregnant women, with greater attention to the role of the provider. A number of participants felt that providers' disinclination to counsel and offer testing presented the greatest barrier to pregnant women's getting tested. The question was raised as to how to create the conditions in which providers are encouraged to test and promote testing to every pregnant woman. Participants suggested these elements to be essential: trust between provider and patient; continuity of care and repeated opportunities to discuss testing during pregnancy in the event the patient refuses; financing of counseling; and provider education. One program administrator at the workshop attributed her program's success with voluntary testing to the education and endorsement of the provider, who ". . . has been the fulcrum. The provider has been the motivating force at getting women to test . . . it required a lot of education on our part . . . for an extended period of time to sensitize providers. Once we did that, we have providers who actually signed on, some sooner, others later, but we eventually had them all sign on."

REFERENCES

American Academy of Pediatrics (AAP). Provisional Committee on Pediatric AIDS. Perinatal human immunodeficiency virus test. *Pediatrics* 95:303–307, 1995.

Centers for Disease Control and Prevention (CDC). U.S. Public Health Service recommendations for human immunodeficiency virus counseling and voluntary testing for pregnant women. *MMWR* 44(RR-7), 1995.

Connor EM, Sperling RS, Gelber R, Kiselev P, Scott G, O'Sullivan MJ, VanDyke R, Bey M, Shearer W, Jacobson RL, Jimenez E, O'Neill E, Bazin B, Delfraissy JF, Culnane M, Coombs R, Elkins M, Moye J, Stratton P, Balsley J. Reduction of maternal–infant transmission of human immunodeficiency virus type 1 with zidovudine treatment. Pediatric AIDS Clinical Trials Group Protocol 076 Study Group. *N Engl J Med* 331(18):173–1180, 1994.

Etzioni A. HIV testing of infants: privacy and public health. When does preserving the right to privacy jeopardize the life of an infant? The policy debate heats up. *Health Affairs* 17:170–183, 1998.

Levin BW, Krantz DH Jr., Driscoll JM, Fleischman AR. The treatment of non-HIV-related conditions in newborns at risk for HIV: A survey of neonatologists. *Am J Publ Health* 85(11):1507–1513, 1995.

WORKSHOP AGENDA

Washington, D.C.
February 11, 1998

9:00–9:15 a.m. Welcome and introductions

9:15–11:00 Scientific and clinical perspectives on the efficacy of interventions for pregnant women and newborns and the accuracy of HIV testing

Counseling, testing, diagnosis of HIV infection in pregnant women
Ruth Tuomala

Determinants of vertical transmission and efficacy of preventive strategies, including retrovirals
Lynne Mofenson

Diagnosis, viral and immunopathogenesis, and therapy in the newborn
Catherine Wilfert

11:00–11:15 Break

11:15–1:00 p.m. Institutional positions regarding prenatal/newborn HIV testing and counseling

Public Health Service
Martha Rogers

American Medical Association
John Henning

American College of Obstetrics and Gynecology
  Michael Greene
American Academy of Pediatrics
  Gwendolyn Scott
National Medical Association
  Rani Lewis

Reactions

Pediatric AIDS Foundation
  Tim Westmoreland

1:00–2:00   Lunch

2:00–3:15   State policies/laws regarding prenatal/newborn HIV testing
                   and counseling

                   Presentation of survey results
                     Zita Lazzarini

                   Reactions

                   AIDS Policy Center for Children, Youth and Families
                     David Harvey

                   Health Care Financing Administration
                     Theresa Rubin

                   National Alliance of State and Territorial AIDS Directors
                     Joseph Kelly

3:15–3:30   Break

3:30–5:00   History and implementation of New York's newborn testing law

                   New York State Assembly
                     Nettie Mayersohn

                   New York AIDS Institute
                     Guthrie Birkhead

                   New York Academy of Medicine
                     Alan Fleischman

                   HIV Law Project
                     Theresa McGovern

                   George Washington University
                     Amitai Etzioni

5:00   Adjourn

APPENDIX

D

Workshop II Summary

Amy Fine

On April 1, 1998, the Institute of Medicine (IOM) Committee on Perinatal Transmission of HIV held a public workshop focusing on the impact of the 1995 Public Health Service (PHS) Guidelines for universal counseling and voluntary testing of pregnant women for HIV. The workshop agenda included five panels, covering the following topics: results from the Centers for Disease Control and Prevention (CDC) surveillance and enhanced surveillance systems; results from the Health Resources and Services Administration (HRSA) data systems; provider practices; results from provider and patient surveys and state data systems; and patient perspectives. Findings and discussion are summarized below.

RESULTS FROM CDC SURVEILLANCE AND ENHANCED SURVEILLANCE SYSTEMS

A panel from CDC—including Pascale Wortley, Martha Rogers, Mary Lou Lindegren, and R.J. Simonds—provided an overview of CDC surveillance findings, including presentation and analysis of basic trend data and an analysis of the chain of events needed to achieve prevention success. Most of the data from the presentation are from six CDC studies: (1) The Survey of Childbearing Women (SCBW) is a 1989–1994 population-based survey conducted in 45 states and the District of Columbia. It is based on anonymous newborn heel-stick blood sample. (2) National Pediatrics AIDS Surveillance is conducted in all states and territories and Pediatric HIV Surveillance is conducted in 31 states. Both are population-based surveillance systems. Pediatric HIV surveillance includes information on perinatally exposed infants and monitors their subsequent HIV infection and

AIDS status. (3) The State Enhanced Pediatric HIV Surveillance Program (STEP) is an enhanced pediatric surveillance system that is conducted in four states (New Jersey, South Carolina, Michigan, Louisiana) with adult and pediatric HIV reporting. This system also includes data on HIV-exposed and HIV-infected children. (4) The Pregnancy Risk Assessment Monitoring System (PRAMS) is a population-based surveillance system based on a sample of women with a recent live birth. Information is gathered through a mailed questionnaire with a telephone follow-up. In 1996, 11 states participated. (5) The Perinatal Guidelines Evaluation Project (PGEP) is an in-depth, ongoing four-site project (Connecticut; North Carolina; Brooklyn, New York; and Miami, Florida) using medical chart reviews and interview data of pregnant and postpartum women. The prenatal study population is restricted to women whose health care providers had discussed HIV with them within the previous 60 days. The postpartum study population was a cross section of women delivering in the study's site hospital. (6) Pediatric Spectrum of Disease (PSD) is an eight-site medical record review of HIV-exposed and infected children in care at participating sites since 1989.

HIV/AIDS Trends in Women

The HIV/AIDS epidemic in women is concentrated in the Northeast and in the South, with the highest rates found in New York, New Jersey, Florida, Maryland, Connecticut, and Puerto Rico. States with the greatest number of cases include New York, New Jersey, Florida, California, and Texas. While the highest rates were first observed in the Northeast, during the past five years the greatest increase in rates has been in the South. African-American and Hispanic women are disproportionately affected. Over time, the number of cases among women attributable to injection drug use has declined, while the proportion attributable to heterosexual contacts has increased.

It is estimated that from 6,000 to 7,000 HIV-infected women delivered infants each year from 1989 to 1995. Trend data from the SCBW showed a relatively steady national rate of HIV seroprevalence for childbearing women between 1989 and 1994. There are, however, important regional variations. In the Northeast, where the epidemic started and peaked earliest, there was a 22% decline in the rate of HIV-infected childbearing women giving birth between 1989 and 1994. In the South, where the epidemic started later, there was a 25% increase between 1989 and 1991, which then leveled off. The West and Midwest have had stable and relatively low rates.

HIV/AIDS Trends in Infants and Children

Perinatal transmission accounts for virtually all new HIV infections in children. It is estimated that more than 15,000 HIV-infected children have been born to HIV-infected mothers in the United States. By the end of 1997, more than

7,000 perinatally acquired AIDS cases were recorded nationwide, the vast majority of which were among African-American and Hispanic children. The distribution of perinatally acquired AIDS is highly concentrated, with three-quarters of cases diagnosed in eight states/jurisdictions: New York, Florida, New Jersey, California, Puerto Rico, Texas, Maryland, and Pennsylvania. Many states have very low prevalence: 23 states account for a total of less than 2% of reported perinatal AIDS cases.

The number of pediatric, perinatally acquired AIDS cases rose rapidly in the late 1980s and early 1990s, peaked around 1992, and subsequently declined 43% by 1996. According to the CDC, this dramatic decline, coupled with other recent trend data, point to the conclusion that preventive efforts in this country have been successful in reducing perinatal AIDS transmission.

Trends by age at diagnosis show that the largest declines are among children diagnosed as infants, with substantial declines also among children diagnosed at ages one to five years. However, for older children, similar levels of decline have not been observed. These findings are consistent with the expectation that efforts to prevent perinatal transmission would be reflected earliest in infants because older children were born before ACTG 076 (AIDS Clinical Trials Group protocol number 76).

PCP (*Pneumocystis carinii* pneumonia) is the most common AIDS-defining condition in children, occurring most prominently in infancy. Since recommendations regarding PCP prophylaxis were evolving during the same period that dramatic declines occurred in perinatally acquired pediatric AIDS cases, it is useful to look at whether declines in pediatric AIDS reflect more than declines in PCP. CDC surveillance findings show substantial declines in AIDS among infants—not only in those with PCP as the presenting diagnosis, but also in those with other opportunistic infections. This indicates that the decline in pediatric AIDS cases is not being driven solely by changes in PCP, but rather appears to reflect declining perinatal transmission rates.

In order to estimate the impact of the ACTG 076 results, Byers and colleagues (1998) compared two sets of estimates of children born with HIV infection and children diagnosed with AIDS by year through 1997. The first series is based on extrapolating data through 1994 from the SCBW, and assumes a gradual decline in the number of HIV-infected women giving birth. These "SCBW" estimates, however, assume a constant transmission rate of 21.43%, representing, as a base case, the effect of no progress in preventing transmission. The second series of estimates is based on the number of children reported with AIDS, adjusted for incubation time and reporting delays. This "surveillance" series, therefore, estimates the number of children born with HIV infection or diagnosed with AIDS that could eventually be observed. The surveillance and SCBW estimates are similar through 1990, but taken together indicate a 42% decrease in the number of HIV-infected births in 1995 and a 65% decrease in 1997. In terms of AIDS diagnoses, the estimates suggest a 16% decrease in 1995 and a 29% decrease in 1997. Byers and colleagues feel that these decreases are consistent with, and in large part reflect, widespread implementation of the ACTG 076 regimen.

CDC scientists feel that, collectively, these trend data point to the conclusion that declines in pediatric AIDS, particularly among infants and particularly since 1994, are principally related to declines in perinatal transmission rates with increasing use of maternal and newborn zidovudine (ZDV). While the declines actually precede some of the PHS recommendations, they likely reflect the impact of pregnant women using ZDV for their own health. In addition, since ACTG 076 results were published in February 1994, four months before the PHS recommendations for use of ZDV to reduce perinatal transmission (published in August 1994), some women may have received ZDV in early 1994 based on the clinical trial findings. Also, women were treated for their own health in the 1990s, including as many as 20% of pregnant HIV-infected women. Other factors such as increasing use of therapy among HIV-infected children may also be playing a role by delaying the onset of AIDS; however, it should be noted that the use of combination therapy with potent protease inhibitors was not the standard of care for children during the period of rapid decline.

Chain of Events for Prevention Success

As a framework for understanding the impact of efforts to prevent perinatal HIV transmission, CDC representatives presented its data in terms of a chain of events or steps that must be taken to ensure prevention success. The chain is based on ensuring timely and complete implementation of the ACTG 076 regimen and includes the following steps: (1) receipt of early prenatal care (depends upon access to and utilization of care); (2) provider offering of counseling and testing (depends upon health care provider knowledge, attitudes, beliefs, and practices); (3) client acceptance of testing; (4) HIV-positive client acceptance of ZDV (depends upon provider offering therapy); (5) ZDV adherence (requires taking ZDV during the antepartum, intrapartum, and postpartum periods); and (6) follow-up care for both mother and baby.

Prenatal Care

Compared to the general population, HIV-infected women are much more likely to receive late or no prenatal care. Provisional STEP data indicate that only 63% of HIV-infected women giving birth received prenatal care prior to the third trimester. This compares to 95% to 97% of women in the general population (based on National Center for Health Statistics 1994 natality data and PRAMS data from 11 reporting states). As in the general population, prenatal care use among HIV-infected women varies by race and ethnicity, with African-American and Hispanic women likely to have fewer prenatal visits. The strongest predictor of inadequate prenatal care among HIV-infected women, however, is illicit drug use in pregnancy. Preliminary STEP data indicate that the proportion of HIV-infected pregnant women who receive no prenatal care is 35% for illicit drug users but only 6% for non-drug users.

Testing Offered

Among childbearing women responding to the PRAMS survey in 1996, approximately 75% said their health care worker talked to them about HIV testing during pregnancy (based on the median for the 11 participating states). PGEP data indicate that pregnant women were offered counseling and testing at an even higher rate: overall 88%. The range for the four sites was from 82% to 92% of women reporting that they were offered testing during prenatal care. Multivariable modeling within each site for factors associated with not being offered an HIV test during pregnancy did not find any predictors except in North Carolina where African-American ethnicity and prior testing history were found to be significant. Finally, a preliminary analysis of PRAMS data indicate that certain groups are more likely to be offered testing than others: African Americans and Hispanics (versus whites); young women aged 15 to 19 (versus women over 35); women with less than a high school education (versus more than 12 years of school); women cared for in public care settings (versus private settings); and Medicaid-eligible (versus non-Medicaid-eligible) women.

Testing Accepted

PRAMS data indicate a high test-acceptance rate among childbearing women, with 83% of women offered testing actually receiving the test (median of data from five states). Preliminary data from PGEP provide some information on the reasons women give for not being tested, despite receiving counseling from a health care provider. Overall, women who perceived that the provider gave testing little to no importance were three times as likely to not get tested as women who thought the providers were neutral to supportive of getting a test. Among 1,142 interviewees in public prenatal clinics, the most common response among women who did not get tested focused on timing (i.e., not a good time to be tested or to hear results). In a separate study of 1,134 postpartum women, most of whom delivered in university hospitals, the most common reason given by the 212 women who did not get tested was the woman's assessment that she was not at risk, and the second most common reason given was that the woman had already been tested. Women in the prenatal sample were more likely to have attended a public clinic; women in the postnatal sample were more representative of the general public. Other less common reasons cited in the two surveys were fear of certain components of the test (the needle, blood drawing); fear of discrimination or consequences related to health and life insurance; and belief that the woman's partner did not want her to get tested.

Overall, STEP project findings indicate that in 1996, 79% of HIV-infected women giving birth in four states had been identified as infected by the time of their delivery (numerator based on state surveillance data; denominator based on newborn data from survey of childbearing women).

Acceptance and Receipt of ZDV by HIV-Infected Women

Findings from an enhanced version of the SCBW, which tested blood spots for ZDV, include the following: (1) the prevalence of ZDV use among childbearing women in the eight study states increased substantially between 1994 and 1995, indicating that treatment was widely adopted soon after it was recommended in 1994; (2) on average, in 1995, more than half of all HIV-positive women giving birth in the eight survey states received perinatal treatment with ZDV during labor/delivery or the newborn period (this is a minimum estimate because only ZDV intrapartum or postpartum was measured); (3) if the transmission rate in women receiving ZDV was reduced from 25% to 8% (as in ACTG 076), more than 150 perinatal HIV infections were prevented in these eight states alone in 1995. Population-based pediatric HIV surveillance data from 29 reporting states for 1993 to 1996 shed further light on the extent to which ZDV is being accepted and received among mothers who were diagnosed as HIV-positive before giving birth. These data show that between 1994 and 1996, the proportion of prenatally diagnosed mother–infant pairs receiving some part of the ACTG 076 regimen increased from 36% to 86%. Preliminary STEP project data based on 1995–1996 chart abstractions for approximately 500 HIV-infected women indicate that only 5% of women offered ZDV refused treatment and another 6% discontinued ZDV during pregnancy. Their reasons for discontinuing included non-compliance, toxicity/side effects, and inability to pay. Data from both the PSD study and STEP point to the conclusion that a major reason for not receiving intrapartum ZDV appears to be that the woman's status is unknown at the delivery hospital. A second reason is insufficient time to administer ZDV at the hospital. Finally, with regard to why newborns do not receive ZDV even when their mothers test positive, in preliminary data from the PSD project it appears the most common cause is that providers are not aware of the mother's test result and the second most common cause is parent refusal.

CDC Summary and Recommendations

In summary, CDC representatives highlighted the following points. Since shortly after the PHS recommendations were published, there have been rapid implementation by health care providers and acceptance of therapies by HIV-infected women, as borne out in several different surveillance studies. This, in turn, has affected perinatal AIDS transmission. Overall, approximately two-thirds of pregnant HIV-infected women are on the ACTG 076 regimen. Among those not receiving ZDV, lack of prenatal care is the major cause, with illicit drug use being the greatest contributor to the lack of prenatal care. The next biggest reason for not receiving ZDV is that not all women are being offered testing (women in certain high-risk categories are more likely to be offered). This points to the need for education and training to improve provider knowledge, attitudes, and beliefs. While the relative contribution is smaller, some women do refuse to be tested, and some of their reasons—such as fears about potential discrimination or not perceiving themselves at risk—could be addressed. Once women are identified as HIV-positive, there does not appear to be a major problem with providers offering therapy or with women accepting it. Finally, while there is not much data yet on adherence to the ZDV regimen, this is a major concern, especially since there is a move to more complicated regimens.

The CDC is currently pursuing two systemic interventions that it hopes will improve the success of prevention efforts: (1) providing states with model Medicaid managed care contract language on prenatal HIV counseling and testing and (2) adding prenatal testing as a HEDIS quality assurance measure for managed care entities.

To achieve greater success in preventing perinatal HIV transmission, CDC presenters recommended that efforts be undertaken to (1) improve prenatal care access and utilization, especially for substance-using women; (2) improve provider knowledge, attitudes, and practices, especially in private care and managed care settings; (3) improve client perception of risk and need for testing, and address fears about testing; and (4) develop interventions to improve adherence to medications.

Discussion

Among the issues raised in the participant discussion was the need to test all women, regardless of their apparent risk, particularly given the increasing numbers of women who become infected through heterosexual relations. This, in fact, is what CDC is working toward. One participant noted that even if the woman herself does not engage in risky behavior, her partner might. Another participant noted the need for a greater focus on factors such as drug use, other addictive behaviors, and multiple partners, all of which can affect infection rates.

A participant pointed out the need to go beyond a focus on the individual woman's behavior to address broad policy issues that might affect the ability of women who use drugs to access prenatal care; for example, state laws that call for jailing pregnant drug users or that take the baby away if the mother screens positive for drugs. In response, Dr. Rogers suggested a multitiered approach to perinatal AIDS issues, which would address (1) political/social/legal factors; (2) health delivery system factors; and (3) client behavioral factors. There was a discussion of the need to review policies outside the public health system that could affect the availability of and access to prenatal care—especially for illicit drug users, but for others as well. For example, national welfare reform legislation may have added more barriers to the ability of women to receive care. A concern was raised about the impact of a shift to Medicaid managed care, which moves women out of public sector prenatal care clinics (where counseling and testing are more likely) and into the private sector, where women may be less likely to receive counseling or testing. A multivariate analysis of factors associated with the receipt of counseling and testing would be helpful in projecting the impact of managed care.

Noting that from a public health perspective, testing prior to pregnancy would be ideal, a participant asked about CDC surveillance data and efforts to promote pre-pregnancy testing. Dr. Rogers noted that a very large percentage of CDC's prevention program goes to publicly funded counseling and testing centers, which include family planning, prenatal care, sexually transmitted disease (STD) prevention, and drug treatment clinics. Dr. Wortley noted that for the STEP project, 33% to 40% of the women who delivered were tested prior to pregnancy.

Discussion focused next on the impact of state statutes on overall outcomes. Are laws that require prenatal counseling and offering of HIV testing rigorously enforced? Perhaps a more salient question is whether the statutes establish a standard of care to which a physician can be held (i.e., does the statute permit lawsuits against the physician?). One participant noted that the California law has resulted in more testing, probably because providers think testing is mandatory. Another participant noted that as cases are litigated, state law and PHS guidelines are both used to establish a standard of care, so that passing state laws gets a message to private providers. The same participant further noted that in many of the cases in litigation, the issue is really perception of risk.

Turning to the impact of prenatal ZDV use on infants, another participant asked if there is any information indicating whether HIV-infected infants born to women who took ZDV in pregnancy actually progress to AIDS more slowly. Dr. Simonds noted that there was not yet enough data from observational cohort studies to really address whether prenatal ZDV exposure prevents or has an effect on the natural history of those children who do become HIV-infected. Ongoing, long-term follow-up studies will provide some of these answers.

It was noted that there is confusion in the field regarding how the guidelines apply to treatment for HIV-exposed infants who did not receive ZDV in the prenatal or intrapartum periods. Discussion focused on the guidelines and what is known about the efficacy of newborn treatment that only begins after delivery. Dr. Simonds responded that both the older and the newer guidelines allow—and in a sense encourage—beginning treatment as soon as possible after delivery, but the efficacy of this approach is not yet known.

Discussion focused on confidentiality being a deterrent to treatment. It was noted that in some policy discussions there is a sentiment that this is a non-issue.

Participants noted, however, that there are instances in which confidentiality makes a critical difference; for example, in one case where a woman was murdered by her boyfriend after finding out she was infected with HIV. Dr. Simonds reported that PGEP will have some data on adverse events such as loss of job, loss of relationships, and domestic violence.

HRSA DATA

Michael Kaiser and Karen Hench presented information from the Health Resources and Services Administration (HRSA), including an overview of HRSA-funded AIDS prevention and treatment; essential components of a care system to reduce perinatal HIV transmission; findings from a range of HRSA-funded projects; and a more detailed review of the Women's Initiative for HIV Care and Reduction of Perinatal Transmission project (WIN). HRSA is the service branch of the Department of Health and Human Services (DHHS), that reaches historically underserved populations, including low-income populations, and racial/ethnic minorities. Among the HRSA programs are Maternal and Child Health Services Block Grant Programs, Healthy Start, Community and Migrant Health Centers, Health Care for the Homeless, Rural Health Programs and HIV/AIDS Programs. Among HRSA's HIV/AIDS Programs are the Ryan White Comprehensive AIDS Resources Emergency (CARE) Act Programs (Titles I–IV), Special Projects of National Significance (SPNS), and AIDS Education and Training Centers (AETCs), which provide training on implementation of PHS guidelines.

While HRSA does not have surveillance data, it does have site-specific service delivery findings that complement surveillance findings presented by CDC. Overall, data from HRSA-funded project sites across the country indicate that (1) with adequate counseling, women accept HIV testing, particularly during pregnancy; and (2) significant advances have been made by HRSA-supported programs in reducing perinatal HIV transmission through voluntary, non-regulated HIV counseling, testing, and perinatal ZDV prophylaxis. Examples were given from select HRSA-funded project sites where 93% to 97% of HIV-infected pregnant women accepted ZDV and where perinatal transmission had been reduced so dramatically that at least three of the project sites have reported no cases of perinatal transmission for periods ranging from six months to four years.

Essential Components of the Care System

Similar to the chain of prevention events noted in CDC's presentation, HRSA outlined "essential components" of the care system to reduce perinatal HIV transmission. These include early identification of HIV infection for women of childbearing age, providing HIV counseling and voluntary testing, linking HIV testing sites and primary care, ensuring access to care, offering ZDV prophylaxis, and maintaining women and infants in care.

Acceptance of Counseling and Voluntary Testing

Findings from a range of HRSA-funded project sites indicate there is a high testing acceptance rate among women in prenatal care. A small survey of obstetricians and gynecologists in New Orleans found that more than three-fourths of providers reported at least 90% acceptance of HIV testing. Of all women who received pre-test counseling through SPNS adolescent care projects, 91% accepted testing, and 94% of *pregnant* women accepted testing. At one Cook County site, a 1996 survey indicated that 70% of prenatal and postpartum women were offered HIV testing. Of those offered pre-test counseling, 82% accepted testing, compared to 61% acceptance among those without prior counseling.

Access to HIV Care

Successful models of care funded by HRSA include: one-stop shopping models in St. Louis, Missouri and Miami, Florida; co-location of a birthing center and a comprehensive care center in New York City; and a publicly funded case management program in northern Virginia that allows women to receive care in a private provider setting.

Offering ZDV

All HRSA-supported programs are expected to routinely offer ZDV prophylaxis to pregnant women living with HIV. In one rural Wisconsin project, 100% of women receiving prenatal case management accepted and received ZDV.

Maintaining Women and Infants in Care

Post-delivery care maintenance is essential both for the mother and for the infant. Some successful strategies include home visits by nurses or case managers, family appointments that allow mother and infant to get care at the same time or place, transportation assistance (bus tokens, cab vouchers, rail passes), and the use of peer advocates to help negotiate the care system.

Reaching Providers

Even if universal access to care is achieved, much would still depend on the provider. HRSA has therefore focused considerable resources on provider preparedness, including provider training and technical assistance, and dissemination of provider and consumer educational materials, including step-by-step protocols for each phase of the ZDV regimen and a guide for perinatal HIV counseling and testing.

Focus Group Findings

Various HRSA-supported focus groups have identified barriers to optimal reduction of perinatal HIV transmission. Clients have identified the following barriers to HIV counseling and testing: distrust of providers, concerns about confidentiality of test results, fear of discrimination, fear of losing custody of children, previous negative HIV test, and the perception of not being at risk. With regard to the use of ZDV, client-identified barriers include: concerns about effects of ZDV during pregnancy, mistrust of information from health care providers, judgmental responses from providers when women elect not to take ZDV, fear of providers pressuring women to take ZDV, fear of legal/social consequences of refusing ZDV, and lack of timely availability of ZDV. Systemic barriers identified include: *lack of* transportation, child care, awareness or understanding of resources, and linkages between providers; limited client knowledge; limited provider knowledge; and a sense of helplessness or hopelessness. Finally, barriers identified by providers include: lack of perceived risk among "private" patients, lack of time, lack of reimbursement for counseling time, and lack of knowledge or training.

Women's Initiative for HIV Care and Reduction of Perinatal Transmission

HRSA's WIN, which includes ten sites across the country, was developed in FY 1995 in response to ACTG 076 findings. WIN goals include encouraging women to learn their HIV status as early as possible, linking women with a continuum of ongoing comprehensive care services, and facilitating strategies that reduce perinatal HIV transmission. Very preliminary WIN data from 1997 client interviews and 1996 provider interviews, along with some medical chart reviews, provide some interesting information on a range of topics. All clients interviewed were HIV-positive and pregnant. On the issue of quality and content of HIV counseling, 72% of clients reported that they were aware the test was going to be done prior to being tested; 6% reported feeling forced to take the test; 56% of clients reported that they received post-test counseling, and of these, 53% felt it was non-directive/non-coercive; and nearly 75% felt counseling information was clear. Among WIN clients, the ZDV acceptance rate has been very high: 92% for prenatal use, 95% for intrapartum use, and 94% for the use in neonatal period. About three-fourths of respondents said they had been counseled about not breast-feeding their babies; however, none of the WIN mothers did breast-feed. The five most needed medical and support services identified by WIN participants include: (1) prescription services; (2) help with money, food, and clothing; (3) transportation; (4) housing; and (5) dental care. Of these, the services least likely to be received were housing, dental care, and help with money, food, and clothing.

Summary

Based on descriptive information from a range of HRSA-supported projects and on preliminary qualitative and quantitative data from WIN, HRSA representatives reported the following conclusions and recommendations: (1) with adequate counseling, women accept HIV testing, particularly during pregnancy; (2) there has been significant progress in reducing perinatal HIV transmission through voluntary, non-regulated responses; (3) an ongoing, comprehensive system of care is critical; (4) services must be provided in settings that are accessible, as well as culturally, age, and gender appropriate; (5) different strategies should be employed for different settings and target populations; (6) provider training opportunities related to reducing perinatal HIV transmission should continue to be offered to assist providers in ensuring the availability of quality, appropriate care; (7) providers must involve clients in personal health care decisions and program planning, implementation, and evaluation; and (8) the perceived barriers of providers and consumers need to be identified and addressed to further reduce perinatal HIV transmission.

PROVIDER PRACTICES

The provider panel included representatives from: the American Academy of Family Physicians (Marshall Kubota); the Association of Women's Health, Obstetric and Neonatal Nurses (Maureen Shannon); the American College of Nurse Midwives (Jan Kriebs); the Association of Maternal and Child Health Programs (Deborah Allen); and the American Association of Health Plans (Johanna Daily). Joseph Thompson from the National Committee for Quality Assurance and Timothy Flanigan from The Miriam Hospital also made presentations.

American Academy of Family Physicians

The American Academy of Family Physicians (AAFP) is the medical specialty organization representing more than 84,000 practicing family physicians, family practice residents, and medical students with an interest in family practice. AAFP representative Marshall Kubota highlighted the following points: (1) family physicians and general practitioners are responsible for more outpatient medical visits than any other specialty; (2) a significant proportion of family physicians include obstetrics and pediatrics in their practices (30.5% provide obstetric care and 91.5% pediatric care); and (3) preventive health services are a high priority for AAFP.

Incorporation of Guidelines

AAFP policies regarding HIV disease have closely followed those set forth by PHS. The academy recommends universal HIV counseling and voluntary testing for all pregnant women, and has adopted as policy the section "Guidelines for Counseling and Testing for HIV Antibody" from the CDC statement "Public Health Service Guidelines for Counseling and Antibody Testing to Prevent HIV Infection and AIDS." In addition, the AAFP supports the enactment of state laws providing for (1) reporting to the appropriate public health authorities of all individuals testing positive for HIV, and (2) public health agencies to conduct appropriate confidential contact identification, notification, and counseling. This does not preclude the physician or patient from notifying the contacts. Finally, HIV education is part of state association meetings, and the two AAFP publications also cover HIV issues.

Implementation

Data from the National Ambulatory Medical Care Survey indicate that in 1993, HIV accounted for only 0.12% of all family practice office visit conditions, and that counseling on HIV transmission was included in 0.54% of office visits. While Dr. Kubota noted that these data are somewhat old, he still felt they reflected important trends. Dr. Kubota offered several observations about why family practice physicians may not be offering counseling and testing. First, he said, family practice physicians' standards are high, so if they include HIV testing they would want to do appropriate pre- and post-test counseling; yet the yield—the number of HIV-positive patients—is low. Time pressures are even greater now with the move to a highly penetrated managed care market. Although other tests, such as phenylketonuria (PKU) and galactosemia, also have a low yield, they do not require intensive pre-test counseling. There is also an issue of mixed messages about whom to test: while in the past, the model has been risk-based testing, suddenly in the area of prenatal care, risk stratification does not matter. This is a contradiction. The rapid changes in HIV treatment also add a new complexity to counseling, so that the models of treatment and care are moving much faster than the average family physician can keep up with. Finally, in many towns there is a lack of expert backup help should a patient test positive. All of these factors mediate against family physicians routinely providing testing and counseling for HIV.

Discussion

During the discussion a participant remarked on the importance of recognizing that pretest counseling recommendations may deter providers from testing. In response, Dr. Kubota pointed out that if the goal is to recommend prenatal testing, then putting HIV on a checklist for routine prenatal tests is probably what physicians want and is likely to be most effective.

Association of Women's Health, Obstetric, and Neonatal Nurses

Maureen Shannon spoke based on her clinical expertise working as a nurse midwife at the Bay Area Perinatal AIDS Center (BAPAC) at San Francisco General Hospital and her participation in the development of guidelines addressing the HIV counseling, testing, and clinical care of women. BAPAC offers "state-of-the-art" services to HIV-infected women and infants by combining access to clinical trials with primary, perinatal, pediatric, and social support services. Services are family-centered, offering integrated maternal/infant/child clinical care, a model that works well for maintaining the health of both mother and child. Since May 1995, only one of sixty-two infants born to HIV-infected women receiving ongoing prenatal care through BAPAC has tested positive. This represents a perinatal transmission rate of less than 2%. Ms. Shannon offered the following observations.

Incorporation of PHS guidelines in California

California statute has incorporated PHS guidelines, requiring every prenatal care clinician to counsel women about HIV and to offer voluntary testing. These activities must be documented in the woman's medical record. The state has also developed and widely disseminated comprehensive clinician education and resource materials (including interactive teaching materials for use with patients) and has made a toll-free clinician help line available. Ms. Shannon noted that the resource materials were of very high quality and recommended that they be evaluated for use in other states, as in the California Perinatal HIV Testing Project described below.

Implementation in California

Clinical implementation of the guidelines is very uneven. In one large HMO (health maintenance organization), there is more than 95% testing in prenatal clinics, but it is not clear how informed these clients are about the test and its implications. In another large medical center in the same area, only about half of the women using a well-known physician-based practice receive testing. Yet in the same center, more than 90% of the women seen by nurses, nurse practitioners, or nurse midwives receive testing. The difference has been attributed to a number of factors, including interactive counseling of women by the nurses compared with a more passive approach by the physician group (which uses an information sheet in the prenatal packet given to all new prenatal clients), and the more consistent incorporation of clinical practice guideline recommendations into practice by nurses compared to physicians. Later, during the discussion, Ms. Kriebs observed that another reason is differing roles and responsibilities, with nurses having more time to devote to counseling and patient education in some settings (this may be decreasing in many centers due to the impact of managed care).

Monitoring Compliance and Updating Guidelines

Ms. Shannon observed that it is reasonable to hold providers, practices, and health plans accountable for HIV guidelines and statutes through the Joint Commission on Accreditation of Health Care Organizations (JCAHO) and National Committee for Quality Assurance (NCQA) mechanisms. Tracking HIV testing rates, however, is problematic because: some hospitals prohibit recording HIV testing in patient charts, some clients opt for anonymous testing, and targeting acceptable rates for HEDIS might lead to coercive testing. In her opinion, it would be preferable to track rates of counseling and make efforts to understand variations in testing rates. She also urged professional organizations to regularly update and disseminate clinical guidelines to their membership.

Primary Care Model

Ms. Shannon advocated a primary care prevention model for women, children, and families. From a prevention perspective, HIV counseling and voluntary testing should be offered well in advance of pregnancy and should be incorporated into primary care for all sexually active individuals (female and male) as part of STD risk reduction, screening, and early treatment. Ms. Shannon noted that while a primary care philosophy is endorsed by American Women's Health Organizaton of Neonatal Nurses (AWHONN) and many other professional organizations, very few programs actually offer this kind of approach to clinical services. An example is the sole targeting of pregnant women for HIV counseling and testing, without providing adequate HIV counseling and testing, access to clinical services, and psychosocial support to other family members. In addition to clinical services that focus on reducing perinatal transmission, it is essential that we expand services in order to provide for the health needs of the mother during and after pregnancy in a continuous and comprehensive fashion. Too often, the health needs of the mother are inadequately addressed after she gives birth.

Clinical Care and Clinical Trials

Ms. Shannon made the following points. (1) Pre-conception counseling should be part of the clinical services offered to HIV-infected women. (2) Participation in clinical trials should be offered to all HIV-infected women, since some of the current investigations may further reduce vertical transmission of HIV and improve maternal health status. (3) Counseling of the HIV-infected pregnant woman should be non-directive regarding the continuation or termination of pregnancy and the use of antiretroviral therapy; ultimately, it is the woman's decision. Experience shows that judgmental or coercive counseling leads to alienation from care and mistrust of the health care system, thus delaying the initiation of therapeutic interventions. (4) HIV-infected pregnant women should be counseled and offered antiretroviral and other HIV therapy as determined by their disease status. The PHS guidelines for the use of antiretroviral drugs in HIV-infected pregnant women should be incorporated into the clinical care of these women. Clinicians with limited knowledge regarding these treatment strategies should establish ongoing collaborative relationships with specialists in the management of perinatal HIV. (5) Regionalization of perinatal HIV services should be seriously considered, so that all women have the opportunity to access state-of-the-art clinical care provided by perinatal experts and to enroll in perinatal clinical trials.

California Perinatal HIV Testing Project

Mori Taheripour and Gail Kennedy provided a brief overview of the California Perinatal HIV Testing Project, funded by the California Department of Health, Office of AIDS, and the Health Care Financing Administration (HCFA) Medicaid Office in March 1997. A direct response to the California law mandating HIV counseling and promoting voluntary testing, the program combines the development and dissemination of provider resource materials with implementation assistance to providers, including managed care programs. It has succeeded in part because of buy-in from programs such as the state Maternal and Child Health Program, which has helped disseminate materials. The project is based on the understanding that for providers, a major barrier to offering counseling and testing is the lack of educational resource materials. The project's resource packet includes a flip chart for providers, a brochure that mirrors the flip chart (available in several languages), and testing and counseling guidelines. The project has been realistic about the limited amount of time providers have for counseling by providing a checklist for an abridged counseling session. Materials went out to approximately 7,000 providers in February 1998. Response has been very positive, with more than 300 requests for additional materials and for Spanish language versions. Work is now under way to help HMOs implement the program's guidelines. The program is being evaluated: data from a provider satisfaction survey should be available in June 1998, along with statewide data on the impact of the California law on HIV testing rates.

American College of Nurse Midwives

Jan Kriebs spoke on behalf of the American College of Nurse Midwives (ACNM), which represents approximately 6,500 certified nurse midwives in practice or in school in this country. Nurse midwives practice in every state as well as in the District of Columbia and Puerto Rico. While nurse midwifery is usually thought of as care for low-risk women, two-thirds of U.S. midwives care for women who are at-risk—socioeconomically, demographically, or medically.

Incorporation of PHS Guidelines

The ACNM has incorporated PHS recommendations into its "ACNM Position on HIV/AIDS," which calls for universal counseling and offering of HIV testing, with informed consent. In addition, the statement specifically (1) opposes mandatory testing; (2) calls for non-directive counseling regarding reproductive choices and pregnancy care; (3) advises that all HIV-positive women should be counseled regarding risks of prenatal ZDV and should be offered the medication; and (4) recommends that all HIV-positive women with access to adequate formula supplies should be advised to avoid breast-feeding. The current ACNM statement is likely to be amended to include a discussion of more complex antiretroviral therapies.

Implementation

Nurse midwives have good compliance with counseling programs because they are taught that risk status alone cannot identify all HIV-infected women, which means that every woman needs to hear the basics of counseling. The ACNM also has a program of continuing education for members, which regularly includes topics relating to HIV.

Clinical Experience

Using universal counseling and voluntary testing, two Baltimore area practices with which Ms. Kriebs has been affiliated have achieved a greater than 95% acceptance of testing and 100% acceptance of ZDV use by HIV-positive pregnant women. As a result, transmission has been less than 10% over four years. The success rate has been attributed to a well-coordinated multidisciplinary team effort that provides smooth transitions between counseling, testing, and follow-up care. Within these practices, there is a growing trend for HIV-positive women to plan pregnancy. These women, like other high-risk mothers, want to minimize the risks for themselves and their infants. Ms. Kriebs noted that comprehensive HIV services are resource intensive, an issue that will need to be addressed particularly in an era of managed care.

Ethical Issues

Ms. Kriebs stated that in her opinion, it is not ethical to screen for a chronic, potentially fatal disease in a vacuum, or by imposing a gender bias in responsibility by testing only pregnant women. Rather, providers have a responsibility to empower women to make good decisions for themselves; then, virtually all will accept testing as part of good care for themselves and their children.

Discussion

Discussion focused on the similarities and differences between counseling and testing for HIV versus other diseases. Ms. Kriebs noted that HIV is different from other STDs because it is still life-threatening. HIV counseling should therefore be more extensive than for other STDs and more comparable to that for heart disease, diabetes, or other chronic, fatal diseases.

Association of Maternal and Child Health Programs

Deborah Allen spoke on behalf of the Association of Maternal and Child Health Programs (AMCHP), which represents state maternal and child health programs. Established under Title V of the Social Security Act, these programs are responsible for the health of all women and children in the state, including children with special health care needs. Responsibilities are met through assessment, policy and program development, and assurance of care.

Incorporation of PHS Guidelines

AMCHP has incorporated PHS guidelines into its policy on HIV counseling and testing, which supports early and routine counseling to enable all pregnant women and others of reproductive age to understand the risk of HIV infection and the benefits of early testing, identification, and treatment. In addition, the statement calls for voluntary testing with informed consent as the standard of practice.

Implementation

State MCH programs are engaged in planning and delivery of appropriate HIV/AIDS-related services through activities such as provider training; incorporation of HIV services into Title V clinical services for pregnant women and children; conducting outreach; providing family support services; and linking specialty care to community-based programs. Title V programs work collaboratively with many other state agencies and programs to build an infrastructure that addresses HIV/AIDS prevention and care.

Massachusetts Title V Program Experience

As in many states, the Massachusetts Title V program uses a range of approaches to address HIV/AIDS, including conducting a needs assessment to identify gaps in services, and developing and obtaining Ryan White Title IV funding for a regionalized care system. Under this system, pediatric HIV specialists provide care in community sites once a month in conjunction with local pediatric primary care providers. This allows families to receive high-level services in their own communities, an approach that reflects the Title V mandate and commitment to providing family-centered, community-based care. One of the lessons learned from interviews conducted by the Massachusetts Title V program is that families say their greatest need is for assistance in dealing with HIV/AIDS-related discrimination and stigma.

Barriers

Among the barriers faced by state Title V programs as well as other providers are organizational/agency "turfism"; the tendency to focus on public providers (where there is more direct clout); and not recognizing the power of the "bully pulpit" in persuading private providers of the value of universally offering counseling and testing.

American Association of Health Plans

Johanna Daily, an infectious disease consultant with a New England HMO, spoke based on her experience and that of colleagues working in managed care environments. She made the following points. (1) Strategies to change managed care practices need to take into account the fact that within any given practice, guidelines of the managed care organization with which they contract may vary tremendously. While some of the larger HMOs have enough staff to write HIV protocols and have nurse practitioners to implement them, others do not. (2) The cost-effectiveness issue needs to be addressed. For many HMOs, decisions are made based on whether universal counseling and testing are cost-effective, and for many the impression is they are not. It would be useful to have data comparing the costs of care for an HIV-infected infant with the cost of offering universal counseling and testing. (3) Dr. Daily noted that in her own HMO, the initial prenatal visit is carried out by nurse midwives, who use a checklist approach to testing and uniformly counsel all pregnant women. This approach seems to work well. (4) HMO collaboration with the NIH or other research programs is very important to clinical practice because it allows HMOs to refer HIV-infected pregnant women to specialized care, including antiretroviral therapy, without incurring additional expenses. (5) Among the centers contacted by Dr. Daily, counseling is consistently offered; however, test acceptance varies, depending upon the "pitch." Patients are less likely to accept testing if they feel it means they are identifying themselves as high risk. They are more likely to accept testing if they see the test as a means of helping providers to better manage their care. It may be helpful to provide specific language to be used in counseling. (6) There is a need for additional HIV funding, since good, comprehensive services are expensive.

Discussion

During the discussion, Dr. Kubota pointed out that in his experience, physicians who treat HIV are frozen out of HMO provider panels, since their care is seen as too expensive.

National Committee for Quality Assurance

Joseph Thompson represented the National Committee for Quality Assurance (NCQA), a private, non-profit organization located in Washington, D.C. The mission of NCQA is to maintain and improve the quality of care within the managed care environment by holding managed care organizations (MCOs) accountable and providing purchasers of care with information on quality. This is accomplished through two NCQA activities: on-site accreditation and the use of standardized HEDIS measures to compare plans. Using HEDIS measures, NCQA last year provided information to the public on the care of 37 million commercial enrollees, all Medicare enrollees, and Medicaid enrollees in 35 states.

In his presentation, Dr. Thompson focused on the clinical measures within HEDIS as the area in which there is the greatest opportunity for NCQA to affect the quality of HIV/AIDS care. In general, NCQA evaluations show great variation across plans in the quality of clinical care. While there are HEDIS measures in place to reflect primary prevention of vaccine-preventable disease (immunization) or early detection of breast cancer (mammography), there are gaps in HEDIS with regard to measures for several chronic diseases, including HIV/AIDS.

With funds from the Kaiser Family Foundation, NCQA has started to look at HEDIS measures for HIV/AIDS care. An expert panel has targeted three potential measures: (1) HIV evaluations, either counseling or screening; (2) PCP prophylaxis; and (3) adequate antiretroviral therapy. Dr. Thompson noted that measures for PCP prophylaxis and adequate antiretroviral therapy are problematic because they require identification of people with HIV/AIDS and therefore run into confidentiality issues. In addition, from the HEDIS perspective, there is a sample size issue because of the small number of HIV-infected individuals in any given plan.

From the perspective of perinatal transmission, the HEDIS focus on HIV evaluations is most relevant. Current thinking within NCQA is that in the absence of universal counseling with a universally accepted and documentable counseling event, it may be very difficult to focus on counseling as a measure. It is possible, though, to document testing, since there are clear CPT-4 codes and there are lab data that can be tracked. Dr. Thompson cautioned, however, that HEDIS is a "two-edged sword." If HIV testing is implemented as a HEDIS measure, there will be financial incentives for the plans to increase testing rates, but this might also lead to coercive testing or testing without informed consent. Concerns about this possible impact may be mitigated if an HIV testing measure is implemented only in those states where counseling is legislatively mandated, so that there is a legal imperative for plans to provide and document that pre-test counseling has occurred.

Discussion

Asked to elaborate on the potential for coercive testing, Dr. Thompson noted that if HIV testing is added as a HEDIS measure, plans with higher percentages of tested women will be viewed by purchasers as providing better care. If universal counseling is not required and limited to testing, some plans may focus only on increasing the numbers tested and ignore the importance of informing the woman and obtaining her consent. Dr. Thompson reiterated the importance of legal requirements for counseling as a means of assuring that plans adequately counsel and inform. Ms. Shannon asked whether there has been any consideration of a HEDIS measure focusing on counseling and testing of men, as a primary prevention measure. Dr. Thompson replied that HEDIS screening measures are limited to those with clear scientific evidence linking primary screening to a specific intervention outcome. Since this is not yet the case for populations other than pregnant women, it is unlikely that HIV testing in the general population would become a HEDIS measure.

Rhode Island State Prison System

Timothy Flanigan, an infectious disease specialist who directs an HIV clinical care practice at The Miriam Hospital in Providence, Rhode Island, and also directs HIV care for the Rhode Island State Prison System, spoke about the relationship of HIV to the correctional system. He focused on the importance of reaching incarcerated populations as a means of dramatically reducing perinatal AIDS transmission both in incarcerated populations and in the community at large. Dr. Flanigan made the following points:

1. Incarcerated men and women represent a substantial portion of HIV-infected individuals in this county. Mainly due to the large number of injection

drug users (IDUs), AIDS is 14 times more common in correctional systems than in the U.S. population overall. There are more drug users in correctional facilities than in all drug treatment centers combined. Nearly half of incarcerated women are in for drug-related charges, which accounts for the fact that among those who are incarcerated, the HIV infection rate among women is almost three times that of men. Correctional populations continue to increase. Between 1980 and 1996, the number of women incarcerated increased threefold.

2. Incarceration offers a unique opportunity to reach hard-to-reach populations. Prevalence of HIV among incarcerated women ranges from less than 1% to 25%. Women tend to have short lengths of stay, and frequently move from incarceration to the community and back again. Generally, these women have little access to health care in the community, so incarceration offers a unique opportunity to counsel, test, initiate treatment, and link to community services.

3. The Rhode Island Prison System provides an example of how a correctional based system of HIV care can impact the broader community. Within the Rhode Island system, all incarcerated individuals are routinely tested upon intake. For infected individuals, comprehensive HIV care is available, including antiretroviral agents, viral load testing, gynecological care, substance abuse counseling, and psychological support. In addition, HIV patients are successfully linked to follow-up care in the community: after release, 83% of HIV-infected women link with initial medical follow-up, and 68% make the initial contact with a community-based drug treatment service. The Rhode Island State Prison HIV program has had a tremendous impact on HIV diagnosis in the state overall: over the past five years, 32% of all persons identified by the health department as HIV-infected were tested through the correctional system. More specifically, 28% of women, 39% of women IDUs, and 38% of all persons with heterosexual HIV infection were identified through the correctional system.

Finally, Dr. Flanigan recommended that: (1) HIV testing and diagnosis of incarcerated individuals always be linked to comprehensive HIV care during incarceration and community care after release; (2) HIV-positive persons be integrated within the incarceration setting without segregation, and institutional confidentiality maintained; (3) "turf wars" between the National Institute of Justice, the corrections system, state departments of health, and Ryan White programs be overcome so that Ryan White resources can be used to initiate diagnosis and treatment within the correctional setting (it may be possible to mandate Ryan White programs to work with the incarcerated population); and (4) standards be promulgated for comprehensive HIV care to incarcerated individuals. At the federal level, this could be done by the National Institute of Justice.

RESULTS FROM PROVIDER AND PATIENT SURVEYS AND STATE DATA SYSTEMS

This panel included presentations from Massachusetts, North Carolina, and New Jersey and from the federal Health Care Financing Administration (HCFA).

Massachusetts

Deborah Allen, from the state's Title V program, reported on the Massachusetts experience.

Incorporation and Implementation of PHS Guidelines

The State of Massachusetts has used a variety of interventions to educate providers and promote counseling, testing, and the use of ZDV for HIV-infected pregnant women: (1) soon after ACTG 076 results were published, the state sent a clinical advisory to obstetric, pediatric, and women's health providers; (2) a pocket guide on counseling and testing has been disseminated; (3) provider training has been undertaken statewide; and (4) a media campaign has also been launched. Provider materials are currently being revised to include additional therapies and to promote a model of specialized HIV care for pregnant women (previously, a primary care model was promoted). The Department of Public Health currently provides HIV counseling and testing to 20,000 to 25,000 pregnant women per year.

Trends and Challenges

Data for 1992 to 1995 indicate two related but separate trends in Massachusetts: (1) the number of HIV exposed infants dropped approximately 44%; and (2) the decline in the number of HIV-infected infants was even greater—approximately 75%. These trends reflect more women knowing that they are HIV-positive, accompanied by a move among HIV-infected women to forgo or delay pregnancy; and the use of ZDV in pregnancy. Despite these gains, challenges remain in the state: (1) in 1995, 15 HIV-infected babies were born in Massachusetts; (2) it is estimated that eight of their mothers did not know their status; and (3) there may be an emerging trend of women opting to become pregnant or to continue pregnancies now that therapies are available.

Provider Survey on Counseling and Testing

Ms. Allen reported the following findings from a 1996 survey of obstetric and midwife practices in Massachusetts. (1) On average, these providers reported that in 1995, they offered testing to about 73% of their pregnant patients; they counseled 67%; and they tested about 39%. It is interesting to note that despite the fact that it is not legal to test in Massachusetts without counseling, clearly this is happening in some practices. Also, it is clear that far fewer women are tested than are counseled or offered testing. (2) Having an HIV clinical practice policy in place is the single best predictor of whether a provider counsels, offers, or performs a test. Client characteristics are also predictors of whether women are offered or receive testing in Massachusetts. Specifically, African Americans are more likely to be offered a test; Hispanics are more likely to be tested; and privately insured patients are less likely to be tested. Ms. Allen noted that these findings indicate that providers continue to use a risk assessment model. She observed that providers do not seem to be getting a clear message about what the PHS guidelines say: that is, they think they are following the guidelines when they counsel based on risk. (3) Survey findings indicate that provider attitudes do not seem to make a difference in whether the provider counsels, offers a test, or tests; however, they do make some difference in the likelihood of the practice having a policy in place.

Patient Survey on Counseling and Testing

In a separate but parallel study conducted among HIV-infected women who had experienced pregnancy, women were asked whether they thought testing should be mandatory. Nearly all—24 of 26 interviewees—said yes, "because of the baby." Ms. Allen noted that this finding should be taken as evidence of the strong feelings HIV-infected women have about their babies, not necessarily as the best public policy to pursue. The patient interview also indicated that HIV-infected women want to have a good relationship with their providers and that providers can greatly influence patients' decisions. However, it appears that often providers do not recognize the importance of this relationship. Finally, Ms. Allen noted that having a case manager can influence women's acceptance of testing, particularly women who are not from the dominant culture.

North Carolina

Rachel Royce, an epidemiologist from the School of Public Health, University of North Carolina, presented an overview of efforts in her state to prevent perinatal HIV transmission through prenatal HIV counseling and testing. She presented results of a survey of prenatal care providers and a study of women offered testing during prenatal care.

Incorporation of Guidelines

Immediately after the ACTG 076 results were reported, North Carolina's health officer sent a letter to all prenatal care providers in the state informing them of the results and giving them a list of consortium centers and providers that could take care of HIV-infected women. In August 1995, North Carolina passed a law requiring providers to counsel women as early in pregnancy as possible, and to offer testing.

Study Findings/Implementation of Guidelines

Several recent evaluations indicate that around 70% of pregnant women in North Carolina are tested for HIV during pregnancy. Data from the Pregnancy, Infection and Nutrition (PIN) study—a prospective cohort study, based on a sample of women attending prenatal clinics in North Carolina teaching hospitals and health department clinics—indicate that 89% of women interviewed were offered an HIV test during pregnancy. Based on study findings, the researchers project that had testing been universally offered, the proportion tested would have increased from 68% to 75%. PIN data also show that women's perceptions of provider recommendations clearly influence the decision to accept or reject testing. Women who perceive that their provider thinks it is important to get tested are much more likely than others to accept testing. Reasons women gave for refusing testing include the following: they did not believe they had HIV/AIDS (68%); had been tested recently (24%); or did not want to know results (5%). Very few women gave fear of the consequence of getting a test as a reason. Finally, PIN study findings indicate that women are not naive about testing prior to the index pregnancy. In fact, 67% in the study sample were tested prior to pregnancy.

Findings from a July 1995 provider survey (conducted prior to passage of the North Carolina law) indicate that while providers said they supported universal offering of testing, their practice varied from this ideal. More specifically, while 93% of respondents said they support universal offering of testing, only 82% of practices had a policy of offering testing to all; 67% of providers reported that they offered testing to all women; and only 54% said they would recommend testing to women with no identifiable risk. The 1995 survey also indicated that providers' HIV testing recommendations and practices are influenced by practice setting and patient's insurance status. Private providers and HMOs were least likely to recommend testing; public health providers were most likely, followed by providers at tertiary care centers. Providers were most likely to recommend testing to public/uninsured and self-pay patients and least likely to recommend testing to privately insured patients.

New Jersey

Sindy Paul, medical director of the Division of AIDS Prevention and Control, New Jersey Department of Health, presented an evaluation of implementation in her state. In addition to CDC surveillance data, findings from four other sources were highlighted: the Survey of Childbearing Women (SCBW); the STEP project; a provider survey; and an assessment of pregnant women's knowledge, attitudes, and beliefs regarding the use of ZDV (convenience sample, 170 pregnant women).

Incorporation and Implementation of Guidelines

Since 1995, New Jersey has had a law requiring mandatory counseling and voluntary testing of all pregnant women. The law stipulates three components: HIV counseling, offering testing, and testing. A physician-to-physician peer education program has been implemented in the state. The New Jersey Department of Health and Senior Services (NJDHSS) funded and collaborated with the Academy of Medicine and the State Medical Society on a statewide symposium on the prevention of perinatal HIV transmission in 1997. The NJDHSS also funds and collaborates with the Academy of Medicine of New Jersey on roving symposia of the topic. Finally, a public education campaign has been undertaken, including the use of posters, postcards, videos, and public service announcements. These discuss the benefits of ZDV in preventing perinatal HIV transmission.

Trends/Findings

Prevention of perinatal HIV transmission is a public health priority in New Jersey, since it is the state with the highest proportion of women among its cumulative AIDS case reports (27%), and it has the third highest number of pediatric AIDS case reports in the nation (695 as of May 31, 1998). Virtually all of New Jersey's pediatric AIDS cases (94%) and HIV-infected pediatric cases (98%) are the result of perinatal transmission.

In New Jersey, HIV seroprevalence among pregnant women peaked in 1991 at 0.56% and declined through 1997, when it was 0.27%. Cumulative seroprevalence rates among childbearing women in New Jersey since 1991 are 1.47% for African Americans, 0.48% for Hispanic women, and 0.10% for whites. While the rate is declining among all racial and ethnic groups, the state's African-American women are disproportionately affected, with rates 14.7 times that of their white counterparts and 3 times greater than that of Hispanic women.

Results from New Jersey's Survey of Childbearing Women (SCBW) indicate that the percentage of HIV-infected pregnant women receiving ZDV increased significantly between 1994 and 1995, from 13% to 48%. An analysis of factors associated with ZDV use indicates that women less than 30 years old were more likely than those 30 and older to have used ZDV in pregnancy. It is estimated that ZDV use in New Jersey prevented perinatal HIV transmission to 28 children in 1995.

STEP provides information on the use of ZDV during the three perinatal phases (prenatal, intrapartum, and postnatal/newborn) and also provides follow-up data on outcome. STEP data for the state indicate that between 1993 and 1996, ZDV use during pregnancy increased from 7.6% to 47%; use during delivery increased from 2% to 35%; and use in neonates increased from less than 1% in 1993 to 64% in 1996. Overall, the proportion of women/neonates who received ZDV during pregnancy, delivery, or the neonatal period increased from 8% in 1993 to 67% in 1996.

Since a significant proportion of HIV-infected women still do not receive ZDV in pregnancy, two surveys were undertaken to determine the reasons. A provider survey of eligible physician members of the Academy of Medicine of New Jersey (52% response rate) indicates that 94% of respondents offer HIV testing to all or almost all of their patients, 90% discuss the benefits of testing, and 77% offer counseling. Overall, only 59% offer all three components. Respondents were more likely to offer counseling if they felt: it fit into the office routine; it resulted in better outcomes; it was easy; they were confident in counseling; the patients appreciated it; it was the standard of care; or it had been actively promoted by the medical community. Dr. Paul noted that findings from the provider survey lead to the conclusion that improved diffusion and implementation of HIV counseling and testing among obstetrician–gynecologists could be accomplished through peer education.

A survey of pregnant women also focused on factors associated with ZDV use. Among a convenience sample of largely young, African-American and Hispanic pregnant women, 57% said they would use ZDV, 41% were unsure, and only 2% indicated they would not use ZDV. Among the factors associated with intention to use ZDV to prevent HIV transmission are positive beliefs about ZDV; recommendation by a doctor or nurse; access to ZDV through the clinic or doctor; and sufficient information to make an informed decision. Evaluators found that conspiracy theories about ZDV were not associated with respondents' reported intention to take ZDV. Based on these findings, Dr. Paul and her colleagues concluded that pregnant women are willing to consider ZDV use if they are given adequate, accurate information.

Dr. Paul summarized as follows: (1) there has been a marked improvement in efforts to prevent perinatal HIV transmission in New Jersey; (2) physicians do offer counseling and testing; (3) pregnant women are willing to use ZDV; (4) surveillance and seroepidemiology studies have documented ZDV use; and (5) mandatory counseling and voluntary testing appear to be working in New Jersey.

Health Care Financing Administration

Theresa Rubin, a regional AIDS coordinator for the Health Care Financing Administration (HCFA) presented information on implementation and evaluation efforts undertaken by the agency.

Incorporation and Implementation of PHS Guidelines

Below are examples of HCFA efforts to incorporate and implement PHS guidelines:

• In March 1994, less than a month after ACTG 076 results were published, HCFA sent a letter to its regional AIDS coordinators informing them of the study results and recommending improved outreach to pregnant women so that they can be evaluated and offered ZDV as early in the pregnancy as possible.

• In a July 1994 "Medicaid Letter," HCFA conveyed its policy of providing an enhanced federal match of 90% for HIV testing and counseling claimed as a family planning service.

• In March 1998, HCFA sent a notice to state Medicaid agencies and welfare offices informing these agencies about Ryan White CARE Act provisions relating to counseling and testing of pregnant women for HIV/AIDS. The notice urged Medicaid agencies to work closely with Ryan White grantees to assure optimal counseling and testing.

• In May 1996, HCFA conducted a survey of regional AIDS coordinators that looked at: state laws addressing HIV counseling and testing of pregnant women; access to HIV testing, counseling and treatment in the state; the nature of HIV provisions in Medicaid managed care contracts; and state Medicaid agency collaboration with other state agencies, providers, and consumers in implementing PHS guidelines. One of the goals of this survey was to help raise awareness of the role of state Medicaid agencies in promoting the PHS guidelines and the need to work with others in the state toward this end.

• Finally, HCFA also has undertaken a consumer information program (CIP), which started with a four-state pilot in January 1996. In its CIP, HCFA has focused on (1) developing informational materials to alert Medicaid-eligible HIV-infected women, pregnant women, and women of childbearing age to the benefits and implications of ZDV therapy; (2) assisting women in making an informed decision about ZDV therapy and (3) informing women that they may be eligible for Medicaid, which covers this treatment. As part of the campaign, HCFA has developed and disseminated consumer information materials in several languages, including posters, videos, and brochures. A preliminary evaluation of the campaign has been undertaken in the pilot states and results are being analyzed.

PATIENT PERSPECTIVES

Laquitta Bowers and Kay Armstrong provided preliminary findings from focus groups they are conducting as part of the AIDS Policy Center for Children, Youth and Families (APCCYF) study on HIV testing of pregnant women and newborns. Joseph Kelly provided an update on a review of state efforts. Rebecca Denison provided her perspective as an HIV-positive woman.

AIDS Policy Center for Children, Youth and Families

Ms. Armstrong briefly reviewed the methodology used in APCCYF focus groups. Efforts were made to get geographic diversity, with representation from areas with high and moderately high incidence rates. Seven of the eight groups include women only; the other group includes men. Participants are of reproductive age and are sexually active. HIV-positive women, Hispanic women and those at high risk for drug and alcohol use are included and targeted for some of the groups. Ms. Armstrong highlighted the following preliminary findings, based on completion of five of the eight focus groups.

• When asked about availability and accessibility of HIV counseling and testing, most participants felt that knowing their HIV status could help them improve their own health and that of their child and partner. There appear to be some gender differences in this response, which will be further explored.

• There appears to be a complex set of factors that influence women's receipt of prenatal care, including current drug and alcohol use and past experience with health care providers. Participants are very concerned about their own health and that of their babies.

• The way in which HIV testing is conducted is very important. Participants told "horror stories" about receiving HIV-positive results over the phone or not being informed in advance that they were being tested. Only a few found out they were infected with HIV during pregnancy. Others discovered their HIV status while seeking other medical care. Participants emphasized the emotional impact of such negative experiences.

• Among participants there is a great fear of HIV disclosure. They do not want to be labeled as HIV-infected. There is stigma and distrust as to how information might be used. Most participants did not trust the government in issues associated with HIV testing. Gender and partner issues were often discussed, with women participants worried about partner and family rejection, as well as partner violence.

State Activities Update

Joseph Kelly reported that in March 1998, as part of the APCCYF study, NASTAD sent a questionnaire to state health departments to update information on four areas of interest: (1) developments in new state legislative policy, regulation, and practice standards; (2) availability of trend/surveillance data on perinatal HIV transmission; (3) availability of follow-up evaluations/surveys on provider practices, HIV counseling and testing acceptance, and implementation of PHS guidelines; and (4) state contacts for further information.

Mr. Kelly also briefly highlighted new information on state legislation, noting that as of April 1, 1998, there was legislation pending in Delaware, Alabama,

South Carolina, and New York that could change existing statutes on the issue of prenatal or newborn testing and counseling. In Indiana, legislation passed in late February that explicitly allows physicians to order confidential HIV testing of newborns if the mother has not been tested and refuses the test and if the physician believes that the test is medically necessary for the newborn. The state health department has been instructed to issue implementation guidance. One consequence of the legislative debate on this topic is a new awareness in Indiana that physicians are not providing HIV counseling to all pregnant women and are not offering tests. As a result, the health department is now pursuing an emergency rule that would try to ensure or compel physicians to counsel pregnant women. Mr. Kelly said it is likely that other states will try to implement similar newborn screening legislation.

Discussion

During discussion, it was noted that Louisiana may have a similar stipulation that allows physicians to test infants or children if they believe it is medically necessary. One participant noted that in New York, before newborn screening became mandatory, physicians testified that they did not need this kind of law because they had the legal right to test in any case.

Rebecca Denison, Respondent

Ms. Denison spoke from her perspective as an HIV-positive woman. She chose to become pregnant and is now the mother of two-year-old twins who are HIV-negative. Ms. Denison directs Women Organized to Respond to Life-threatening Diseases (WORLD), an organization started by and for HIV-positive women. In this capacity, she has worked closely with and assisted many HIV-positive women.

Ms. Denison started by noting that it is remarkable and heartening to hear meeting participants take seriously the notion of providing medical care to HIV-positive women who want to become pregnant or continue pregnancy. She observed that this is a moving tribute to those who have been willing to look beyond the conventional wisdom and understand what is in the hearts of people who want to become parents. She also reminded participants that beyond all the statistics, there are a lot of emotional issues tied into HIV/AIDS that will never be captured in numbers, but that profoundly affect people's lives.

Ms. Denison followed with a series of observations on a number of issues:

• Expanding therapy options: Ms. Denison noted that it is important to recognize that in practices such as BAPAC in San Francisco, treatment options go well beyond the ACTG 076 protocols. For example, in the past two years, BAPAC has provided clinical care that incorporates the clinical evaluation of pregnant women for evidence of disease progression with the offering of appropriate combination therapy. In addition, as a pediatric ACTG site, BAPAC has been able to offer pregnant women and their infants access to perinatal/neonatal research trials that improve maternal health and further reduce perinatal transmission rates.

- Mandatory versus universal testing: It is important to define terms. It is Ms. Denison's impression that most women will accept testing and most prefer being asked rather than being forced. She believes testing should still remain voluntary, even though this is an imperfect approach.

- Standards of care needed: For many basic obstetric procedures, there is no standard of care established for HIV-infected women; for example, there are no standard recommendations or cost-benefit analyses on cesarean sections, amniocentesis, and fetal scalp monitoring for the HIV-positive mother.

- Testing does not equal care: Ms. Denison cited several examples of known HIV-positive women receiving unacceptable care from poorly informed physicians.

- ZDV issues: There are many issues around the use of ZDV, including women's fear of long-term side effects. Ms. Denison noted that of all the women she has talked to, none was told about the National Cancer Institute study findings on potential long-term risks to the children whose mothers took ZDV prenatally. She stressed that women need to be told about the study and then be told that the potential benefit outweighs the risk. It is also important to acknowledge that some infants are still becoming infected even though their mothers took ZDV during pregnancy.

- Violence: Issues around domestic violence need to be taken seriously. Disclosure can lead to a life-or-death situation for some women with violent partners.

- Prevention gaps/men's role: There are serious gaps in prevention, particularly with regard to the male role. Current efforts put the burden for prevention on the woman, which is unfair. There is also a need for support groups for heterosexual men who are HIV-positive or who have HIV-positive partners.

- WIC: The WIC program can be a source of infant formula for some HIV-infected mothers; however, it does not pay the full cost of formula. A more significant problem is that WIC programs "push" breast-feeding, but do not adequately screen for or counsel regarding the HIV status of the mother. Ms. Denison noted that this approach is frightening and needs to be addressed.

- Welfare reform and immigrants: With welfare reform, undocumented immigrants are cut off from publicly assisted prenatal care. Ms. Denison cited an example from California of an HIV-positive pregnant immigrant who was afraid that accessing care would lead to deportation.

- Trust is essential: Ms. Denison stressed the importance of trust in the provider-patient relationship. Providers can be extremely judgmental in their attitudes toward HIV-positive women. Women need to feel comfortable going to their providers when they have problems with complex therapies for themselves or their babies. They need to be supported in the difficult process of caring for themselves and their children.

• Funding: Finally, noting the importance of access to high quality, specialty care, Ms. Denison stressed the need for sustained and increased funding for comprehensive perinatal HIV/AIDS services such as those provided by BAPAC in San Francisco.

REFERENCE

Byers Jr. RH, Caldwell MB, Davis S, Gwinn M, Lindegren ML. Projection of AIDS and HIV incidence among children born infected with HIV. *Stat Med* 17:169–181, 1998.

WORKSHOP II AGENDA

Washington, D.C.
April 1, 1998

8:30–8:45 a.m.   Welcome and introductions

8:45–10:15   Impact of the Public Health Service voluntary testing
                     recommendations: Results from CDC's surveillance and
                     enhanced surveillance systems
                         Pascale Wortley
                         Martha Rogers
                         Mary Lou Lindegren
                         R.J. Simonds

10:15–10:30   Break

10:30–11:30   Results from CDC's surveillance and enhanced
                     surveilance systems, (*continued*)

11:30–12:30 p.m.   Impact of the Public Health Service voluntary testing
                     recommendations: Results from HRSA data systems
                         Michael Kaiser
                         Karen Hench
                         Moses Pounds
                         Lori DeLorenzo
                         Amelia Birney

12:30–1:30	Lunch

1:30–3:00   Provider practices
American Academy of Family Practitioners, *Marshall
  Kubota*
Association of Women's Health Obstetric, and Neonatal
  Nurses, *Maureen Shannon*
American College of Nurse Midwives, *Jan Kriebs*
Association of Maternal and Child Health Programs,
  Deborah Allen
American Association of Health Plans, *Johanna Daily*
National Committee for Quality Assurance, *Joseph
  Thompson*
The Miriam Hospital [prison health], *Timothy Flanigan*
California, *Mori Taheripour*
California, *Gail Kennedy*

3:00–3:15   Break

3:15–4:30   Impact of the PHS voluntary testing recommendations:
Results from provider and patient surveys and state data
systems
    Massachusetts, *Deborah Allen*
    North Carolina, *Rachel Royce*
    New Jersey, *Sindy Paul*
    Health Care Financing Administration, *Theresa Rubin*

4:30–5:30   Patient perspectives: AIDS Policy Center for Children,
Youth and Families focus groups
    APCCYF, *Laquitta Bowers*
    APCCYF, *Kay Armstrong*
    NASTAD, *Joseph Kelly*

                   Respondent:
                   WORLD, *Rebecca Denison*

5:30   Adjourn

APPENDIX

E

New York/New Jersey Site Visit Summary

Miriam Davis

INTRODUCTION

The Institute of Medicine (IOM) Committee on Perinatal Transmission of HIV visited five HIV prevention programs in the New York metropolitan area to obtain a firsthand account of the implementation of the Public Health Service (PHS) guidelines. The New York metropolitan area accounts for 38% of all perinatal AIDS cases in the United States (see Chapter 3). The programs were selected to illustrate a variety of approaches to prevention of perinatal HIV transmission. As publicly supported health care providers in urban settings, their pregnant patients were predominantly low-income women of African-American or Hispanic origin. Many were immigrants with poor command of the English language.

The programs that were visited reported dramatic success at preventing perinatal transmission of HIV. This summary highlights what program administrators judged to be the elements of their success, as well as the barriers they encountered. These publicly supported programs were required either by law (New Jersey) or by regulation (New York) to counsel all pregnant women.* This summary also delves into the more intractable problems posed by special populations, such as adolescents and immigrants. Finally, it presents experiences with implementation of the mandatory newborn testing legislation in New York State.

---

*New York State requires its state-regulated facilities, such as hospitals, clinics, and HMOs, but not its private practices, to counsel pregnant women about HIV and perinatal transmission. New Jersey requires all pregnant women to be counseled regardless of where their treatment is rendered.

SUCCESSES WITH IMPLEMENTATION OF
PUBLIC HEALTH SERVICE GUIDELINES

The programs attributed their success to the following elements: infrastructure and research funding; counseling emphasis on newborn and maternal health; health care financing; and routine incorporation of counseling into care. These elements are discussed further below.

Infrastructure and Research Funding

Programs repeatedly ascribed their success to the vigorous efforts of specially trained counseling staff (i.e., nurses, counselors, and social workers). These were the professionals responsible for the bulk of HIV counseling to encourage patients to accept testing and treatment. Counselors' work was often time-consuming because they were trained to approach patients, repeatedly if necessary, and not be deterred by the patient's initial refusal of an HIV test. It was not uncommon for some patients to delay for months the decision to accept testing or treatment (see patient profiles). The duration of a typical counseling session was reported to vary greatly, but consumed up to one hour for some high-risk women. A number of programs reported that the effectiveness of their efforts—in terms of patients' acceptance of testing and treatment—depended greatly upon the experience, training, and motivation of individual counselors.

To be effective, prenatal counseling generally includes outreach, because the women who are hardest to reach are considered to be at highest risk for HIV. An illustration of how labor-intensive outreach and counseling can be was provided by the Francois Xavier Bagnoud Center at the University of Medicine and Dentistry of New Jersey. When a pregnant patient misses an appointment, the center's policy is to mount an elaborate outreach effort. First, staff call the patient, then send a letter, followed by a registered letter. If there is still no reply, they send an outreach worker to the patient's home who is instructed to wait until the patient comes home. Their last option is to track the mother through the child, if the child receives medical care at their center, or to pursue the mother through her insurer. A program administrator summed up the program as "going through extraordinary lengths to get these women in."

Obtaining funds to hire counseling staff was a dominant concern of many programs. Federal research funds were deemed to be essential. Since programs had many of their patients actively enrolled in ongoing research, they were able to use counselors hired with funding for research, patient recruitment, and related purposes. At one program, for example, two of the four HIV counselors were hired with research funds. In light of the pivotal role played by counselors and other staff, program administrators were continually concerned that cutbacks in research or program funds would force them to scale back on their staff. One administrator remarked, "We have created a house of cards . . . as we lose research components, we are not prepared financially. If we don't have research, we don't have resources."

Counseling Emphasis on Newborn and Maternal Health

Counselors reported finding pregnant women to be generally receptive to HIV testing, even more receptive than women who are not pregnant. In their experience, the most persuasive arguments for patient acceptance of testing and treatment emphasized health benefits, first to the newborn and then to the mother. One counselor said, "We tell them [the pregnant women] that it's right for their baby, and what's best for the baby is also best for you." The experience of the counselors was confirmed by the patients who were interviewed. Virtually all patients described their newborn's health, before their own, as their overarching reason for proceeding with testing and treatment (see patient profiles). They described their experience as mothers as the best time of their lives. A number of them chose to proceed with subsequent pregnancies despite being HIV-positive.

Financing of Health Care

Most programs reported state and federal programs to be indispensable to financing health care. For low-income pregnant women, Medicaid was the premier program that paid for medications and medical care. Medicaid financed laboratory tests, antiretroviral therapy and other medications, primary care, and hospitalizations, including labor and delivery. Medicaid is relatively easy for pregnant women to obtain, if they meet federal and state eligibility requirements. Most programs helped their patients to fill out applications. Low-income women who are awaiting Medicaid approval or who do not qualify for Medicaid are eligible for supplementary coverage through a program called ADAP (AIDS Drug Assistance Program) that receives funds under the federal Ryan White Comprehensive AIDS Resources Emergency (CARE) Act. This program covers, free of charge, HIV-positive patients' medications, primary care, and home care.

Routine Incorporation of Counseling into Care

Programs regarded another ingredient of their success to be the incorporation of counseling, testing, and treatment procedures into routine clinical practice. Well-established clinic policies and management support were seen as key. Programs understood that counseling, while labor- and time-intensive, was pivotal to patient acceptance of testing and treatment. Some programs also had policies for repeat testing to ensure that patients did not seroconvert later in pregnancy. One program reported testing patients every three to four months if the patient was seen early in the prenatal period.

BARRIERS TO IMPLEMENTATION OF PHS GUIDELINES

The programs encountered the following barriers to implementation of the PHS guidelines: lack of prenatal care; lack of perceived risk; lack of rapid HIV test; family ostracism and domestic violence; some resistance to antiretroviral therapy; and resistance to HIV counseling by private physicians. These topics are discussed further below.

Lack of Prenatal Care

The lack of prenatal care was seen as one of the greatest barriers to the prevention of perinatal transmission of HIV. Without prenatal care, there simply is no opportunity to counsel, test, and treat women prior to labor and delivery. For instance, there were four HIV-positive newborns born at Bellevue Hospital Center in 1997, to mothers whose HIV status had not been known until the baby was identified. Three of the four were born to mothers who had not received prenatal care. The fourth was born to a mother who had declined to be tested prenatally. These four infants were part of a cohort of 20 HIV-positive newborns born that year, 16 of whom were born to mothers whose infection was detected during pregnancy.

Programs estimated that about 10% to 15% of women giving birth did not receive prenatal care. Lack of access was not considered to be a major factor, because New York and New Jersey heavily subsidize prenatal care and outreach activities. One administrator described his program's outreach efforts as an "ongoing battle" to bring women into care. Most programs deemed injection drug use as the overriding explanation for women not accessing prenatal care. Injection drug users (IDUs) are considered to be the most difficult to reach group of pregnant women. They are thought to avoid prenatal care out of a mixture of apathy, shame over their drug use, and fear that their children may be removed from their custody. The lack of prenatal care is one of the key factors fueling the demand for a rapid HIV test for use in the labor and delivery setting. Bellevue Hospital Center, for example, has proposed a rapid testing program, with results available within hours (see below). The availability of a rapid test paves the way for intrapartum administration of zidovudine (ZDV) and continued treatment of the mother and infant.

Lack of Perceived Risk

Women who do not perceive themselves to be at risk are believed to account for a large share of those who refuse HIV testing during pregnancy. For instance, at New York's Bellevue Hospital Center, where prenatal HIV counseling is mandatory under the state's health regulations, about 20% of pregnant women refuse HIV testing.

The single greatest reason appears to be the lack of perceived risk. Many of the women are undocumented immigrants in what they perceive to be monogamous relationships. They view HIV as affecting only prostitutes and homosexuals, not themselves. Other women who do not view themselves at risk may be in denial about their own risky behavior.

Lack of Rapid HIV Test

An accurate, rapid test, with results available in hours, is considered to be an important HIV prevention tool. While a Food and Drug Administration (FDA) approved rapid test is commercially available, its rate of false positives is regarded as too high for widespread use. Conventional HIV testing, using enzyme-linked immunosorbent assays (ELISA) and confirmatory testing takes about one to two weeks for results. This is a crucial gap for adolescents and other groups of patients who commonly do not return to receive test results in the prenatal setting. It is seen as an even more crucial gap in the labor and delivery setting, which offers the last opportunity to interrupt HIV transmission via administration of intrapartum antiretroviral therapy and advice to avoid breast-feeding.

Bellevue Hospital Center has applied for permission to launch a voluntary, rapid testing demonstration program for all women in labor and delivery who previously have *not* been tested for HIV. Since women who do not agree to prenatal testing, or who did not obtain prenatal care, are considered to be an "enriched" population with high HIV prevalence, the commercially available rapid test is less likely to be beset by false positives. When the rapid test is positive, antiretroviral therapy is to be offered beginning immediately in the intrapartum period, even though the rapid test must be confirmed by more definitive tests. If such tests later find the mother not to be infected, the protocol permits the interruption of therapy to mother and infant. Program administrators acknowledged that the labor and delivery setting is not an ideal time to obtain informed consent and hoped to counsel patients in as sensitive and thoughtful a manner as possible under the circumstances.

Family Ostracism and Domestic Violence

Many pregnant women fear taking an HIV test for the devastating impact of disclosure of positive results on their sexual partner or families. Many are single women often living at home with a parent(s). One HIV-positive mother admitted that if her family learned of her HIV status, she would be evicted (see patient profile). She would lose more than just shelter, since families often provide emotional, economic, and baby sitting support. Programs also spoke of patients' fears of domestic violence committed by sexual partners. Males who are ignorant of their own HIV status or are unwilling to be tested may blame the woman for having sex with someone else, however true or untrue, and may be prone to violence from jealousy. Alternatively, if males are HIV-positive, they may become violent toward the woman they blame for infecting them—again, whether or not this is true. For women who are striving to conceal their HIV status, the fear of family desertion or domestic violence affects far more than their decision to be tested. It extends through the treatment period and affects their ability to comply with a demanding medication regimen, as discussed below.

Resistance to Antiretroviral Therapy

While programs described pregnant patients' overwhelming acceptance of antiretroviral therapy, this was not universally true. Some patients needed persistent encouragement by motivated counseling staff. These patients were often in such shock or denial after the diagnosis that it sometimes took them months to confront the need for and accept the medication. This was especially true of adolescents (see later section).

Among the reasons given for patients' reluctance to accept, or comply with, antiretroviral therapy were concerns that it was a "poison" and might have long-term effects on the child; the side effects; the demanding regimen of administration, especially for babies; and fear of disclosing their HIV status to family members by virtue of the frequent administration of medications for themselves or their newborn. Patients sometimes resorted to removing prescription labels. One patient, a former injection drug user, admitted to the IOM visitors her fears that the medication was addictive and actually caused AIDS, although she realized in retrospect that her fears were unjustified (see patient profiles).

Managed Care

The advent of managed care, in both public and private health insurance programs, was considered to be detrimental to the prevention of perinatal transmission of HIV. While program administrators acknowledged that managed care is receptive to prevention in general, the reality was more ominous because of competing priorities. Their major concern was with managed care's emphasis on shorter hospital stays. The labor and delivery process has become so compressed that program administrators complained of the difficulty of finding the appropriate time to counsel and test women who never received prenatal care. Even if the program had succeeded in motivating the mother to be tested, test results would not be back in sufficient time before patient discharge. Outreach efforts seemed futile because in many cases, patients were not reachable, having provided a false address.

Another problem is encountered in the prenatal setting, where there are strong pressures to increase patient load by reducing the time spent with each patient. This is seen as leaving insufficient time or financial incentives for HIV counseling by physicians who receive flat fees per patient or are on salary. Many program administrators expressed concerns that if managed care organizations established HIV counseling requirements, counseling would be done too hastily, or testing might be performed without consent.

Resistance to HIV Counseling by Private Physicians

Through their active outreach efforts and professional contacts, many of the programs were able to shed light on why HIV counseling does not seem to be occurring in private obstetrical practices. Program administrators confirmed the widespread failure on the part of private physicians to offer HIV counseling, even in New Jersey where counseling is mandatory for all patients. The most common explanation was that counseling is seen as too burdensome, particularly when most of their patients are not at risk. One program administrator relayed the experiences of a colleague in private practice who had counseled and tested about 600 pregnant patients without finding one to be HIV-positive. In the judgment of private physicians, HIV counseling consumes too much time in relation to the rarity of infection. While other administrators acknowledged pre-test counseling to be unnecessarily onerous, they thought it presented an important opportunity to educate the patient more generally about HIV rather than perinatal transmission per se.

Physician discomfort was deemed to be another important factor deterring counseling in private offices. Not only did physicians seem to be uncomfortable discussing sexual practices with patients, but they also were uncomfortable with the possibility of implying—however erroneously—to a patient that she might be at risk. One administrator put it starkly, "Doctors don't want to offend private patients. In a competitive health care environment, they're afraid of losing them." Another administrator, however, observed that patients' reactions depend upon the manner in which testing is offered. He noted that patients would not be offended when the testing message is presented as a policy that applies uniformly to all patients. The singling out of at-risk patients was what offended patients, according to this view.

Other reasons offered for private physicians' disinclination to counsel pregnant patients and encourage HIV testing were lack of financial incentives for counseling; lack of physician knowledge about complex HIV therapies and side effects; lack of referral networks; discomfort with counseling in general; and ignorance of the details of their state's counseling, testing, or consent laws and regulations.

SPECIAL POPULATIONS

This section examines the additional problems in preventing perinatal HIV transmission in adolescents and immigrants. Two of the programs visited by the IOM specialized in counseling and/or caring for these special populations. Other special populations, touched upon throughout this summary, are the homeless and IDUs.

Adolescents

Adolescents are a critical, yet underrecognized, population for the prevention of perinatal HIV transmission. Although the nationwide seroprevalence of HIV infection among adolescents appears to be relatively low, urban areas are disproportionately affected: New York, for example, is estimated to have 20% of the nation's adolescents with AIDS. An estimated 25% of HIV-infected adults nationwide acquired their infection as adolescents (Rosenberg et al., 1994). Adolescents infected with HIV pose unique problems in identification, consent to testing, and entry into care. Traditional HIV "risk assessment" by health care providers misses a significant percentage of cases. There is also a lack of ready access to systems of care by the most disenfranchised adolescents who are most vulnerable to HIV. Consequently, many teenagers are unaware of their HIV infection, having neither been recommended for, nor received, testing. And an HIV-positive test does not ensure access to care. All of these problems may be compounded in pregnancy because of the added social stigma against adolescent pregnancy.

A comprehensive treatment program for adolescents in the Bronx visited by the IOM, the Adolescent AIDS Program of Montefiore Medical Center, has been successful at reducing perinatal transmission of HIV in adolescents. At any given time about one-third of the adolescents in this referral program are pregnant, and virtually all accept antiretroviral therapy. Of 12 babies born to HIV-positive adolescents in 1997, 11 were HIV-negative. The one baby who did test positive was born to a mother in the late stages of AIDS who was non-compliant with the ZDV treatment. The program attributes its success to these features: labor-intensive outreach to adolescents and health care professionals to encourage testing with linkage to treatment; lack of financial barriers to testing and treatment through sliding fee scales and help with obtaining Medicaid and other public financing programs; accessibility through subsidized transportation to the program; a "one stop shopping" approach enabling teenagers to receive counseling, testing, treatment, and medications for HIV at the same site—both during and after pregnancy (although obstetrical services are available through referral); and understanding the special needs and fears of adolescents.

Among the barriers to HIV testing of pregnant adolescents are physicians' discomfort with discussing sexuality; physicians' lack of awareness that consent to testing (in New York and many other states) can be given solely by the adolescent and need not require the parent; and adolescents' fears of being reported, despite assurances of confidentiality. Among the barriers to acceptance of, and compliance with, treatment are the lack of linkages between testing and treatment programs; adolescents' perception of invincibility and difficulty in understanding the abstract concepts of disease latency and probabilities of transmission; and injection drug use and homelessness. Apart from the multiplicity of problems created by homelessness, frequent changes of address or no home address jeopardizes their ability to receive Medicaid.

Immigrants

Immigrant women face a number of barriers in relation to prevention of perinatal HIV transmission. The most formidable are cultural, financial, and legal, including denial of residency or citizenship, as discussed further below. Insight into the experiences of Hispanic immigrants was offered to the IOM committee by a community organization serving Dominicans, the Community Association of Progressive Dominicans (ACDP). This organization counsels women and refers them to testing and treatment, among its other services to the community.

With a population approaching 500,000, Dominicans represent the second largest Hispanic group in New York City. The vast majority (68%) are immigrants whose flight from the Dominican Republic was the result of deteriorating economic conditions over the past decade. In New York City, 46% of Dominicans live below the poverty rate, a proportion higher than that of any other ethnic group in New York City (Hernandez and Rivera-Batiz, 1997). The proportion of undocumented Dominicans is not fully known, but was estimated in 1994 by the U.S. Immigration and Naturalization Service at less than 1% (Hernandez and Rivera-Batiz, 1997). From the perspective of ACDP, however, which serves the neediest, the figure is much higher.

For many Hispanic women, motherhood represents the pinnacle of their lives. It is a sacrosanct right of passage that imbues women with a sense of purpose, achievement, and bolsters their self-esteem and optimism about the future. Children are viewed as a "creation of God," according to one program administrator. With this cultural and religious mindset, the idea of prenatal testing for HIV is thought, in some cases, to verge on the preposterous.

The problem is exacerbated early in pregnancy by women's reluctance to seek prenatal care. Prenatal care is seen as a lesser priority than housing and employment, which frequently are more problematic. Further, many immigrant women distrust the health care system. The foreignness of the language and the institutional atmosphere inspire fears of deportation and death. Equating hospitals with death is not uncommon among other minority groups as well (see patient profiles, and workshop testimony from the National Medical Association from Appendix C). Another obstacle is the women's perceived inability to pay for prenatal care. Many providers and programs offer free care or care at reduced cost, but federal law explicitly prohibits undocumented immigrants and certain categories of legal immigrants from receiving Medicaid. Instead of seeking prenatal care, women often engage in self-care, through home remedies, or seek the aid of unlicensed doctors who are paid in cash.

Those bold enough to seek prenatal care are commonly resistant to counseling and testing for HIV. Many Hispanic women are uncomfortable discussing sexual matters. Sometimes the subject is fraught with shame and guilt, especially for women who prostituted themselves to secure the funds to emigrate to the United States. For these women, discussion of sexuality is not only taboo, but it is also laden with fear about a husband or partner learning of their past. "It's even difficult to admit this to other women," observed a program administrator, who claimed that women who are not pregnant, yet seeking his organization's help, took an average of two and a half years to talk openly about their sexuality and the possibility of HIV testing. The program's policy is not to ask, but to wait for women to raise the subject on their own, a policy designed not to disenfranchise them. The consequences of disclosure of HIV test results to the husband or partner are dire: women are concerned about domestic violence, abandonment, and divorce. Divorce is feared because it may affect their immigration status and, consequently, their eligibility for Medicaid. Furthermore, HIV-infected individuals, by federal law, are excluded from entry into the United States (Immigration and Nationality Act, Section 212a).

Denial of HIV risk abounds. Women do not see themselves at risk, either because they do not engage in risky behavior or because they deny the possibility of their partners being at risk. From their perspective, "If a man is clean, then he can't be positive," according to a program administrator. Denial extends to the HIV status of their offspring. Under the assumption that children are God's creation, they can only be seen as perfectly healthy. Therefore, testing for HIV is viewed as completely unnecessary. Yet the women who ultimately agree to HIV testing and treatment do so out of motivation to help their child—not themselves—according to program administrators.

Paying for treatment is yet another deterrent to prevention efforts. Few of the women seen by the programs have private insurance or Medicaid. Being barred from Medicaid eligibility, the only avenue for undocumented women to pay for the exorbitant costs of care is through programs such as ADAP in New York (described earlier), designed for low-income, Medicaid-ineligible people infected with HIV. Newborns born to undocumented immigrants, however, are covered under Medicaid by virtue of being born in the United States, which confers U.S. citizenship.

IMPACT OF NEW YORK STATE
MANDATORY TESTING LEGISLATION

In New York, unlike New Jersey, newborn testing for HIV is mandatory under State law. The New York testing program has been in effect since February

1997. Program administrators at New York sites shared with the IOM committee their experiences with the first year of the mandatory testing program.

Programs inform pregnant patients during standard prenatal HIV counseling that their newborns will be tested for HIV. They nevertheless find their patients' retention to be erratic. At postpartum visits, many seem unaware of the law, either because they had forgotten or because they were not told at another site where they had received prenatal care. The information was devastating, especially for those women unaware of their HIV-positive status until newborn testing. Programs described women being so traumatized from the news that they were unable to cope. For some, it took months to agree to treatment for themselves, but they agreed to medication for their infants much sooner (see patient profiles).

Because of the seeming lack of widespread knowledge of newborn testing, programs did not find the newborn testing law to deter women from receiving prenatal care or from delivering in a hospital. They noted, however, the difficulty of drawing this conclusion because they have such limited, if any, contact with these women. Their patients did express concerns about a breach of confidentiality to agencies outside the health care system and about being intimidated in taking their medication. These women were concerned that if they declined therapy for themselves or their infant, even out of legitimate concerns over long-term effects, they might be coerced through the courts.

PATIENTS' EXPERIENCES

Patient 1: Tanya

Tanya (a pseudonym) is an African-American woman who describes herself as a former injection drug user (IDU) with four children. She learned of her HIV infection seven years ago when she was pregnant with her second child. Her first child had been removed from her custody as a consequence of her drug use. It took two to three months of active encouragement from a dedicated Bellevue Hospital nurse to convince her to be tested. She elected to be tested because of the nurse's assurances that she was not alone and could get help for herself and her baby. Tanya declared, "If it weren't for my nurse, I wouldn't have gotten tested."

Upon learning she was HIV-positive, she was reluctant to accept medication. She was afraid of the medication because she linked—mistakenly she now realizes—her brother's death from AIDS to his medication, rather than to the disease. Having been a former IDU, she also was fearful of the medication being addictive. She ultimately accepted medication, again after vigorous counseling, and has since given birth to two children who are uninfected. She takes a cynical view of IDUs and sees drug abuse treatment as a necessary prerequisite for HIV testing and treatment of IDUs. When she was under the influence of drugs, she claims to have been even more eager to get high as an escape from the possibility that she might be infected with HIV. In her judgment, testing of pregnant women should be voluntary for all women except those using drugs. "If you're on drugs," she said, "I think they should just test without asking. . . . When I was on drugs, I didn't want to find out."

Patient 2: Rita

Rita, an African-American mother of two girls, was diagnosed with HIV around the time she learned of her second pregnancy. Her health clinic asked her to take an HIV test immediately after they diagnosed the pregnancy. Rita agreed to the HIV test thinking that the results would be negative. "I was so surprised by the results that I spent one to two months in denial. . . . Once I adjusted, I was able to cope, take my medicine." With the support of her counselor at Bellevue, she started antiretroviral therapy at five months of pregnancy and encountered no side effects. Her decision to proceed with therapy was based on her concern for her child. Her newborn daughter is HIV-negative, as is her older, nine-year-old daughter.

She felt compelled to conceal her HIV status from her family, with whom she lives, for fear of "being thrown out of the house." To disguise the true purpose of the medication for her newborn daughter, she told her family that it was for sickle cell disease. She did, however, notify the father and unsuccessfully urged him to get tested. Said Rita, "I told him to get the test, but he won't."

Patient 3: Janet

Janet is an African-American woman who was told she was HIV-positive early in her first pregnancy. She was stunned by the news because she did not know she even had been tested. "I would have preferred them to ask me," she reflected, "because I would've said yes." Despite the receipt of antiretroviral therapy before, during, and after delivery, her one-year old child is HIV-positive. Janet became pregnant again soon after the birth of her first child. Her second child also received an aggressive regimen of antiretroviral therapy. The HIV status of the second child, who was only three weeks old at the time Janet spoke to the committee, is not yet known. The father of her children died of AIDS, as did her sister. When advising her friends to get tested for HIV, she said, "They get offended. They say, 'You're crazy, girl.' "

Patient 4: Elina

Elina is a 26-year-old Hispanic mother of two daughters. Her first child, born five years ago, is autistic. She found out that she and her second daughter were

HIV-positive through New York State's mandatory newborn testing program. She was called back to the hospital one month after the delivery. The news was incomprehensible to her, for she had no reason to think she was infected, having gone regularly for prenatal care. She had even taken a breast-feeding class. She said, "I was never counseled about HIV, never offered an HIV test, never told about the risk of HIV transmission, and never told my baby would be tested." After absorbing the news, she rushed to put her daughter on antiretroviral therapy. Her baby's health, not her own, was foremost on her mind. It took her months to come forward and get treated herself. She reflected, "Women won't come in for themselves, only for their child." She is anguished to think she might have prevented infection by avoiding breast-feeding. "My biggest concern is that my daughter could have been infected with HIV unnecessarily," said Elina.

Patient 5: Maria

Maria is a Hispanic immigrant and former obstetrician in her home country who sees herself as having been victimized twice: once by her American husband, who infected her with HIV, and a second time by the legal system that bars her not only from U.S. residency (owing to her HIV status), but also from receiving her husband's benefits as a veteran. She nursed her husband for two years before he died of AIDS, only to learn that he had infected her. Upon applying for his veteran's benefits, she discovered that six months before her marriage he had married another woman, whom he also infected. The marriage licenses had been issued in the same building and same office. The first marriage invalidated her claim for widow's benefits, leaving her virtually penniless.

Because of her HIV status, she has faced discrimination in housing and employment. Her salvation has been New York's ADAP program which provides medications and medical care for HIV-positive people. As difficult as it has been in the United States, returning to her country would be far worse. Speaking through an interpreter, she said, "If I returned to my country it would be sure death." Her family has rejected her, and medications and services are unavailable to those in her country without the means to pay for them.

She has devoted herself to educating other Latina women to prevent them from spreading infection. Despite fears of deportation, she is determined to speak out about the plight of undocumented immigrants. "We need help for the sake of human rights," Maria lamented. "We live in limbo. . . . We have nothing to be able to survive."

POLICY OPTIONS

The following policy options were recommended by programs that were visited by the IOM committee.

Prenatal Period

- Shorten pre-test counseling for all patients, yet expand post-test counseling for those who test positive.
- Make counseling procedures routine for all patients.
- Ensure continued funding for prenatal HIV counseling staff (without reliance on grants).
- Make available an accurate rapid test for use with select patients deemed unlikely to return for results (e.g., adolescents, IDUs, patients with disordered lives, etc.).
- Support case finding of adolescent infected with HIV.
- Provide skills training to women to help them avoid high risk behaviors.
- Ensure availability of culturally and linguistically appropriate information and materials for immigrant women.

Labor and Delivery

- Make an accurate rapid test available for at-risk women whose HIV status is unknown.

Training of Private Physicians

- Disseminate educational materials for physicians and patients including an interactive CD-ROM (already developed for another purpose) and laminated card for breast pockets that indicates the key points to convey to patients.
- Seek help from medical malpractice insurers in educating physicians to make HIV counseling a routine part of care for prenatal patients.

REFERENCES

Hernandez R, Rivera-Batiz F. Dominican New Yorkers: a socioeconomic profile, 1997. Dominican Research Monographs, The CUNY Dominican Studies Institute, The City College of New York, 1997.

Rosenberg PS, Biggar RJ, Goedert JJ. Declining age at HIV infection in the United States. *N Engl J Med* 1994;167:1096–1099.

SITE ADDRESSES AND PARTICIPANTS

The IOM committee members who visited the programs in New York and New Jersey were Susan Cu-Uvin, Ellen Mangione, Robert Fullilove, and Douglas Morgan. Others present from IOM were Michael Stoto, Study Director, Donna Almario, and Miriam Davis (consultant).

Community Association of Progressive Dominicans
2268 Amsterdam Ave.
New York, NY 10033
  Carmen Chavez, Director of HIV/AIDS Services
  Felix Rivera, Coordinator of HIV/AIDS Services
  Rosa Benitez, Health Educatior
  Mildred Zeno, Outreach Worker, Women's Project
  T. Givins, Director HIV Prevention Services, Iris House Inc.
  Carla Basinat-Smith, Director SSHP, Iris House Inc.
  Hilda N. Melore, Volunteer, Latina Roundtable on Health and Reproductive
    Rights
  Kimberly Hutchenson, Kirkland and Ellis Fellow, HIV Law Project
  Maria Luisa Mirando, Obstetra Peer Educator, Latino Commission on AIDS
  Seydi Vazquez, Clinical Coordinator, Columbia Presbyterian Medical
    Center
  Julio Dicent-Talpierre, Director, Alianza Dominicana

The Francois Xavier-Bagnoud Center
University of Medicine and Dentistry of New Jersey
University Hospital
150 Bergen St.
Newark, NJ 07103
  Mary Boland, MSN, RN, FAAN, Director, Francois Xavier Bagnoud Center
  James Oleske, M.D., MPH, Director, Division of Pulmonary, Allergy, Im-
    munology and Infectious Diseases
  Theodore Barrett, M.D., Director, University OB/GYN Associates
  Joseph Apuzzio, M.D., Director of Maternal-Fetal Medicine
  Tzong-Jer Wei, M.D., Acting Director, Division of Neonatology
  Paul Palumbo, M.D., Principal Investigator, CDC HIV Perinatal Cohort
    Study
  Deborah Storm, Ph.D., RN, Research Program Manager, Pediatric-Perinatal
    HIV Studies
  Judy Barros, MSN, CPNP FXB Center
  Ruth Fleshman, MSW, LCSW, Director of Social Work Services

Lower New York Consortium for HIV-Affected Families
Bellevue Hospital Center
First Avenue and 27th Street
New York, NY 10016
  Keith Krasinski, M.D., Director

Model Comprehensive Health Care Program for Adolescents/ Adolescent AIDS
    Program
3514 Wayne Avenue
Bronx, NY 10467
    Donna Futterman, M.D., Director
    Neal D. Hoffman, M.D., Medical Director
    Alice Myerson, N.P., Primary Care Coordinator
    Mayris Webber, Ph.D., Montefiore Hospital, AIDS Research Program, De-
    partment of Epidemiology and Social Medicine

Northern Manhattan Women and Children HIV Demonstration Project
Columbia School of Public Health
600 West 168th St. and Broadway on 168th
New York, NY 10032
    Dr. Mahrukh Bamji, M.D., Metropolitan Hospital
    Cyra Borsy, Columbia School of Public Health
    Chris Cynn, HIV Law Project
    Danielle Greene, M.P.H., Columbia School of Public Health
    Cheryl Healton, Dr.P.H., Columbia School of Public Health
    Lynn Jackson, Metropolitan Hospital
    Mary Ellen Kelly, M.P.H., Metropolitan Hospital
    Stephanie Taylor, M.P.H.. Columbia School of Public Health
    Nancy VanDevanter, Dr.P.H., Columbia School of Public Health

Alabama Site Visit Summary

Amy Fine

On April 27, 1998, a site visit to Alabama was conducted on behalf of the Institute of Medicine (IOM) Committee on Perinatal Transmission of HIV. Its purpose was to seek input from public health officials, practitioners, and patients on the implementation of the Public Health Service (PHS) recommendations on perinatal HIV transmission and on any additional efforts/means to reduce perinatal transmission. Alabama was chosen for a site visit because it is a southern state with a large rural population, and, as such, represents the region with the greatest recent increases in perinatal HIV transmission rates. Site visit discussions were held both in Birmingham (in Jefferson County) and in Eutaw (a small community in rural Greene County). Participants included representatives from the University of Alabama at Birmingham's 1917 Clinic, the University of Alabama's Department of Obstetrics and Gynecology, the Alabama Department of Public Health, Jefferson County Department of Health, the Children's Hospital of Alabama, St. George's Clinic at Cooper Green Hospital, and patients and staff of West Alabama Health Services.

HIV/AIDS TRENDS IN ALABAMA

The number of reported HIV/AIDS cases in Alabama rose dramatically in the 1980s, and has since peaked, or at least plateaued, in the mid-1990s, with approximately 1,100 cases reported annually between 1995 and 1997. A total of 9,646 HIV/AIDS cases (5,028 AIDS cases and 4,618 HIV infections) had been reported statewide through May 25, 1998. While HIV/AIDS cases have been reported in all but one county in the state, infection rates in southern Alabama are about twice those in the northern part of the state. In general, the epidemic in the southern part of the state reflects a disproportional HIV/AIDS frequency among African-American women, while in the northern part of the state it is more an epidemic among white, homosexual men.

Through May 25, 1998, a total of 1,933 female HIV/AIDS cases were reported in Alabama. HIV/AIDS seroprevalence rates among childbearing women in the state are approximately 1/1,000, similar to the national rate. Among African-American childbearing women, however, the seroprevalence rate is 1/250, considerably higher than national rates. Thus, the state's racial disparity among HIV-infected women is particularly large. The rate of HIV/AIDS infection among women has increased steadily since 1986.

A total of 105 pediatric HIV/AIDS cases have been reported in Alabama since 1985. In contrast to trends for the adult population, the annual number of reported pediatric cases in Alabama peaked in the early 1990s (with 17 HIV/AIDS cases reported in 1990 and 16 in 1991), declined to 11 cases in 1995, and then to 4 cases in 1996 and 1 in 1997. It is important to note that reported pediatric HIV/AIDS cases have declined, even though the number of infants reported as perinatally exposed to HIV has continued to increase steadily—from 51 in 1994 to 67 in 1997. Among those infants known to be perinatally exposed, the proportion receiving zidovudine (ZDV) at delivery has increased from approximately 6% in 1994 to 63% in 1997. The number of infants receiving ZDV after delivery rose as well, from 20% in 1994 to 96% in 1997. These findings are consistent with the implementation of PHS recommendations for perinatal HIV exposure. One emerging trend cited by perinatal care providers is that over the past 18 months there has been an apparent increase in the number of HIV-infected women who choose to continue their pregnancies, rather than opt for termination.

In Alabama in 1997, the greatest percentage of reported HIV counseling and testing was performed in family planning clinics (41%), followed by STD (sexually transmitted disease) clinics (35%), and prenatal care sites (12%). Prisons accounted for only 3% of counseling and testing performed, community health centers for 2%; TB (tuberculosis) programs for 2%, and private physicians for only 4% of the total.

Data on receipt of prenatal care indicate that in 1996, 5.6% of live births in Alabama were to mothers who received inadequate prenatal care, as measured by the Kessner index. Adequacy of care varied considerably between the two counties visited by the committee, with 12% of births in rural Greene County considered to have had inadequate care, but only 4% of births in urban Jefferson County. These data are important in considering potential barriers to and solutions for improving perinatal HIV transmission rates.

IMPLEMENTATION OF PHS GUIDELINES

The site visit team sought information on the extent to which the July 1995 PHS recommendations for universal counseling and voluntary HIV testing of pregnant women have been implemented in Alabama. More specifically, participants reported on (1) incorporation of PHS guidelines into other guidelines or protocols; (2) provider implementation of counseling and testing guidelines; (3) the proportion of pregnant women tested at different sites and reasons for variations; (4) acceptance of treatment and reasons for refusal; and (5) reactions to possible variations in guidelines.

Incorporation of Guidelines

Participants noted that Alabama Department of Public Health (ADPH), the Jefferson Country Department of Health (JCDH), and West Alabama Health Services (WAHS) (a private, non-profit community health provider), have all incorporated the PHS guidelines into their own guidelines or protocols. The ADPH has undertaken several measures. First, shortly after the AIDS Clinical Trials Group protocol number 76 (ACTG 076) was published, the state health officer and the state perinatal advisory committee sent out a joint letter to all health care providers in Alabama recommending that they follow the PHS recommended protocol. The ADPH has also incorporated PHS guidelines into guidelines for public health clinics throughout the state. (Local public health clinics throughout the state are actually operated by the ADPH. Only Mobile and Jefferson counties have relatively autonomous local health departments.) The ADPH guidelines, *Comprehensive Health Record Instruction Manual (CHR)*, require HIV counseling and the offering of HIV testing within the first two prenatal visits. Additional HIV testing will be offered in later visits if clinically indicated. During the postpartum visit, offering of HIV test and counseling are required. Finally, the ADPH supported legislation being considered by the Alabama legislature at the time of the IOM site visit. The legislation, which did not come up for a vote during the recent legislative session, would have given the state board of health the authority to require routine testing for specified notifiable diseases. If the law had passed, then the board of health would likely have required routine HIV testing of all pregnant women, with the patients having the right to refuse testing.

The JCDH has incorporated the PHS recommendations into its clinical management protocols for care of its maternity patients. The JCDH protocol currently in use was developed in June 1995 and includes the following components: (1) a risk assessment at the initial visit for all maternity patients, with risk status recorded in the county's automated record system maintained by the JCDH and the University of Alabama at Birmingham Department of Obstetrics and Gynecology; (2) a strong recommendation that all prenatal patients receive HIV serology testing; (3) routinely obtained written informed consent for confidential HIV serology testing on admission; (4) clear notification to patients that any HIV information obtained will be shared with the hospital responsible for delivery and with the high-risk obstetrics clinic; (5) required pre-test counseling, with components specified; (6) required post-test counseling, regardless of results; and (7) referral of all HIV-infected women to the county's special HIV prenatal clinic.

The WAHS provides an example of how PHS recommendations have been incorporated in clinical guidelines for a private, non-profit agency serving a large number of pregnant women in a rural setting. WAHS offers a comprehensive prenatal care program that incorporates routine HIV/AIDS education/counseling and voluntary testing.

Guideline Implementation and Test Acceptance

Despite incorporation of guidelines at state and county levels and within some parts of the private sector, those interviewed were in agreement that provider implementation of HIV counseling and testing appears to be quite uneven in both the public and the private sectors, and that this variation is probably the most important factor in determining test acceptance. Participants believed that in clinics where providers routinely offer testing and educate women about the health benefits, particularly for the baby, the proportion of women tested was extremely high. Participants, however, thought that some providers offer testing based on assessed risk while other providers (particularly within the private sector) routinely test without pre-test counseling or informed consent. Some providers routinely provide a comprehensive HIV education/counseling program, while others inform patients by leaving brochures in the waiting room. Interviewees reported that some physicians refuse to see maternity patients unless they are tested for HIV, thus making the test mandatory. At the other extreme, some physicians refuse to treat women once they test positive.

Participants expressed the opinion that further provider education is needed to make practice more consistent with the PHS guidelines. In addition, some believed that routine testing (i.e., including HIV as part of a regular prenatal test panel, with patient opt-out provisions) was the best way to improve test rates. Finally, participants agreed that although current implementation of the PHS recommendations on counseling and testing is less than ideal, the trend is favorable.

With regard to test acceptance, participants felt that if properly counseled, the overwhelming majority of pregnant women would accept testing. Barriers to acceptance include lack of trust in the provider, fear of blood tests, late entry into prenatal care, religious beliefs, fear of the disease itself, and the legacy of the Tuskegee syphilis study.

Proportion of Childbearing Women Tested

Public health officials noted that statewide, only 55% to 65% of public health maternity patients were tested or knew their HIV status. In several counties, maternity patients are referred to STD clinics for HIV counseling and testing. Asked whether this might be a barrier to testing because of the stigma associated with STDs, they responded that it may be a barrier and this is a local decision.

In Jefferson County, testing among the county's eight clinic sites has been uneven as well. The percentage of JCDH maternity patients tested increased from 45% in July 1995–June 1996, to 69% in November 1997–March 1998; however, rates vary by site. Recent data from the county's Obstetrical Automated Record (OBAR) system indicate that among the eight clinic sites, the proportion of maternity patients *not* tested ranges from 2% to 66%. To address variations in testing across sites, in November 1997 the health department held an in-service education program aimed at changing provider behavior.

It is important to note that on an annual basis, clinics provide maternity care to about 5,000 pregnant women in Jefferson County, and to 30,000 women state-wide (roughly half of all childbearing women in each jurisdiction). Changes in implementation of counseling and testing practices in the public sector could thus have a profound impact on overall perinatal HIV transmission in Alabama.

With regard to testing at WAHS, the director stated that under its comprehensive counseling/education program, 99% of WAHS maternity patients voluntarily accept testing. Finally, although no data were available on the proportion of private maternity patients in Jefferson County or in the state who received HIV counseling and testing, public health officials noted that private providers clearly are testing, using state labs, and reporting cases to the state.

Acceptance of Therapy

On the issue of acceptance of ZDV and other, complex therapies (combination, protease inhibitor-containing regimens), all those interviewed agreed that once HIV-infected pregnant women receive test results, most accept therapies. Reasons given for non-acceptance include fear of loss of confidentiality for those being in small communities; fear of domestic violence; and fear, denial, and depression about the disease itself. Participants noted the importance of providing a smooth transition from testing to treatment, offering comprehensive primary care to the HIV-infected woman and her infant, establishing a trusting provider–patient relationship, and providing needed mental health and social services.

Participants indicated that both ethical and resource issues impact whether mono- or combination antiretroviral therapy is offered. In Jefferson County, while the HIV high-risk centers are offering complex therapies, the JCDH reimburses only for ZDV, primarily because of resource constraints. Some providers also are concerned that multiple therapies may be considered experimental, and so are reluctant to prescribe them for ethical reasons or fear of liability.

Participants pointed to a growing need for resources to sustain care. They were particularly concerned about insufficient funding to pay for care and medications (especially combination therapies) for HIV-infected mothers once they are six weeks postpartum and no longer Medicaid-eligible. Interviewees stressed that federal Ryan White funds had been essential to building and maintaining current services and to meeting future need.

On the issue of general barriers to care, particularly among poor, rural African Americans, the following observations were offered. There is not a culture of accessing primary care in general and maternity services in particular. Rather, birthing is something that "mama and grandmama" used to assist with; family members' attitudes continue to have substantial influence over whether or not a woman seeks prenatal care. In addition, for many, educational levels are very low, so health education must be tailored to make sure patients can understand and follow through with care.

Reactions to Possible Variations in Guidelines

At several points during the site visit, participants were asked their opinions regarding possible changes in the PHS guidelines. Most providers felt that mandated testing is not desirable. One participant said, "I don't think we have to resort to that." Others noted that mandatory testing could exacerbate the problem of women being tested without their knowledge, which in turn could seriously undermine patient–provider trust.

It was pointed out that the real focus should not be on mandatory testing, but rather on how the term "voluntary" is defined and implemented. Most participants preferred maintaining a voluntary approach through routine testing (as part of a standard prenatal test panel), with a patient opt-out provision. The Emory University protocol calls for universal counseling and routine testing, with an exclusion consent. One participant expressed concern that if offered a list of tests from which they could opt out, some patients would refuse syphilis testing. In rural Alabama, people refuse some testing because of the Tuskegee history. Others refuse prenatal genetic testing because they will not terminate the pregnancy regardless of the test outcome. Finally, one participant suggested that financial incentives or disincentives might prod providers to routinely include HIV testing.

MODELS THAT WORK

Throughout the site visit, participants provided examples of how innovative programs are successfully addressing perinatal HIV transmission. Among the highlights are the following:

• In Jefferson County, through a concerted outreach effort to the faith community, a network of AIDS care teams has been established. The Care Team Network project has a two-pronged focus: (1) intensive education and outreach to local clergy (aimed at changing the role of church communities from "among the least supportive" of people with HIV/AIDS to among the most supportive); and

(2) organizing church/synagogue-based AIDS care teams to provide emotional support and assistance to people with AIDS. Recently, the AIDS teams have been "mainstreamed" into a general care team network that assists victims of other chronic conditions such as Alzheimer's disease.

• Again in Jefferson County, a broad range of HIV care providers working in a variety of clinical settings has developed a well-coordinated system of care for HIV-infected women and their children. These programs serve local HIV/AIDS patients as well as those referred from northern and southern Alabama. Patients travel as much as four to five hours to receive integrated care in Birmingham's HIV centers. For all patients, whether local or referred, attention has been given to assuring smooth transitions from testing to primary and specialty care; providing long-term follow-up care; and providing an array of support services including transportation, emotional support, and funding for needed medications. Included among the collaborating institutions are the "1917 Clinic" at the University of Alabama at Birmingham, the JCDH, St. George's Clinic at Cooper Green Hospital, and the Children's Hospital of Alabama.

• In rural Greene County, WAHS has integrated HIV/AIDS education, counseling and testing into a well-developed comprehensive prenatal care program. Using a model developed under a Ford Foundation grant, program components include outreach and home visiting, the use of clearly laid out educational protocols, and monitoring of quality assurance. WAHS achieves near universal prenatal testing among its maternity patients.

SITE ADDRESSES AND PARTICIPANTS

The IOM committee members who visited the programs in Alabama were Lorraine Klerman and Sten Vermund. Others present from the IOM were Michael Stoto, study director, Donna Almario, and Amy Fine (consultant).

1917 Clinic
908 South 20th Street
189 CCB
Birmingham, AL 35294-2050
    Malcolm L. Marler, Chaplain Education Specialist, Infectious Disease
    Phyllis Percy, NP
    Michael Saag, MD, 1917 Clinic Director, Professor, Infectious Disease
    Kathleen Squires, MD, Associate Professor, Infectious Disease

Alabama Department of Public Health
201 Monroe Street, Suite 1400
Montgomery, AL 36104
    Jane Cheeks, MPH, Director, Division of HIV/AIDS,
    Richard Holmes, MPH, Director, HIV/AIDS Surveillance

St. George's Clinic, Cooper Green Hospital
1515 6th Ave. S.
Birmingham, AL 35233
    Jane Mobley, MD

University of Alabama at Birmingham
618 South 20th Street
560 OHB
Birmingham, AL 35294-7333
    Robert L. Goldenberg, MD, Professor and Chair, OB/GYN

West Alabama Health Services
P.O. Box 599
Eutaw, AL 35462
    Sandral Hullett, MD, MPH, Director

South Texas Site Visit Summary

Donna Almario

On May 10, 1998, the Institute of Medicine's Committee on Perinatal Transmission of HIV visited San Antonio, Texas, to examine issues regarding the perinatal transmission of HIV in South Texas. Compared to previous site visits in New York, New Jersey, and Alabama, South Texas had similar issues with regard to providing care for pregnant women and their babies. Unlike the other sites, though, South Texas encountered additional barriers in providing care because of its vast area, low prevalence of HIV in women, and proximity to Mexico.

DEMOGRAPHICS OF HIV IN SOUTH TEXAS

Geographically, South Texas is a large yet sparsely populated area that includes 54,000 square miles (about the size of New York State). Included in this area is the region around the Texas-Mexico border, also known as La Frontera. The population includes about 55% to 60% Mexican Americans and 7% African Americans. Economically, this area has an unemployment rate of 20% to 25%, and three of the poorest counties in the nation.

The primary mode of HIV transmission in women in this area is through sex. Few cases (less than 2%) are directly due to injection drug use. HIV-positive men usually do not know they are infected and some are closeted bisexuals. When families come in for care, fathers are rarely seen.

IMPLEMENTATION OF PHS GUIDELINES

Prior to 1995, about two-thirds of children diagnosed with AIDS had mothers who were identified previously as being HIV-positive. Since the release of the

Public Health Service (PHS) guidelines, birth certificates record whether or not an HIV test was done prenatally and during delivery. Additionally, the Texas State legislature passed a law in February 1996 requiring routine HIV testing with notification of all pregnant women at the first prenatal visit and during delivery, except for those who specifically opt out. Since 1995, the number of children diagnosed with AIDS has dropped.

A provider from the University Health Center who cares for diabetic and other complicated pregnancies reported that about 99% of these women are tested for HIV. In Centro del Barrio, a clinic that provides services to poor women in San Antonio and Bexar County, ten women (95%) are tested per month, and so far no one has tested positive. Family Health Services, part of the city's health department, delivers 4,000 of the 20,000 births in the county. They report that all pregnant women are offered the HIV test and 90% to 95% of these women accept testing. However birth certificates record that only 85% of pregnant women were tested. One of the physicians who provides care for HIV-infected women reported that 95% of women who are offered the test accept it. The other 5% refuse to be tested because of stigma, discrimination, fear of breach of confidentiality, and belief that they are not at risk.

Of the pregnant women tested and notified of their positive result, 5% refused zidovudine (ZDV) therapy during pregnancy and very few refused postnatal ZDV treatment for their babies. Most physicians use ZDV alone, although an increasing number use triple combination therapy.

When informed of the danger of breast-feeding to the baby, most HIV-positive women refrain from breast-feeding. The WIC program provides formulas to HIV-positive mothers.

Overall because of the AIDS Clinical Trials group protocol number 76 (ACTG 076), more HIV-infected women are having babies. They are aware of the ACTG 076 results and believe they can safely deliver the baby.

PROGRAMS REPRESENTED

Unlike Dallas and Houston, San Antonio has little local tax funding for HIV care so it relies heavily on Title I–IV funding. Because of the low prevalence of HIV in South Texas, there is strong competition for a small pot of federal money. One participant mentioned that there is no strong will to direct the money into prevention. However, despite this, there are connections that enable the present system to work. HIV-infected women in San Antonio are getting into care.

Many people who are HIV-infected are referred to the following sites: South Texas AIDS Center for Children and Families (STAIDS), Valley AIDS Council (VAC), Community First Health Plans, Centro del Barrio, and the San Antonio Metropolitan Health District. All except for Community First Health Plans (an HMO, health maintenance organization) receive federal funding from Health

Resources and Services Administration (HRSA's) HIV Bureau (Title I-IV) and/ or the Centers for Disease Control and Prevention (CDC). Besides providing care, STAIDS also conducts research.

The following are programs in South Texas that provide care for HIV-positive people. STAIDS was established at Santa Rosa Children's Hospital in San Antonio in 1988, primarily to treat hemophiliacs. Within a few years, children infected perinatally were increasingly being admitted and more children from the surrounding areas were coming in for care, even as far south as the Lower Rio Grande Valley (LRGV), which is about 270 miles away. Eventually, additional service sites were established in the towns of McAllen, Harlingen, and Corpus Christi in the LRGV.

STAIDS is part of the Division of Community Pediatrics of the Department of Pediatrics, University of Texas Health Science Center at San Antonio. It was founded in the late 1980s as part of the original 17 Title IV sites. In the last four to five years, the center has received funding to conduct several projects:

• The *Salud y Unidad en la Familia* is a SPNS (Special Projects of National Significance) project that is intended to develop the delivery system of care for children and mothers in South Texas. The project works with organizations that provide HIV services in Corpus Christi and the LRGV; it collects data on families to study the quality of life for HIV-positive women and barriers to care.

• *La Frontera* is another SPNS project that includes working with VAC (located at the Texas-Mexico border) and the United Medical Center (in Maverick County). The project studies the migrant and rural population to better understand the patterns of HIV disease, transmission, and case finding in these areas of the state.

• The Texas Department of Health funds a project to study education and prevention for youth in detention facilities.

• Two other grants provide funds to study the management of chronic diseases in the valley and the impact of Medicaid managed care of children with special health needs.

VAC is the primary AIDS clinic in the LRGV. Since 1995, it has expanded to include a medical clinic. The program has provided an array of services, including medical services, case managers, referrals to dental services, and transportation to help people keep their medical appointments. Case managers assist families so that children reach appointments on time. They also have funds to provide emergency medication, care for migrant women, and an educational program on HIV testing in the valley. There is a walk-in testing clinic where turnaround is fast. VAC also works with other nearby hospitals.

Much of the obstetric care in the valley for HIV-infected women is provided by the Family Residency Program. Private obstetricians initially did not treat these women, but the situation has improved. Now a limited but increasing number of physicians are demonstrating an interest in helping out. Most of the women treated do not have the resources to pay for care.

Community First Health Plans is the first public HMO in Texas. It was established in 1997 and is a tax-exempt Texas corporation sponsored by the University Health System. The HMO was established in response to the changing marketplace, especially the move to managed care for Medicaid populations. Community First Health Plans tries to identify plan members who are at risk for HIV infection through their claims data. Members with HIV infection are assigned a case manager who facilitates members into infectious disease services and tracks health status. Members with HIV are allowed to choose their infectious disease provider as their primary care physician.

Centro del Barrio is a private non-profit community health center that provides HIV testing and offers free obstetric and gynecologic services. Counselors are registered nurses, educators, certified nurses, and social workers. HIV testing is free, and an on-site laboratory provides results within two or three days. More than 95% of the women who receive prenatal care through the Centro del Barrio are tested. Pregnant women who are in shelters have outreach workers who link them to care. The center also collaborates with the hospital district.

The San Antonio Metropolitan Health District's Family Health Services Bureau sees 4,000 prenatal patients per year out of the 20,000 births in Bexar County. Most of the women are indigent, and since 1996, four women have been diagnosed with HIV.

BARRIERS TO CARE

Some of the barriers to implementing the PHS counseling and testing guidelines in South Texas are: counseling and informing patients in a low prevalence area, obtaining and correctly analyzing test results, notifying patients of the test results, the distance some must travel to obtain care, providing care for undocumented residents, and cultural stigma.

The low prevalence of HIV in the South Texas region makes it difficult to educate physicians to counsel and inform their patients of HIV. Patients with HIV make up less than one percent of the typical physician's workload. Because of the low percentage, keeping up to date with the current literature can be considered inefficient, counseling may impede a doctor's workload, and seeing fewer patients may decrease revenues. There are training classes for HIV counseling offered at the AIDS Training Center in Houston, but few physicians attend; instead, social workers and nurses usually attend. One participant recounted an incident that demonstrates providers' lack of training: a medical resident who notified a pregnant patient of her positive result was unable to answer the patient's questions about HIV, the effect of the medication on the baby, or refer her to STAIDS. When the patient asked for a retest, the resident incorrectly answered, "the tests are accurate and there is no need for retest."

Obtaining and analyzing test results can also be very difficult. In one system, the physicians themselves must call the lab directly to obtain test results. Some tests may not be returned because the physician forgets or the patient forgets to remind the doctor to obtain the results. At one site to counteract this problem, a nurse practitioner obtains all the lab results and reads through them to find an HIV-positive result. Once she finds a positive result, she determines which physician has seen the woman most often and then asks the doctor to contact the woman.

The analysis of the test results are sometimes misinterpreted. In a number of cases, women with a positive ELISA and indeterminate Western blot were incorrectly informed that they were HIV-positive. Although all were eventually re-tested, this lack of attention to important facts about HIV testing may result in the patients' mistrust of their care providers and may contribute undue stress in the women's lives. In one such situation, a woman told her husband of her positive status, and he left her immediately. When her initial results were found to be false positive, it was already too late.

Some doctors seem misinformed of the standard procedure for administering the ACTG 076 regimen or assume that pharmacies automatically have injection ZDV in stock. For example in Harlingen, one physician requested administration of ZDV during labor of an HIV-positive woman, not knowing that the Harlingen hospital did not automatically stock ZDV. Unfortunately by the time the medication arrived from San Antonio, the woman had already delivered the baby. The participants believed that this situation is seen in many other smaller towns where there is a low prevalence of HIV/AIDS. Some doctors do not know the proper administration of ZDV during labor. One doctor reportedly said, "We don't use injection form here."

The distance to travel for health care is also an issue. For example, one grandmother must travel 150 miles both ways so an infant can take part in a drug trial. One of the patients interviewed said that if she were to take public transportation to her clinic, it would take her two hours. Considering the importance of complying with the ZDV regimen, transportation can be considered a barrier when caring for HIV-positive pregnant women. Some providers around the LRGV must travel 1400 miles in less than a month to deliver the results to people. Transportation is "expensive, labor intensive, and time consuming."

Finally, there is difficulty in notifying the woman of a positive result. Many women are lost because they provide false addresses (often because of immigration concerns). Others are lost because of the effects of a provider's unsympathetic notification of the positive result.

Texas Law

In response to the lack of preparation in dealing with HIV and delivering medications, the Texas legislature passed a law in February 1996 that requires routine HIV testing with notification of all pregnant women at the first prenatal visit and during delivery, except for those who specifically opt out. Counseling is supposed to be offered and pamphlets about HIV/AIDS from the Texas Department of Health given to all women in prenatal care.

The participants saw a number of benefits of the law. Most importantly, more women, especially those considered at low risk, were getting tested. However although more women were being tested, the participants cited several gaps in the law's implementation. First, there is no tracking system to know which and how many women stayed away from care because of the testing policy. Second, although the law requires counseling, no funds are set aside for counseling nor is counseling tracked. Third, although testing is required, there is no enforcement of the law. Remarkably, many providers and patients, even those interested enough in perinatal HIV to attend the committee's site visit, seemed ignorant of the law's specific provisions.

Special Populations

Undocumented Women

Because of Texas' close proximity of the Mexican border, many Mexican women cross the border to deliver their babies in South Texas. Many of these women have not received prenatal care because they are ineligible for Medicaid.

Several dilemmas may arise for these women. One is providing care for other sick family members who are not U.S. citizens. According to one participant, there was a case where an HIV-infected Mexican woman delivered her baby in the United States. The woman has six other children who are not U.S. citizens, all who have tested positive for tuberculosis (TB), and one who is HIV-positive. The provider must then decide between treating other sick family members despite their lack of U.S. citizenship or not treating them at all, which may lead to death or in the cases of the TB infected individuals, be a threat to others. In these situations providers must be creative, often relying on limited charity funds, in finding solutions to treat sick family members.

Another dilemma arises when providing care for a baby who is a U.S. citizen and dealing with a mother who is not. In one such situation, there was a choice between deporting the mother along with the baby, thereby depriving U.S. care for the HIV-infected baby or deporting only the mother and leaving the baby behind to be enrolled into a drug trial. Luckily, the baby was able to remain in the United States with her grandmother.

South Texas also has a large migrant population. To access health care and since they do not have a permanent address, migrants must return to the state where they originally applied for Medicaid. If they access their health care elsewhere they risk losing their Medicaid eligibility. Thus, pregnant migrant women living in Texas who are HIV-infected must deliver in the state where they originally applied for Medicaid. That state may not have routine HIV testing during pregnancy, and then the women ends up returning to Texas without accessing HIV care.

Culture

The family unit is very important and highly regarded in the Hispanic culture. HIV infection, however, is seen as a threat to the cohesiveness of the family. One patient noted that the worst thing for a Hispanic family is having a member who is homosexual, uses drugs, or is promiscuous. In the Hispanic culture, HIV encompasses those aspects and so one who has HIV is considered "not good." Some positive women, then, are reluctant to tell their families of their HIV infection. Single women who are pregnant and have HIV must also deal with the additional stigma of being a single unwed mother.

Since "family" is so important in the Hispanic culture, many women do not use birth control. For instance, women feel that they cannot ask a man to put on a condom because as his wife or partner, she would not be satisfying him. Because of the importance of the family, on the other hand, a pregnant woman will work out of her culture and seek early prenatal care and take medications if she understands there is a benefit to her baby. Usually, the women are more compliant in using formula if they know that breast-feeding may harm the baby. All of the patients who were interviewed stressed the importance of taking the medication "because of the baby."

PATIENTS

Patient 1: Theresa

Theresa (a pseudonym) is a Hispanic woman who was tested for HIV in 1994 and was negative. In 1998 she was tested again after signing forms for a test she thought was routine. She was 6.5 months pregnant at time of diagnosis, and she had never received information on how HIV transmission from mother to child can be prevented.

Upon receiving the positive test result from her provider, who is a medical resident, Theresa at first did not believe it. She asked questions about HIV, the medication, its side effects and potential harm to the baby, yet the resident was unable to answer the questions or refer her to specialized care in San Antonio.

Theresa felt "dirty, not worthy, trashy, and filthy." She perceived that HIV-positive people were prostitutes and drug users, and that people would see her in the same light. Luckily a nurse practitioner overheard the conversation between Theresa and the resident, consoled Theresa, and told her about Community Pediatrics. Unfortunately Theresa was still distraught and contemplated suicide on her way home. However the counselors at Community Pediatrics were very helpful and caring and referred her to other providers. She did not want to return to her first provider.

Initially she went to the Family Focus AIDS Care Treatment and Services Clinic (FFACTS), found that it primarily treated homosexual men, and consequently felt uncomfortable. There were also HIV/AIDS signs in the clinic, and she believed that her confidentiality was being threatened.

Two months prior to delivery, she developed shingles and was hospitalized. Her providers wore full masks and gowns when they entered the room, and she assumed that they were protecting themselves from HIV, not the shingles. No one had told her why.

Her mother knows her HIV status, and both are learning more about the disease. Theresa used the HIV brochures that she received from her providers to explain the disease to her mother, who is very supportive. On the other hand, Theresa's two sons do not know her HIV status, and she fears that they will discover it. When she administered the ZDV to her newborn, Theresa told her sons that they were vitamins. There are support groups in the evenings, but it is difficult for her to attend since her children do not know she has HIV. She also has a roommate who helps support her and the children. Without him, she and her family would be out on the streets. She does not receive support from the baby's father because she believes that he feels guilty.

After her diagnosis, she began to lose her concentration at work, and her performance deteriorated. She believed that having her baby in daycare while she was at work and administering ZDV would put her confidentiality at stake. She quit her job but eventually found a new one. Upon bring hired, though, she will have to relinquish her Medicaid status since her salary is now over Medicaid's earning requirements. She is concerned that people will find out at work. At a previous job, one woman knew and treated her differently. She is afraid of getting sick at her job or even cutting herself.

Theresa's providers helped her find a pharmacy where no one knew her. She is now on triple therapy and is very compliant to the medication regimen. Her doctor told her two months before the site visit that she would live five or ten more years. Two weeks before the site visit, the doctor said that she will live eight to twenty more years. He said that as long as she takes her medication, she would live longer.

She reports that she "takes the medication for her [baby] and myself. . . . I may not see her wedding or prom, but will see her everyday until it [death] comes."

Patient 2: Loretta

Loretta was five months pregnant when she was diagnosed with HIV. She did not know about the HIV testing law, and her nurse told her that it was mandatory. However, when Loretta questioned the nurse about the informed consent form which had boxes of "yes" and "no," the nurse restated, "It's the law."

Her private obstetrician/gynecologist (she's covered by Medicaid) told her on the phone that her tests came back abnormal and that it was important to see both her and her husband immediately. Once in the office, the doctor told Loretta that she had HIV and showed her the lab results. She was in disbelief and thought, "I'm no lab technician, how am I supposed to read this?" The doctor then gave her a prescription of ZDV and a copy of several pages from a book about AIDS.

Her first thought was that she was going to die immediately, and both she and her husband were distraught and overcome by tears. Loretta's second concern was for her baby. Her husband demanded a retest, but the doctor at first refused but later relented. The doctor referred her husband to the Health Department to be tested.

At the Health Department, they began to get answers and support. The counselors explained the test procedures, the medication, and then referred them to the FFACTS clinic. When she returned to her private obstetrician/gynecologist to get the second test results, she felt uncomfortable with him and thought that he did not know how to handle her situation. He asked if she was taking ZDV, and Loretta replied that she had not started because she did not know what it was.

What she initially knew of ZDV was through a homosexual friend who had HIV. He took ZDV, still deteriorated, and later died. She believed that ZDV caused her friend's death and so assumed that HIV led to AIDS with ZDV, and that led to death.

Her first thought was how were people going to treat her. She believed that only homosexuals and drug users were infected with HIV. She felt alone, ashamed, and dirty. She thought that people would not want to be around her and no one would take care of her baby if she was not around.

However once Loretta began seeing her current physician from the FFACTS clinic, she began to understand the benefits of ZDV. When she began learning more about the disease, she informed her family. Her baby is negative and now she is on triple therapy.

Patient 3: Olivia

Olivia was diagnosed with HIV after donating blood. One month later, the blood drive's sponsor tracked her down and informed that she had HIV. She contacted her mother, but at that point, she felt she had nowhere to turn. Her fourteen-year-old son and her partner were both found negative.

Upon notification, physicians in her hometown of Seguin where the blood bank was located, told her that they "didn't know how to help." They referred Olivia to other several places. She finally contacted the health department in Seguin, and they referred her to the FFACTS clinic. At that point, one month after she donated blood, the physician told Olivia that she was four months pregnant. Olivia wanted to have an abortion, but the doctor said that she was too far along in her pregnancy and could not have an abortion. At that point she started feeling scared.

Olivia was immediately placed on ZDV and informed that the ZDV was to benefit the baby's health. She was very compliant with treatment and kept every appointment. Her baby is negative.

Her partner's family reacted negatively because of her status. She, however, was not afraid to tell her own family and receives strong support from her family, which she attributes to the family's closeness. When Olivia's younger niece worries that Olivia would die and would not be able to take care of the baby or that the baby would die, Olivia responds, "You just have to pray."

She is now on triple therapy and Prozac because of her depression.

Patient 4: Tina

Tina who is six months pregnant, originally grew up in Puerto Rico and was probably infected there by an abusive boyfriend who later died of AIDS. After being tested while still living in Puerto Rico, a nurse called to say "you have to come down. It doesn't look good." She hung up, and did not get retested until after moving to San Antonio.

After complaining about migraines, she was admitted to the hospital, where it was determined that she was pregnant. For her prenatal care, she visited the health department and found out that she was 2 weeks pregnant and had HIV. She began to cry upon receipt of the news, but the physician comforted her by saying that "a positive status doesn't mean you're going to die." This gave Tina some hope.

Tina told her cousin about her HIV status, and her cousin told her whole family. Her family was not supportive, and Tina felt they were treating her like "trash." Her father, though, was very supportive.

Tina's partner also attended the meeting and reported that Puerto Rico is backwards compared to the United States in HIV care and understanding of the disease. HIV patients are not treated with dignity and there is condescension of the lifestyle these patients have led. Most people, he thinks, believe, "You did it, you deserve it."

Tina did not know that medications can help her baby until she saw her partner taking his medication.

She does not like being pushed and if testing were mandatory, she would go somewhere else for prenatal care.

SITE ADDRESSES AND PARTICIPANTS

Representing the committee were Katherine Luzuriaga and Stephen Thomas and IOM staff were Michael Stoto (study director) and Donna Almario.

Centro del Barrio
7420 Blanco Road Suite 200
San Antonio, TX 78216
　　Jay Sanchez, Program Director

Community First Health Plans
7420 Blanco Rd. Suite 200
San Antonio, TX 78216
　　Susan Lomba, Director of Health Promotion and Wellness

San Antonio Metropolitan Health District
Bureau of Family Health
332 West Commerce
San Antonio, TX 78205-2489
　　Maurine Porto, M.D., Interim Chief

South Texas AIDS Center for Children and Their Families
Division of Community Pediatrics—Department of Pediatrics
University of Texas Health Science Center at San Antonio
7703 Floyd Curl Drive
San Antonio, TX 78284-7817
　　Victor F. German, M.D., Ph.D., Program Director
　　Terence Doran, M.D., Ph.D., Clinical Medical Director
　　Rachel Davis, R.N., Assistant Director
　　Yolanda Cantu, M.P.H., Planner, Evaluator
　　Yvonne del Bosco, M.P.H.

Valley AIDS Council
2220 Haine Suite 45
Harlingen, TX 78550
　　Lydia Benavides, Director of Client Service
　　Lisa Casas, Case Manager

APPENDIX

H

Florida Conference Summary

Michael Stoto

On April 16, 1998, the Institute of Medicine (IOM) Committee on Perinatal Transmission of HIV held a public hearing in conjunction with the Florida HIV Conference in Orlando. Florida Title IV program directors and others were notified about the hearing in advance of the meeting, and others were told of the hearing at the meeting itself. The comments and views expressed below are those of the participants.

COUNSELING AND OFFERING OF HIV TEST

In October 1996, Florida enacted a law requiring that all women in prenatal care be counseled and offered an HIV test. For those who refuse, a document of the patient's refusal and signature must be obtained and entered into the patient's record. The offering and acceptance of an HIV test are different in the public and private sector. Almost all women in public sector prenatal care are offered an HIV test, and less than 5% of these women refuse testing. Women who receive prenatal care in the private sector, on the other hand, are less likely to be offered a test.

According to the participants, prenatal tests are offered in the private sector, but in different ways. Some women are given a blanket consent form for all prenatal tests, including the HIV test, although this practice is illegal according to one participant. In other areas, nurses counsel women about the HIV test, as part of the setup for their first prenatal care visit with a physician.

One participant said that she had mixed feelings about such "routine" test-

271

ing; pre-test counseling is important, she says, but so is getting tested. She suggests a shortened version of pre-test counseling, covering only essential points.

A Ryan White-funded program in the Tampa area provides nurse case managers, and has 100% compliance with HIV testing in public settings. In contrast, 85% to 90% of the women in the private sector accept the test. The program also works with private sector physicians and group practices to improve compliance with the state law. The nurses visit offices, do chart audits, and make recommendations on how to improve testing rates. Only about ten group practices have been visited to date, but these were chosen because of the large number of births they are responsible for. The nurses are viewed partly as people who can help the practices with HIV testing and link them with specialized HIV care when necessary, and partly as government auditors. The program also provides services to pregnant women in the private sector. It provides case management services for private prenatal patients (two patients so far), programs to help the baby's transition into a Title IV program, and supplementary services in conjunction with care from their private prenatal providers.

MANDATORY NEWBORN TESTING

One participant suggested that mandatory newborn testing to detect babies whose mothers were not tested under the voluntary system be considered. Another responded that a colleague of hers from New York had said that the "unblinding" of newborn tests in that state was supposed to expand access to care for both mothers and babies, but that resources were not available for this purpose.

UNDOCUMENTED WOMEN

"Undocumented" women (illegal aliens) make up a substantial part of the prenatal HIV caseload. At the University of Miami Hospital, every woman giving birth is offered an HIV test, and many of the HIV-positive women identified in this way are undocumented women who were not tested in pregnancy. Such women do not seek out prenatal care because they presume that they are not eligible for services and, more importantly, they fear discovery of their status. In Miami, they are no longer covered by Medicaid. Some cities, however, are making an effort to provide care for undocumented women. Officials in Miami have found ways to get most of these women into care through Ryan White resources, drug companies' compassionate care programs, and charitable organizations. The Title IV program in Orlando brings undocumented women into care through community fund-raising, churches, the United Way, and so on. The Tampa program, in contrast, does not have resources to treat undocumented women.

PRISONS

Florida prison officials make a special effort to ensure that all pregnant women are tested for HIV, and believe that almost all of them are tested. Testing is not, however, strictly required. Incarcerated women are given pre-test counseling in a group before their first physician visit.

BARRIERS TO CARE

Participants said that domestic violence is one of the most important barriers to testing. Many women do not disclose the results of their HIV test to their partners. They fear the results and lack the skills to negotiate sexual behavior, and there are no resources to guarantee women a safe environment. One participant said there needs to be consideration of whom to tell and how to tell them, and an escape plan for when partners become violent.

Participants feel that few HIV-positive mothers in Florida are injection drug users, although many of their partners are. Some use non-injection drugs such as crack.

Outside of the Miami and Tampa areas, perinatal HIV care is less intense than in other areas. In the Gainesville area, for instance, one small HIV center deals with cases from 13 counties. The doctors in this area rarely see HIV cases, and hence are not proficient at pre-test counseling. There are, however, two or three new HIV cases (in adults) per week, about one quarter of whom are seen by private physicians. Despite the presence of a state university medical center, the system has nothing to offer to these private patients.

There is an increasing number of repeat pregnancies in HIV-infected women in Florida, according to participants, and some of these are planned. Women see themselves as having more options since the ACTG 076 (AIDS Clinical Trials Group protocol number 76) results have been made public. In Orlando, there are few abortions among HIV-infected women, in large part because there are no resources to pay for them.

SITE ADDRESSES AND PARTICIPANTS

Representing the committee were Ezra Davidson, Jr., committee vice-chair, and Michael Stoto, study director.

Florida Department of Corrections
Office of Health Services
2601 Blair Stone Road
Tallahassee, FL 32399-2500
    Sara A. Straub

Florida Family AIDS Network
College of Public Health
University of South Florida
Tampa, FL 33612-3805
    Jennifer Allen, Managed Care Coordinator
    Marylin Merida, Program Coordinator

Orlando Regional Healthcare System
Nurse Educator
600 Courtland Street
Suite 500
Orlando, FL 32804
    Suellen T. Cirelli, R.N., B.S.N., ACRN

St. Joseph's Women's Hospital
HIV Obstetrical Liaison/ Perinatal HIV Prevention Program
Social Services Department
3030 W. Martin Luther King Jr. Boulevard
Tampa, FL 33607
    Julie Baltzell, R.N.

Shands Hospital
Department of Obstetrics and Gynecology Women's Clinic
Box 100383 JHMHC, University of Florida
Gainesville, FL 32610
    Diane Biernacki, R.N., RDMS

University of Miami
Department of Family Medicine
1400 NW 10th Avenue
Suite 603B
Miami, FL 33136
    Diana Travieso-Palow, M.S., R.N.

University of South Florida/CMS Department of Pediatrics
One Davis Boulevard, Suite 502
Tampa, FL 33505
    Maite McLeod, R.N., B.S.N., HIV Perinatal Nurse Case Manager

HIV Testing and Perinatal Transmission: Thoughts from an HIV-Positive Mother

Rebecca Denison*

Who Am I and Why Am I Here?

I am the HIV-positive mother of 2-year-old HIV-negative twin girls. I don't have data, graphs, or slides to present. What I do have is my own experience of having HIV for 15 years, and seven years' experience listening to the experiences of other women with HIV/AIDS.

In November 1995 I went public at a conference and in the WORLD newsletter about being a pregnant woman with HIV. Since then, I have spoken with over 100 HIV-positive women about HIV and pregnancy. Some were positive and newly pregnant or considering pregnancy. Others were pregnant and had just been diagnosed HIV-positive. I hope that what I share here can help us all focus on how we can improve the health and welfare of HIV-positive women and their babies.

The Case for Universal Testing

Every pregnant woman should be offered an HIV test. Whether or not a provider perceives a woman to belong to a "high-risk group," the fact that she is pregnant should be evidence enough that she has engaged in high-risk behavior. Even if she is monogamous and has never shared needles, there is no way to know the sexual history of her current or previous partners.

---

*Ms. Denison is the founder and executive director of the Women Organized to Respond to Life-Threatening Diseases (WORLD). The following statement was presented on April 1, 1998 to the Committee on Perinatal Transmission of HIV, Institute of Medicine, National Academy of Sciences.

In my experience, many providers are still thinking in terms of high-risk groups rather than behaviors. The data presented today bear this out, in the number of women who were educated and counseled by their doctors, yet chose not to test because they did not perceive themselves to be at risk.

The majority of positive women I've talked to were told by a medical provider that they were not at risk, only to discover their infection when they became severely symptomatic. Most women accept their providers' assessment of risk. During the first seven years of my own infection, from 1983 to 1990, no medical provider ever brought up the subject of HIV or testing. Had I not gone to a test site (to support a friend who was afraid to get tested), I likely would not have been tested until I was pregnant. It frightens me to think that even then, I might have been discouraged from testing.

Voluntary Versus Mandatory Testing

Whenever I am around HIV-positive women and the issue of mandatory testing during pregnancy comes up, they usually say, "It *should* be mandatory." This should be explored further, however, because the average person does not distinguish between "universal" offering of "voluntary" testing and "mandatory" testing.

I recently sat in a group with three HIV-positive mothers. One was diagnosed HIV-positive when her ex-husband died of AIDS, one was diagnosed when she and her baby were simultaneously hospitalized with PCP [*Pneumocystis carinii* pneumonia], and the third was diagnosed during her pregnancy upon the death of her first child due to a "mysterious" illness. All said they believed testing should be mandatory. When I asked these women if they would have accepted testing if it had been offered during pregnancy, all three said "yes." When I ask if they'd rather be invited or told to test, they say they'd rather be invited.

Positive women, whether pregnant or not, tell me they feel more comfortable when their doctor offers choices, listens, and responds to their questions and concerns, and respects their treatment choices. Likewise, those whose doctors tell them what to do without soliciting or acknowledging the patient's concerns, consistently tell me that they don't like going to the doctor and that they are afraid to tell (and don't tell) when they aren't following the treatment regimen prescribed.

Testing is not an end in itself. For testing to save lives, it must lead to care. My concern with mandatory testing is that it may lead the minority who don't want to be tested to avoid prenatal care altogether, while undermining the doctor–patient relationship for the majority who do want to know their status. If the majority of women are going to agree to be tested, isn't it better that the woman and doctor work together as a team? In my opinion, universal offering of voluntary testing is the best way to identify infected mothers and at-risk babies while enhancing the woman's trust in the medical provider and system.

It's interesting to note that many women with infected children have told me, "I'll always wonder if I'd been tested during pregnancy if my child would have AIDS now." Universally they say they would have taken AZT [azidothymidine;

now called zidovudine (ZDV)] if offered. Occasionally, a mother will tell me, "I'm glad I didn't know, because I might have had an abortion and even though my child has AIDS, I'm glad he/she was born."

Reasons Why Women Might Not Test

Why would any woman choose not to test? If we want to save lives, we need to understand the reasons women might not test, and seek ways to address these concerns.

• Some think they are not at risk. ("I've only ever been with my husband.") We need them to understand that by virtue of being pregnant, they have engaged in a high-risk behavior with someone whose history cannot be known with certainty.
• Some fear that the anxiety of waiting for results (or of testing positive) will drive them to use drugs or alcohol. I have met many women who gave up drugs or alcohol when they found out they were pregnant, but whose ability to abstain was not very stable. If such a woman begins to use drugs but also takes AZT, how will this affect the fetus? If the woman begins to use drugs and avoids prenatal care altogether, how will this affect the fetus?
• Some fear violence, rejection or abandonment by a partner or family members if their HIV status is discovered (which it likely would be if she started taking AZT five times a day). One woman in our community did in fact die when she fell from a fourth story window while trying to escape an abusive partner. Another told us, "My husband hasn't touched me at all or shared dishes with me in the two years since my baby and I were diagnosed." Another became destitute (her baby was born into poverty) when her partner abandoned her.
• Some fear that their babies will be taken away by the authorities because of their HIV status. Whether this fear is perceived or real, it needs to be addressed. One woman I know went through six pregnancies that all ended in miscarriage. She did not seek prenatal care for the first five, afraid that being homeless *and* HIV-positive would result in her child being taken away at birth.
• Some fear that they will be forced to take AZT against their will. While most women are grateful that a drug exists that can reduce transmission, there is also a lot of fear and mistrust of AZT in many communities that can't be dismissed. There have been rumors of a woman who was required to take AZT during pregnancy as a condition of her parole, and of others reported to Child Protective Services for refusing AZT.

Testing Does Not Equal Care

Identifying positive women during pregnancy will save lives only to the degree that identification leads to care for both mother and baby. Unfortunately, I know of many examples of gaps in connecting testing to care.

- For example, in the "East Bay," we have no obstetrician or perinatologist specialized in the care of HIV-positive pregnant women. This means that if a woman from Oakland, Richmond, Berkeley, or Fremont (all high-incidence cities) wants specialty care, she must travel; across the Bay Bridge to BAPAC [Bay Area Perinatal AIDS Center] at San Francisco General Hospital (an hour by public transportation).

- "Sandra" delivered her baby in a high-incidence city to a doctor and medical team who knew she was HIV-positive. They—not just the doctor, but—the entire team forgot to administer intravenous AZT.

- "Alicia" recently delivered a baby prematurely, in her seventh month of pregnancy. Her HIV status and pregnancy were known to medical providers, but she did not keep medical appointments. As of the date of delivery, she had never taken any antiretrovirals.

- "Meg" tested positive at five months of pregnancy in a rural town. Her doctor handed her the results of her blood work and said, "You're HIV-positive. I can't treat you. Here are your lab results (T-cell counts, etc.) but I can't tell you what they mean."

- When "Kim" asked her doctor if he knew how to manage an HIV pregnancy he said, "Oh, yes. Don't worry. We use gloves during the delivery with everyone." This same doctor, who knew she was HIV-positive, asked her three times, "Now, tell me again why you're not planning to breast-feed?"

- "Natalie" had an undetectable viral load on a combination of two drugs when she found out she was pregnant. An obstetrician who had no experience with HIV told her to go off her drugs immediately because she was in her first trimester. Almost immediately her viral load went from undetectable to over 130,000 [copies/mL].

- "Kelly" tested positive at age 22, during a planned pregnancy. Within an hour of her diagnosis she was told, "We can schedule the abortion today." It was only after she terminated her pregnancy that she learned that there would have been a good chance of the baby being born HIV-free.

- "Sheila" knew she was HIV-positive when she became pregnant by accident. Her doctor put her on AZT and d4T (a combination that is contraindicated in any HIV-positive person, pregnant or not). When her baby was four weeks old, her doctor administered the RNA PCR [polymerase chain reaction] test (which gives a number value) for the baby instead of the DNA PCR test (Which shows "positive" or "negative"). The viral load count of 100 that was reported by the lab may be a false positive, or it may not. Because of her doctor's lack of experience and knowledge, she has either gone through an unnecessary scare, or lost valuable time in which she could have had the option of intervening with a combination of antiviral drugs.

- "Andrea" asked me if she should go to BAPAC and pay out of pocket because she was concerned that her HMO [health maintenance organization] was not qualified to manage her pregnancy. I told her I thought specialty care was valuable, but that I could not assess for her whether she could afford it. She stayed with her HMO. At the delivery, there were problems, which she believes BAPAC could have handled. The baby died a few days after birth, having tested negative by DNA PCR.

  • "Celeste" begged for a C-section [cesarean section] after her bag of waters had been ruptured for over eight hours, but her doctor refused. The baby was born after 22 hours' labor, with two broken bones.

  • "Karen" called me two days after her diagnosis, in the fifth month of pregnancy. She already had her AZT but didn't know what a T-cell was, or the difference between HIV and AIDS. Given her overall lack of understanding of her diagnosis, it is hard to imagine that the decision to start AZT was an informed one.

Specialty Care Does Save Lives, So Why Isn't It Adequately Funded?

For me, all the political debate about testing pregnant women feels disingenuous. During the past couple of years as universal offering of voluntary testing has been implemented in California, BAPAC (the only specialty clinic providing care to HIV-positive pregnant women in Northern California) has undergone cut after cut after cut in their funding. It makes no sense. Here we have a program that we know works, that we know saves lives, that we know has reduced transmission rates to nearly zero, and yet they struggle for funding and staffing.

If the real goal is saving lives, then regional centers such as BAPAC need to be adequately funded and staffed, to provide direct services to HIV-positive pregnant women, and to provide training and consultation to providers of women who choose to stay with their regular obstetrician or perinatologist.

Where Is the Procedural Standard of Care?

Finally we have guidelines on the use of antiretroviral therapy in pregnancy. Women have been clamoring for them (for this reason we published a "translation" in the April 1998 WORLD).* But the guidelines leave much unsaid. What about C-sections? Amniocentesis? Fetal scalp monitors? Rupturing membranes?

I know that the research is confusing and at times contradictory, but this should not justify silence. Providers attempting to care for HIV-positive pregnant women who cannot afford the luxury of being specialists need guidance.

---

*WORLD. HIV and pregnancy: The basics. *WORLD Newsletter* 84, April 1998.

Where's the Research?

There's a lot we don't know, that we need to know ASAP. Like how these drugs will affect our babies, in the long and short term. Like how choosing a strategy for reducing perinatal transmission will affect treatment choices for ourselves.

One study presented at the National Women and AIDS Conference in May showed that Viracept reduced certain hormones found in birth control pills. Does this mean we may begin to see unplanned pregnancies in women taking Viracept who use the pill for contraception? What about the seven "unplanned" pregnancies reported in the new antiviral guidelines for women taking Delavirdine? We may wish everyone was using condoms, but if in reality some are using "the pill" and there are antivirals or other HIV drugs that reduce its effectiveness, we'd do better to find out sooner than later.

Harm Reduction Models Are Needed for HIV-Positive People Who Want to Be Parents

Medical providers consulted about HIV and pregnancy face an ethical dilemma. No one wants to feel responsible for encouraging a couple to take action that could result in a child being born HIV-infected. However, we must come to terms with the fact that many couples are determined to conceive a baby, and acknowledge that there are ways to help them reduce the risk of partners or infants from becoming infected. In my experience, many couples are desperate for pre-conception counseling. They have questions like:

- "How can I conceive with the least risk of infecting my partner (or of my partner infecting me, or of either becoming re-infected, possibly with a drug-resistant strain)?" Some couples time ovulation and have sex only once a month, others poke holes in the condom or have insertive sex only when the man is ready to ejaculate; however, many who lack information about any other way just have unsafe sex until the time the woman conceives.
- "Does my husband's viral load affect the risk of the baby getting HIV? (These women have rarely considered the risk that they might become infected with a protease inhibitor-resistant strain of HIV.)
- "If my viral load is high, what's the safest drug combination for me to be on at the time of conception and during the first trimester?" (Wouldn't it be better for women to plan this ahead of time rather than experiment with switching drugs during pregnancy?)
- "If my husband is HIV-positive but I am not, should I take AZT to prevent becoming infected when we have sex to conceive? Should he take medications to reduce his viral load to reduce the risk of infecting me?"

Often providers are so uncomfortable about answering these questions that their patients shut down, stop asking questions, and proceed with conceiving without the benefit of potentially harm-reducing measures.

Other Prevention Needs

I support "universal" testing, because too many medical providers dismiss the risk of their patients actually testing positive. This is evident in the very common practice of telling wornen, "Don't worry about it. We'll call you if there's a problem."

Well, I've spoken to the ones who were unexpected "problems." All too often they got a call from a shocked doctor's nurse at 5 p.m. on a Friday afternoon saying, "Your test is positive. You should see a specialist. I can't see you." Or a nurse calls to say, "The doctor wants to see you right away." Without saying anything more, the woman knows her diagnosis, and all too often it comes when she is at home caring for children, or at work surrounded by co-workers. Imagine trying to "keep it together"—find a baby-sitter, drive a car, talk to your teenage children arriving home from school—under these circumstances.

We want pregnant HIV-positive women to stop using drugs, but how many programs allow them to keep custody of their children? How many are AIDS-sensitive? I have heard of many in which staff require residents known to be positive to use their own dishes and utensils. How appealing is that to a woman who is HIV-positive, addicted, and scared?

Preventing Perinatal Infection Should Begin by Preventing HIV in Women

Most pregnant women are infected by men, yet there is very little social marketing that clearly tells men who have sex with women that condoms are their responsibility. Most prevention programs, posters, brochures, etc., tell women to "make" men use condoms. Let's be honest. Hasn't society kind of given up on men? If we hadn't, we'd tell *them* to wear condoms, instead of their partners.

For men to take steps to protect women, they need to value their lives and the lives of their partners. Yet there are few programs designed for men who self-identify as heterosexual to get support to come to terms with their diagnosis (and issues like drug use history or sexual orientation), and to take responsibility for protecting their health and others.

Women Are Interested in Protecting Their Babies

When I first tested positive, I thought women who got pregnant knowing they had HIV were selfish and irresponsible. It took a long time to admit that I was jealous that they had the courage to do the one thing I wanted to do. Now that I've done it, I get calls from women from all over the country and literally around the world. A small minority are in denial, but most are deeply concerned about protecting the health of their babies. One couple saved up money to fly from the Midwest to consult with BAPAC. In another case, my agency provided Greyhound tickets to a woman and her husband who traveled over 12 hours by bus so that she could deliver at BAPAC. This woman had a substance abuse problem, no money, no place to stay, and social workers who regarded her as an unfit mother, but she was willing to do whatever it took to protect her baby from being born infected.

Other Services Must Be Included in the Strategy to Reduce Perinatal Transmission

Substance abuse is one of the main factors in women avoiding prenatal care. To enhance the likelihood of HIV-positive pregnant women seeking care, we need HIV-sensitive treatment programs that will take pregnant women.

Breast-feeding is contraindicated in the United States for HIV-positive women. Yet when we go to WIC [Special Supplemental Nutrition Program for Women, Infants, and Children] to get formula (my formula bill for twins was $250 a month), we have to go through a nutrition class that pressures everyone to breast-feed without acknowledging that those with HIV shouldn't. My nutrition consultation was held in a room with an open door, and 10 other women sitting outside who could hear everything. I disclosed, but what would another woman do? WIC should include HIV education and awareness in their program. Also, WIC does not cover the full cost of formula. Perhaps in the case of poor HIV-positive women who do not have other ways of feeding their children, it should.

Prenatal care is critical in reducing the risk of transmission. But it's difficult for a woman with no car or child care to trek across town (or across the state) with her kids for medical appointments. Oakland did not allocate Ryan White funds to respite care until after I moved to another city where family could help with child care; and recently mothers who have since received that service have been informed that the hours available have been cut.

Doctors Should Be Supported to Provide Universal Testing

I've been a trainer at several state-sponsored trainings on the new pregnancy testing legislation. Doctors don't come. They send nurses and secretaries. They're too busy. They don't think their patients are at risk. They mostly want to know how to comply with the law without losing a lot of time.

Who can blame them? They've been mandated to offer testing, but don't have a mechanism to get paid for what it really takes to do good pre-test counseling and education. It makes no sense to me. It's like telling restaurants that sell BBQ ribs, "You have to serve a dinner salad first, because it's good for people's health, but you can't bill for it." There needs to be a mechanism for reimbursing the cost of HIV education and testing, with protections to avoid coercion. And there needs to be widespread dissemination of educational materials for providers and their patients. Toward this end, the flip chart and materials presented today from California are very helpful.

Like It or Not, Everything Is Political

Health care is political. This could be a paper in itself, so let me just say that threatening to turn HIV-documented women who seek health care in to the Immigration and Naturalization Service, or to deny them prenatal care, can't possibly be in the best interest of the baby that will be born a U.S. citizen (and thus our responsibility).

Trust Is the Foundation on Which All Else Is Built or Collapses

When we look at data, slides, and numbers, it is easy to lose track of factors that are difficult to measure. In my experience, trust between a patient and provider is the most important element. With it, all things are possible. Without it, the patient probably won't even get prenatal care, let alone engage in other health interventions. Whether a woman's fears (of being judged, of having her child taken away, of her confidentiality being violated) are true or false is irrelevant; until proven otherwise, her fears are 100 percent real to her.

In many communities there is a great distrust of AZT. I have heard of providers who respond to a patient's fear by saying, "OK, then, we'll give you ZDV or retrovir instead." These are, of course, all the same drug. When the patients discover what's happened, trust is undermined.

I went eagerly to every prenatal appointment, despite tremendous inconvenience and having to travel from another city, because of my trust in my providers, and because of the respect I felt from them. Rather than treat me as a potential vector or threat to my unborn child, they treated me as a woman with the power to protect my child. In contrast, when "Angela" became pregnant, she told me she was afraid to seek prenatal care because the doctor in the clinic who cares for her HIV-infected child had told her she'd better not get pregnant again. He meant well, but her fear of being judged or criticized by him led to a dangerous situation for her unborn child.

When I couldn't get any babies to take Septra, despite all kinds of tricks including hiding it in formula during 2 a.m. feedings, I told my providers. At BAPAC they were disappointed, but continued to work with me, and talked to me about symptoms that should prompt an immediate call. In contrast, my regular pediatrician treated me like a bad person, and refused to answer my questions or discuss my concerns. When I eventually got my children's files (it took over two months and $20 to get about six pages), all it said under family history was, "Mother is HIV-positive" in big bold letters. When my child got sick, I was afraid to take her in for care. Now that's a dangerous situation.

I was honest about the fact that I gave up trying to give my babies Septra. That's just the kind of person I am. Well, a lot of women called me to say that they had given up too, but that they had never shared this information with their pediatricians. I encouraged them to discuss it with their providers, but most are afraid.

What will happen to the babies that are positive whose mothers are afraid to have a frank discussion about compliance with their pediatricians? Missing a couple of doses of Septra is not a disaster, but with so few choices available to children with AIDS, missing a few doses of a triple drug combination that includes a protease inhibitor could wipe out their treatment options for life.

Pregnancy is an emotional time in a woman's life, a time of reflection, of learning to trust one's own body, and of having to trust one's inner voice. Regardless of HIV status, the choice to become pregnant is rarely a rational one. (The planet is not underpopulated. Few people suffer from too much free time or money. Morning sickness is not pleasant. Neither are diapers.) Women who choose to become pregnant or continue a pregnancy are usually acting mostly on their emotions, and they will pursue prenatal care and treatment decisions in the same way. I knew all the great facts about AZT's ability to reduce perinatal transmission, but I was afraid to take it until another woman with HIV told me how she did a blessing ritual with hers first. Hokey as it sounds, that worked for me.

If I had been forced to take AZT before I was ready, I likely would have gone running away from prenatal care rather than feel drawn to it. How many of you like to be told what to do? How many respond to orders with an urge to do just the opposite? I could be wrong, but I'm inclined to think that we should offer HIV testing to every woman who is pregnant. I also think that rather than forcing her to do it, we should focus our efforts and money on addressing the issues that will motivate women to want to get tested and get prenatal care. Then, hopefully, she'll be drawn to the benefits of trustworthy and qualified prenatal care, and the rewards that a respectful partnership between provider and patient can offer.

A poster I saw by the Pediatric AIDS Foundation provides a good example of this. It shows all kinds of beautiful babies and the text reads: "All healthy. All HIV free. It's amazing what a mother can do." It's positive, encouraging, respectful, and inspiring. When approached in this way, what woman wouldn't want to test?

Planned HIV Pregnancies May Increase Along with Increased Life Expectancies

In 1994 I enrolled in a study at the NIH [National Institutes of Health]. When I was told that my PCR test came back "undetectable" a whole world opened up for me. For years I had not dared to imagine a future beyond 6–12 months. When this test result led me to dream of actually having a future, the fact that I wanted to be a mother more than anything else in the world became undeniable. In 1994, "undetectable" viral load tests were practically unheard of, but in 1998 they are very common. Women call me on a weekly basis who are having this same experience. For many, if there's a future awaiting them, they want a baby to be part of it.

Conclusion

My pregnancy and prenatal care lasted 9 months. I threw up for 5 months, and spent the other 4 on bed rest. I had a scare with premature labor that had to be stopped with medicines that made me feel crazy. Big deal. It was only nine months.

I'll be a mother—rocking, dressing, teaching, feeding, nurturing, disciplining, and loving my children—for the rest of my life. There are lots of babysitters, foster parents, grandparents, and adoptive families out there, but nobody will ever love my children the way I do. And while my children deeply love and trust many adults, none of them can take my place. So please, let's remember as we all work so hard to protect babies from being born with HIV, to work equally hard for the health of their mothers, so we can be there for them, care for them, and see them grow up.

Thank you for letting me share my thoughts with you today. I realize I didn't always focus directly on the issue of testing, but I felt compelled to share some of the "real-life" stories that can tell us a lot about how to save lives. Make the best decision you can about testing. But remember, when that decision is made there's a lot more that needs to be done to ensure that those who test positive have access to the kind of care that will ensure the well-being of women and their children. Thank you.

Human Immunodeficiency Virus Antibody Testing Among Women 15–44: Results from the 1995 National Survey of Family Growth

Maria Hewitt

National estimates of the use of HIV tests among women of reproductive-age are available from the 1995 National Survey of Family Growth (NSFG) conducted by the National Center for Health Statistics (NCHS, 1997). As part of this survey, 10,847 women were interviewed in their homes from January to October 1995. The survey response rate was 79%. Interviews lasted an average of 103 minutes and covered the following topics: pregnancy and birth history, marriage and cohabitation history, sexual partner history, contraceptive use, diseases related to fertility (e.g., pelvic inflammatory disease, sexually transmitted diseases [STDs]), HIV-related behaviors, and use of HIV tests. To ensure the confidentiality of responses to potentially sensitive questions, a small part of the interview was self-administered. Women listened over headphones to questions on topics such as abortion, sex partner history, and HIV-related behaviors and entered answers directly into laptop computers. This technique, called audio-CASI (computer-assisted self-interviewing), improves reporting of sensitive behaviors (NCHS, 1997).

The tables that follow show HIV test use among women of childbearing age by selected sociodemographic characteristics, pregnancy status, and HIV risk status. HIV test use is shown for women who were pregnant at the time of the interview, had completed a pregnancy in the last year, or had received pre- or postnatal care within the last year (1,472 women representing 13% of the population were pregnant, or recently pregnant using these criteria; these women are referred to as "pregnant" in the tables).

HIV test use is also shown by HIV risk status. A total of 691 women representing an estimated 6% of the population report specific risk behaviors (e.g., injection drug use or sex with an injection drug user), or a moderate to high self-perceived risk of being HIV-infected themselves or of having had sex with someone infected with HIV.

HIV test use is shown in three ways: (1) "all HIV tests" includes self-reported HIV tests and any mentions of blood donation since 1985; (2) "any self-reported HIV test" excludes mentions of blood donation when the respondent does not specifically report having had an HIV test; and (3) "HIV test in last 12 months" is limited to self-reported HIV testing.

All rates and population counts are weighted to provide national estimates. Variance estimates for these HIV test use rates and logistic regression model parameters were calculated using the Taylor series method taking into account the complex design of the survey (STATA statistical software).

PRELIMINARY FINDINGS

Self-Reported HIV Test Use Among Reproductive-Age Women

- From 1990 to 1995, self-reported HIV test use increased from 26% to 35% among reproductive-age women (Table J.1).
- In 1995, pregnant women were almost twice as likely as non-pregnant women to have been tested for HIV (60% versus 31%) (Table J.2).
- Women at high-risk for HIV are almost twice as likely as those at low risk to have been tested for HIV (64% versus 33%). Similarly, there are high rates of HIV testing among women reporting at least one STD in their lifetime (53%) and women reporting six or more lifetime sex partners (49%) (Table J.3).
- Nearly nine of ten pregnant women (87%) at high risk for HIV report having been tested for HIV. HIV testing occurred within the year for two-thirds of high-risk pregnant women (67%) (Table J.4).

Location of Self-Reported HIV Tests

- The most common sites of HIV testing among reproductive-age women are private doctor's offices or heath maintenance organizations (HMOs) (46%), public health department or other clinics (27%), and hospitals (16%). Teenagers, those with lower educational attainment, and the poor are more likely to use public health department and other clinics than private doctor's offices or HMOs (Table J.5).
- Pregnant women are more likely than non-pregnant women to have been tested in the last 12 months at a doctor's office or HMO (62% versus 48%) (Table J.8).

TABLE J.1 Number of Women 15–44 Years of Age and Percent Ever Tested for HIV, by Source of Test Information and Selected Demographic Characteristics: United States, 1990 and 1995[a]

Characteristic	Number of Women (thousands)		Percent Ever Tested					
			Self-Reported Tests[b] (standard error)		All Tests[c] (standard error)			
	1990	1995	1990	1995	1990	1995		
All women[d]	58,381	60,201	25.6	34.7 (0.6)	34.9	47.9 (0.6)		
Race and ethnicity								
Hispanic	5,547	6,703	23.8	38.9 (1.8)	29.8	46.6 (1.5)		
Black, not Hispanic	7,526	8,210	28.5	45.5 (1.3)	34.8	50.8 (1.4)		
White, not Hispanic	42,836	42,521	25.4	32.2 (0.7)	35.8	48.1 (0.7)		
Education								
Less than 12 years	5,618	15,151	24.6	29.9 (1.2)	31.0	36.1 (1.2)		
12 years	17,247	19,987	23.1	35.1 (0.9)	31.3	47.5 (1.0)		
13 years or more	27,033	24,763	28.6	37.3 (0.9)	39.9	55.6 (0.86)		
Marital status								
Never married	20,123	22,679	26.0	31.1 (0.9)	35.7	44.2 (0.9)		
Married	31,417	29,673	23.6	34.2 (0.8)	32.5	48.4 (0.8)		
Formerly married	6,841	7,849	33.5	46.9 (1.3)	43.4	56.8 (1.3)		

Age						
15–19	8,483	8,924	21.5	20.9 (1.3)	28.7	29.0 (1.4)
20–24	9,154	8,946	27.0	40.3 (1.4)	40.8	55.5 (1.5)
25–29	10,637	9,795	33.4	44.6 (1.4)	40.9	60.1 (1.4)
30–34	11,091	10,982	27.5	42.0 (1.5)	37.1	54.6 (1.4)
35–39	10,111	11,297	22.0	33.3 (1.3)	31.5	46.0 (1.3)
40–44	8,905	10,014	20.3	26.4 (1.0)	28.5	41.3 (1.2)
Residence in metropolitan area						
MSA, central city	12,727	18,551	31.9	39.8 (0.9)	39.9	51.3 (0.9)
MSA, other	29,981	29,303	26.1	33.5 (0.8)	36.4	47.7 (0.8)
Non-MSA	11,979	12,348	21.4	30.0 (1.5)	32.4	43.2 (1.5)
Region						
Northeast	11,226	11,496	28.2	32.1 (1.2)	36.9	45.2 (1.5)
South	18,603	20,241	28.0	38.9 (1.1)	39.5	51.6 (1.0)
Midwest	14,453	14,525	23.8	29.4 (1.1)	34.0	44.3 (1.2)
West	10,405	13,938	25.4	36.3 (1.5)	33.5	48.5 (1.3)
Poverty-level income						
0–149%	7,918	13,588	28.1	41.8 (1.2)	35.5	49.6 (1.2)
150% or more	41,980	46,613	25.9	32.6 (0.7)	36.0	47.4 (0.7)

NOTE: MSA = metropolitan statistical area.

[a]Data from 1990 from Wilson, 1993.

[b]Includes only test reported in response to the question: "Have you ever had your blood tested for infection with the AIDS virus?"

[c]Category includes all tests for HIV infection, including those done in connection with blood donation (i.e., all reporting a blood donation since March 1985).

[d]Includes women classified as "other" races, not shown separately because of small sample size.

TABLE J.2 Number of Women 15–44 Years of Age by Pregnancy Status, and Percent Tested for HIV, by Selected Demographic Characteristics: United States, 1995[a]

Characteristic	Number of Women (thousands)		HIV Test Last 12 Months (percent/standard error)		Any Self-Reported Tests[b] (percent/standard error)	
	Pregnant	Not Pregnant	Pregnant	Not Pregnant	Pregnant	Not Pregnant
All women[c]	7,789	52,141	41.9 (1.4)	13.7 (0.4)	59.9 (1.5)	30.9 (0.6)
Race and ethnicity						
Hispanic	1,245	5,448	47.4 (4.2)	16.1 (1.2)	60.3 (4.1)	33.9 (1.8)
Black, not Hispanic	1,166	7,032	55.5 (3.1)	24.3 (1.2)	71.4 (2.7)	41.2 (1.4)
White, not Hispanic	5,020	37,268	37.8 (1.8)	11.5 (0.5)	57.5 (2.1)	28.7 (0.7)
Education						
Less than 12 years	2,025	13,081	54.5 (3.0)	13.0 (0.7)	69.2 (2.8)	23.8 (1.0)
12 years	2,655	17,250	42.1 (2.3)	14.0 (0.7)	59.4 (2.8)	31.3 (0.9)
13 years or more	3,075	21,545	33.6 (2.0)	13.8 (0.6)	54.2 (2.2)	34.9 (0.9)
Marital status						
Never married	2,039	20,593	51.3 (2.8)	15.7 (0.7)	65.4 (2.8)	27.7 (0.9)
Married	5,024	24,457	36.1 (1.8)	10.2 (0.6)	55.2 (1.8)	29.8 (0.8)
Formerly married	726	7,092	55.8 (4.9)	19.8 (1.1)	77.1 (3.9)	43.8 (1.3)
Age						
15–19	957	7,953	55.3 (4.0)	9.9 (0.9)	68.7 (4.2)	15.2 (1.1)
20–24	1,813	7,086	45.3 (3.1)	18.6 (1.2)	61.2 (3.2)	34.9 (1.5)
25–29	2,293	7,443	39.8 (2.9)	18.7 (1.2)	58.1 (2.8)	40.4 (1.6)

30–34	1,802	9,126	40.1 (2.9)	14.5 (0.9)	61.5 (3.1)	38.1 (1.5)
35–39	710	10,544	28.9 (4.2)	13.0 (0.8)	47.5 (5.0)	32.4 (1.3)
40–44	213	9,748	33.8 (8.2)	9.6 (0.8)	55.5 (8.2)	25.8 (1.0)
Residence in metropolitan area						
MSA, central city	2,617	15,891	48.1 (2.6)	16.8 (0.8)	66.7 (2.4)	35.3 (0.9)
MSA, other	3,631	25,499	38.5 (2.0)	12.9 (0.6)	55.9 (2.3)	30.2 (0.8)
Non-MSA	1,542	10,750	39.4 (3.5)	11.0 (0.8)	57.8 (4.1)	26.0 (1.4)
Region						
Northeast	1,431	10,009	40.2 (3.2)	12.9 (0.9)	58.6 (2.7)	28.3 (1.3)
South	2,587	17,569	51.6 (2.8)	16.0 (0.8)	70.3 (2.3)	34.3 (1.1)
Midwest	1,870	12,553	34.3 (2.3)	10.6 (0.8)	51.9 (3.2)	25.9 (1.1)
West	1,901	12,011	37.5 (3.2)	14.2 (0.9)	54.8 (3.7)	33.3 (1.4)
Poverty-level income						
0–149%	2,306	11,250	51.1 (2.5)	17.6 (1.0)	66.5 (2.3)	36.7 (1.3)
150% or more	5,483	40,892	38.0 (1.7)	12.6 (0.5)	57.1 (1.8)	29.3 (0.7)

NOTE: MSA = metropolitan statistical area.

[a] A total of 1,472 survey respondents reported that they either were pregnant at the time of the interview (430), had completed a pregnancy within 12 months of the interview (1,039), or had received pre- or postnatal care in the last 12 months (1,140). Women referred to as "pregnant" in this table are women who were pregnant, or recently pregnant, at the time of the interview.

[b] Includes only tests reported in response to the question: "Have you ever had your blood tested for infection with the AIDS virus?" Mentions of blood donation since 1985 are not included.

[c] Includes women classified as "other" races, not shown separately because of small sample size.

TABLE J.3   Number of Women 15–44 Years of Age Reporting AIDS Risk Behaviors, and Percent Ever Tested for HIV: United States, 1995

		Percent Ever Tested	
Characteristic	Number of Women (thousands)	Any Self-Reported Test[a] (standard error)	All Tests[b] (standard error)
All women	60,201	34.7 (0.6)	47.9 (0.6)
HIV risk			
Moderate/high HIV risk[c]	3,672	63.9 (2.0)	68.5 (1.8)
Low HIV risk	56,528	32.8 (0.6)	46.6 (0.6)
STD history			
At least one STD reported in lifetime[d]	6,218	53.2 (1.8)	66.2 (1.7)
No STD in lifetime	53,983	32.6 (0.7)	45.8 (0.6)
Number of sexual partners in lifetime			
None	6,196	6.8 (0.8)	20.0 (1.6)
One	13,838	25.3 (1.0)	39.1 (1.1)
Two–five	22,655	37.5 (0.9)	50.6 (1.0)
Six–more	16,209	48.9 (1.0)	62.2 (1.0)

[a]Includes only tests reported in response to the question: "Have you ever had your blood tested for infection with the AIDS virus?"

[b]Category includes all tests for HIV infection, including those done in connection with blood donation (i.e., all reporting a blood donation since March 1985).

[c]Women reported whether they had a high, moderate, low, or no chance of being currently HIV-infected and whether they had a high, moderate, low, or no chance of having had sex with someone HIV-infected. Anyone indicating "high" or "moderate" on either question was categorized as at HIV-risk. In addition, during the audio-CASI portion of the interview, women reported whether they injected drugs in the last year, shared needles in the last year, or had a sex partner in the last year who had male partners, injected drugs, or shared needles. Any respondents answering yes to these questions were also categorized as at-risk. Using these criteria, 6% of women were categorized as at-risk (i.e., either self-identified as at-risk or reporting risk behaviors).

[d]Includes mention of gonorrhea, chlamydia, syphilis, genital warts, and genital herpes.

Reason for Self-Reported HIV Tests

- The most common reason for HIV testing among reproductive-age women is "just to find out" (36%), as part of prenatal or pregnancy care (25%), and for a hospital procedure, referral by a doctor or other health provider contact (16%) (Table J.6).

- Two-thirds of pregnant women (67%) cite pregnancy as the reason for HIV tests performed within the last 12 months (Table J.8).

Source of Referral for Self-Reported HIV Tests

• When asked whose idea it was to get tested, 42% of reproductive-age women report a doctor or other health care provider, 39% report self, and 7% report an insurer (Table J.7).

• Pregnant women are more than twice as likely as non-pregnant women to report that they were recently tested for HIV upon the recommendation of a health care provider (70% versus 30%) (Table J.8).

Factors Contributing to Test Use among Pregnant and Non-Pregnant Women

• According to multivariate analyses, different factors are predictive of HIV test use for pregnant and non-pregnant women. Among women who are *not pregnant*, being at HIV risk, African American, poor, living in a metropolitan area, being age 20–39, highly educated, and having been formerly married increase HIV test use. Decreased HIV test use occurs among teenagers and residents of the Northeast and Midwest. Being at HIV risk triples the odds of HIV test use among non-pregnant women (Table J.9).

• Among *pregnant* women, many of the sociodemographic predictors of HIV testing observed among non-pregnant women lose significance (i.e., age, race, poverty, and metropolitan area residence). This suggests that pregnancy is serving as a triggering event for testing, irrespective of the woman's characteristics. The role of education is reversed for pregnant women. Here, *lower* educational attainment is predictive of HIV testing. Different geographic patterns emerge for pregnant women, with residents of the South more likely to be tested than residents of other areas. Being at HIV risk quadruples the odds of HIV testing among pregnant women (Table J.9).

REFERENCES

National Center for Health Statistics. Report of final mortality statistics, 1995. *Monthly Vital Statistics Report* 1997; 45(11:Suppl 2).

Wilson JB. Human immunodeficiency virus antibody testing in women 15–44 years of age: United States, 1990. *Advance Data from Vital and Health Statistics.* Number 238, Hyattsville, Md.: National Center for Health Statistics, 1993.

TABLE J.4 Number of Women 15–44 Years of Age by Pregnancy Status and Percent Tested for HIV by Selected Measures of HIV Risk: United States, 1995[a]

Characteristic	Number of Women (thousands)		HIV Test Last 12 Months (percent/standard error)		Any Self-Reported Test[b] (percent/standard error)	
	Pregnant	Not Pregnant	Pregnant	Not Pregnant	Pregnant	Not Pregnant
All women	7,789	52,141	41.9 (1.4)	13.7 (0.4)	59.9 (1.5)	30.9 (0.6)
HIV risk						
Report HIV-risk[c]	595	3,064	66.7 (4.5)	32.3 (2.4)	87.2 (3.6)	59.3 (2.3)
No report of HIV risk	7,194	49,078	39.9 (1.5)	12.5 (0.4)	57.6 (1.6)	29.1 (0.6)
STD history						
At least 1 STD reported in lifetime[d]	1,022	5,162	44.3 (4.4)	21.1 (1.5)	69.3 (3.9)	50.0 (2.0)
No STD in lifetime	6,767	46,979	41.6 (1.5)	12.9 (0.5)	58.5 (1.5)	28.8 (0.7)

Number of sexual partners in lifetime

One	2,063	11,672	34.4 (2.7)	8.4 (0.7)	48.6	21.1 (0.9)
Two–five	3,416	19,142	43.7 (2.6)	15.0 (0.7)	60.6	33.4 (0.9)
Six–more	2,090	14,048	45.5 (2.8)	20.9 (0.9)	68.8	45.9 (1.0)

[a] A total of 1,472 survey respondents reported that they either were pregnant at the time of the interview (430), had completed a pregnancy within 12 months of the interview (1,039), or had received pre- or postnatal care in the last 12 months (1,140). Women referred to as "pregnant" in this table are to women who were pregnant, or recently pregnant, at the time of the interview.

[b] Includes only tests reported in response to the question: "Have you ever had your blood tested for infection with the AIDS virus?"

[c] Women reported whether they had a high, moderate, low, or no chance of being currently HIV-infected and whether they had a high, moderate, low, or no chance of having had sex with someone HIV-infected. Anyone indicating "high" or "moderate" on either question was categorized as at HIV-risk. In addition, during the audio-CASI portion of the interview, women reported whether they injected drugs in last year, shared needles in the last year, or had a sex partner in the last year who had male partners, injected drugs, or shared needles. Any respondents answering yes to these questions were also categorized as at-risk. Using these criteria, 6% of women were categorized as at-risk (i.e., either self-identified as at-risk or reporting risk behaviors).

[d] Includes mention of gonorrhea, chlamydia, syphilis, genital warts, and genital herpes.

TABLE J.5 Number of Women 15–44 Years of Age Self-Reporting Test for HIV and Percent Tested at Specific Locations for Most Recent Test, by Selected Demographic Characteristics: United States, 1995

Characteristic	Number of Women (thousands)	Location of Most Recent HIV Test (percent/standard error)			
		Private Doctor's Office or HMO	Public Health or Other Cline[a]	Hospital or Emergency Room	Other Location[b]
All women[c]	20,889	46.4 (0.1)	26.8 (0.9)	15.9 (0.7)	10.9 (0.6)
Race and ethnicity					
Hispanic	2,606	41.8 (2.0)	36.6 (2.2)	14.1 (1.6)	7.6 (1.2)
Black, not Hispanic	3,734	40.1 (1.8)	38.6 (1.8)	15.0 (1.2)	6.3 (0.9)
White, not Hispanic	13,675	49.1 (1.3)	21.8 (1.1)	16.6 (0.9)	12.5 (0.8)
Education					
Less than 12 years	4,533	36.7 (1.9)	41.3 (1.9)	16.8 (1.4)	5.2 (0.8)
12 years	7,014	48.1 (1.5)	26.0 (1.3)	15.9 (1.1)	10.0 (0.9)
13 years or more	9,244	49.8 (1.3)	20.2 (1.2)	15.6 (1.0)	14.4 (1.1)
Marital status					
Never married	7,058	39.9 (1.8)	38.3 (1.7)	13.6 (1.2)	8.2 (0.9)
Married	10,149	50.9 (1.3)	18.6 (1.0)	16.6 (1.0)	13.9 (0.9)
Formerly married	3,682	46.3 (2.3)	27.7 (1.9)	18.3 (1.5)	7.7 (1.3)

Age					
15–19	1,864	39.2 (2.9)	41.0 (2.7)	14.3 (2.1)	5.5 (1.2)
20–24	3,607	41.9 (2.3)	38.3 (2.1)	13.3 (1.6)	6.5 (1.2)
25–29	4,372	51.6 (2.0)	25.7 (1.9)	13.0 (1.6)	9.7 (1.1)
30–34	4,614	51.8 (1.8)	22.6 (1.6)	14.8 (1.4)	10.9 (1.2)
35–39	3,763	44.6 (2.1)	21.5 (1.7)	20.6 (1.6)	13.2 (1.6)
40–44	2,643	41.6 (2.3)	18.2 (2.0)	20.8 (1.9)	19.4 (1.9)
Residence in metropolitan area					
MSA, central city	7,378	44.1 (1.5)	31.7 (1.5)	15.6 (1.0)	8.6 (1.0)
MSA, other	9,802	48.7 (1.3)	22.6 (1.1)	15.5 (0.9)	13.2 (0.8)
Non-MSA	3,709	44.8 (2.5)	28.4 (2.2)	17.8 (1.9)	9.0 (1.5)
Region					
Northeast	3,686	42.5 (2.7)	25.4 (2.7)	18.2 (1.6)	13.8 (1.7)
South	7,876	46.4 (1.5)	29.4 (1.4)	15.3 (1.0)	8.8 (0.8)
Midwest	4,269	44.6 (2.5)	24.4 (1.8)	20.2 (2.0)	10.8 (1.5)
West	5,058	50.7 (1.4)	25.8 (1.5)	11.6 (1.0)	11.9 (1.0)
Poverty-level income					
0–149%	5,685	36.5 (1.5)	41.1 (1.7)	16.1 (1.2)	6.4 (1.0)
150% or more	15,204	50.1 (1.1)	21.5 (1.0)	15.9 (0.8)	12.5 (0.7)

NOTE: MSA = metropolitan statistical area.

[a]Includes community clinics, family planning, public health, and other clinics.

[b]Includes other places such as school or college, military facility, home, job site, laboratory, or donation site.

[c]Includes women classified as "other" races, not shown separately because of small sample size.

TABLE J.6 Number of Women 15–44 Years of Age Self-Reporting Any Test for HIV and Percent Tested by Reason for the Last Test, by Selected Demographic Characteristics: United States, 1995

Characteristic	Number of Women (thousands)	Reason for Last HIV Test (percent/standard error)				
		HIV Test Only Reason for Visit	Pregnant, Prenatal Care	Hospital Procedure/ Referred by Doctor[a]	Health/ Life Insurance	Other Reason[b]
All women[c]	20,889	35.8 (0.8)	25.0 (0.8)	15.5 (0.7)	8.5 (0.5)	15.2 (0.7)
Race and ethnicity						
Hispanic	2,605	34.9 (2.5)	29.5 (2.5)	13.3 (1.4)	8.4 (1.3)	13.9 (1.6)
Black, not Hispanic	3,735	46.3 (1.6)	20.5 (1.4)	18.1 (1.2)	5.4 (0.8)	9.7 (1.0)
White, not Hispanic	13,674	33.6 (1.1)	25.3 (1.0)	15.3 (0.9)	9.6 (0.7)	16.2 (0.8)
Education						
Less than 12 years	4,533	39.2 (1.8)	29.5 (1.6)	17.4 (1.3)	2.0 (0.5)	11.9 (1.3)
12 years	7,015	36.6 (1.5)	27.8 (1.4)	15.4 (1.1)	7.6 (0.8)	12.6 (1.0)
13 years or more	9,245	33.3 (1.4)	20.8 (1.0)	14.7 (1.0)	12.4 (0.9)	18.8 (1.1)
Marital status						
Never married	7,058	50.8 (1.5)	17.7 (1.2)	15.1 (1.2)	4.0 (0.5)	12.5 (1.1)
Married	10,148	20.1 (1.1)	33.5 (1.3)	15.8 (0.9)	13.0 (0.9)	17.6 (1.0)
Formerly married	3,682	50.3 (2.3)	15.7 (1.6)	15.3 (1.4)	4.9 (1.2)	13.8 (1.4)

Age					
15–19	1,866	47.3 (3.0)	24.3 (2.4)	16.3 (1.9)	1.5 (0.8)	10.6 (1.9)
20–24	3,606	40.2 (2.4)	32.8 (2.3)	10.5 (1.3)	3.0 (0.7)	13.5 (1.7)
25–29	4,373	36.3 (1.9)	31.5 (2.0)	12.4 (1.4)	6.9 (0.9)	13.0 (1.2)
30–34	4,614	28.8 (1.6)	29.1 (1.6)	15.9 (1.4)	10.8 (1.2)	15.5 (1.4)
35–39	3,765	33.0 (2.0)	17.5 (1.5)	20.3 (1.8)	11.9 (1.3)	17.3 (1.6)
40–44	2,644	37.0 (2.4)	7.8 (1.3)	19.5 (1.7)	15.1 (1.8)	20.5 (1.7)
Residence in metropolitan area					
MSA, central city	7,377	39.5 (1.4)	24.5 (1.3)	15.3 (1.2)	6.6 (0.7)	14.1 (1.1)
MSA, other	9,803	33.7 (1.2)	24.7 (1.1)	14.9 (1.0)	10.2 (0.8)	16.6 (0.9)
Non-MSA	3,708	33.8 (2.3)	26.7 (2.3)	17.7 (1.7)	8.0 (1.3)	13.9 (1.6)
Region					
Northeast	3,686	38.3 (1.9)	22.1 (1.9)	11.3 (1.2)	13.3 (1.5)	15.0 (1.5)
South	7,875	35.6 (1.3)	26.0 (1.4)	18.5 (1.0)	6.5 (0.7)	13.3 (1.1)
Midwest	4,268	30.5 (2.1)	26.8 (1.7)	16.6 (1.5)	8.2 (1.0)	17.9 (1.6)
West	5,058	38.6 (1.6)	24.0 (1.4)	12.9 (1.7)	8.5 (0.9)	16.0 (1.3)
Poverty-level income					
0–149%	5,686	39.0 (1.7)	30.2 (1.6)	17.5 (1.4)	1.9 (0.4)	11.4 (1.2)
150% or more	15,204	34.6 (0.9)	23.1 (0.9)	14.8 (0.8)	11.0 (0.7)	16.6 (0.8)

NOTE: MSA = metropolitan statistical area.

[a]Includes being part of routine or general physical exam, and to start or renew birth control.

[b]Includes being part of a marriage license application, for employment, because potentially exposed to HIV, for immigration or visa application, and for school or college.

[c]Includes women classified as "other" races, not shown separately because of small sample size.

TABLE J.7 Number of Women 15–44 Years of Age Self-Reporting Any Test for HIV and Percent Tested by Referral Source for the Last Test, by Selected Demographic Characteristics: United States, 1995

Characteristic	Number of Women (thousands)	Referral source (percent/standard error)			
		Self	Health Care Provider[a]	Insurer	Other[b]
All women[c]	20,889	39.3 (0.9)	42.4 (0.9)	7.3 (0.5)	10.9 (0.6)
Race and ethnicity					
Hispanic	2,606	40.5 (2.5)	42.7 (2.2)	6.7 (1.0)	10.1 (1.1)
Black, not Hispanic	3,734	44.0 (1.8)	44.2 (1.9)	4.0 (0.7)	7.7 (0.9)
White, not Hispanic	13,675	38.2 (1.1)	41.9 (1.1)	8.5 (0.7)	11.4 (0.8)
Education					
Less than 12 years	4,533	38.5 (1.8)	49.2 (1.7)	1.8 (0.5)	10.5 (1.2)
12 years	7,015	40.0 (1.6)	44.4 (1.5)	6.5 (0.7)	9.1 (0.9)
13 years or more	9,244	38.9 (1.2)	37.8 (1.2)	10.7 (0.9)	12.5 (0.9)
Marital status					
Never married	7,057	49.7 (1.5)	36.3 (1.6)	3.2 (0.5)	10.7 (1.0)
Married	10,148	26.8 (1.2)	49.9 (1.4)	11.5 (0.8)	11.8 (0.8)
Formerly married	3,683	54.0 (2.2)	33.2 (2.0)	3.8 (1.0)	9.0 (1.3)
Age					
15–19	1,865	42.8 (3.0)	41.9 (3.0)	1.5 (0.8)	13.9 (2.3)
20–24	3,606	41.9 (2.2)	44.8 (2.3)	2.9 (0.7)	10.5 (1.6)
25–29	4,372	39.2 (2.1)	46.9 (2.3)	5.9 (0.9)	8.0 (1.0)
30–34	4,615	35.7 (1.7)	45.3 (1.8)	9.0 (1.0)	10.0 (1.0)
35–39	3,764	37.9 (2.3)	39.5 (2.2)	9.8 (1.3)	12.8 (1.4)
40–44	2,643	41.8 (2.4)	31.5 (2.0)	13.7 (1.7)	13.0 (1.7)
Residence in metropolitan area					
MSA, central city	7,378	42.4 (1.4)	41.6 (1.4)	5.9 (0.7)	10.1 (1.0)
MSA, other	9,803	38.8 (1.3)	40.9 (1.3)	8.7 (0.7)	11.5 (0.8)
Non-MSA	3,708	34.6 (2.3)	47.9 (2.1)	6.6 (1.2)	10.9 (1.4)
Region					
Northeast	3,687	43.8 (2.1)	35.0 (2.0)	10.1 (1.2)	11.2 (1.3)
South	7,875	37.4 (1.3)	47.1 (1.4)	5.5 (0.7)	9.9 (0.9)
Midwest	4,268	33.2 (1.9)	45.3 (1.9)	7.4 (1.0)	14.0 (1.4)
West	5,057	44.2 (2.1)	38.0 (1.7)	8.1 (0.9)	9.8 (1.1)
Poverty-level income					
0–149%	5,685	40.3 (1.6)	48.4 (1.6)	1.5 (0.4)	9.7 (1.1)
150% or more	15,203	39.0 (1.0)	40.1 (1.0)	9.5 (0.6)	11.4 (0.7)

NOTE: MSA = metropolitan statistical area.

[a] Includes women for whom the idea for testing came from a doctor, health department, and hospital or medical policy.

[b] Includes employer or school, government policy, sexual partner, and family or friends.

[c] Includes women classified as "other" races, not shown separately because of small sample size.

TABLE J.8   Number of Women 15–44 Years of Age by Pregnancy Status and Percent Tested for HIV In Last 12 Months by Location of Testing, Reason for Test, and Source of Referral for HIV Test: United States, 1995[a]

	HIV Test Last 12 Months (percent/standard error)	
	Pregnant (n = 3,266)	Not Pregnant (n = 7,139)
Location of test		
Private doctor's office or HMO	62.0 (2.1)	48.4 (1.6)
Public health or other clinic[b]	28.8 (1.9)	30.2 (1.5)
Hospital or emergency room	7.2 (1.2)	11.1 (1.0)
Other locations[c]	2.0 (0.6)	10.4 (1.0)
Total	100.0	100.0
Reason for test	(n = 3,265)	(n = 7,139)
HIV test only reason for test	19.3 (1.8)	49.5 (1.5)
Pregnant, prenatal care	66.9 (2.1)	3.4 (0.5)
Hospital procedure/doctor referral[d]	7.3 (1.1)	22.0 (1.4)
Health/life insurance	2.9 (0.8)	9.1 (0.8)
Other reason[e]	3.6 (0.8)	16.0 (1.1)
Total	100.0	100.0
Source of referral for test	(n = 3,265)	(n = 7,139)
Self	24.6 (1.8)	51.0 (1.5)
Health care provider[f]	70.0 (2.0)	30.1 (1.4)
Insurer	2.3 (0.7)	7.6 (0.8)
Other[g]	3.1 (0.8)	11.3 (1.1)
Total	100.0	100.0

[a]A total of 1,472 survey respondents reported that they either were pregnant at the time of the interview (430), had completed a pregnancy within 12 months of the interview (1,039), or had received pre- or postnatal care in the last 12 months (1,140). Women referred to as "pregnant" in this table are to women who were pregnant, or recently pregnant, at the time of the interview.

[b]Includes community, family planning, public health, and other clinics.

[c]Includes other places such as school or college, military facility, home, job site, laboratory, or donation site.

[d]Includes being part of routine or general physical exam, and to start or renew birth control.

[e]Includes being part of a marriage license application, for employment, because potentially exposed to HIV, for immigration or visa application, and for school or college.

[f]Includes women for whom the idea for testing came from a doctor, health department, or hospital or medical policy.

[g]Includes employer or school, government policy, sexual partner, and family or friends.

TABLE J.9 Logistic Regression Model, Predictors of Any Self-Reported HIV Test Among Women by Pregnancy Status, United States, 1995[a,b]

Model Parameter	Odds Ratio Coefficient (95 percent confidence interval)			
	Not Pregnant	Pregnant	Not Pregnant	Pregnant
Intercept	−1.2975	−0.4283		
Race/ethnicity				
Black	0.4234[*]	0.2025	1.53 (1.33–1.76)	1.22 (0.86–1.74)
Hispanic	0.0777	−0.1010	1.08 (0.89–1.31)	0.90 (0.61–1.35)
Other race	−0.1686	−0.0903	0.84 (0.59–1.21)	0.91 (0.50–1.68)
White, not Hispanic	—	—		
Marital status				
Never married	−0.0476	0.0857	0.95 (0.82–1.12)	1.09 (0.77–1.55)
Formerly married	0.4834[*]	0.8050[*]	1.62 (1.42–1.86)	2.24 (1.36–3.68)
Married	—	—		
Residence in metro area				
MSA central	0.3227[*]	0.2823	1.38 (1.16–1.65)	1.33 (0.88–2.00)
MSA other	0.2110[*]	−0.0058	1.23 (1.03–1.47)	0.99 (0.66–1.51)
non-MSA	—	—		
Residence-region				
Northeast	−0.2373[*]	0.1695	0.79 (0.66–0.94)	1.18 (0.80–1.74)
Midwest	−0.3624[*]	−0.0715	0.70 (0.59–0.82)	0.93 (0.61–1.43)
South	0.0078	0.5909[*]	1.01 (0.86–1.18)	1.81 (1.20–2.71)
West	—	—		
Poverty				
0–149%	0.1634[*]	0.0156	1.18 (1.03–1.34)	1.02 (0.75–1.37)
150% or more	—	—		
Years of education				
Less than 12 years	−0.2251[*]	0.4254[*]	0.80 (0.67–0.94)	1.53 (1.03–2.26)
12 years	−0.2379[*]	0.1374	0.79 (0.71–0.87)	1.15 (0.86–1.53)
13 years or more	—	—		
Age				
15–19	−0.4555[*]	0.2697	0.63 (0.46–0.88)	1.31 (0.52–3.29)
20–24	0.5249[*]	0.1734	1.69 (1.37–2.09)	1.19 (0.55–2.55)
25–29	0.6969[*]	0.1901	2.01 (1.69–2.39)	1.21 (0.56–2.61)
30–34	0.5974[*]	0.4478	1.82 (1.54–2.14)	1.56 (0.75–3.28)
35–39	0.3486[*]	−0.2564	1.42 (1.21–1.65)	0.77 (0.35–1.70)
40–44	—	—		

TABLE J.9   Continued

| | Odds Ratio Coefficient (95 percent confidence interval) | | | |
| | Not | | Not | |
Model Parameter	Pregnant	Pregnant	Pregnant	Pregnant
HIV risk				
Moderate/high HIV risk	1.2189*	1.4694*	3.38 (2.77–4.13)	4.34 (2.25–8.41)
Low HIV risk	—	—		

NOTE: MSA = metropolitan statistical area.

[a]Both logistic regression models provide a significant fit to the data ($p < .00001$). For not pregnant women, the model classifies 71 percent of the observed values correctly. For pregnant women, the model classifies 63% of the observed values correctly. Starred coefficients (*) denote statistical significance at $p = .05$.

[b]A total of 1,472 survey respondents reported that they were either pregnant at the time of the interview (430), had completed a pregnancy with 12 months of the interview (1,039), or had received pre- or postnatal care in the last 12 months (1,140). Women referred to as "pregnant" in this table refer to women who were pregnant, or recently pregnant, at the time of the interview.

APPENDIX

K

Details of the Committee's Models and Assumptions

Michael Stoto and *Maria Hewitt*

The conclusions and recommendations in this report rely, partly, on statistical calculations of the predictive value of prenatal HIV testing, economic evaluations of prenatal HIV screening programs, and process evaluations of strategies to reduce perinatal transmission. This appendix is intended to provide detailed information about the models and assumptions that the committee used to support its conclusions in Chapters 6 and 7.

PREDICTIVE VALUE OF HIV TESTING AND COST-EFFECTIVENESS OF HIV SCREENING AND TREATMENT IN PREGNANCY

Although the methods for testing pregnant women for HIV are the same as for other individuals, the relatively low prevalence of HIV in pregnant women in most areas (compared to individuals who seek or are referred for testing) affects the predictive value of the test—the lower prevalence rates correspond to higher false positive rates. In addition, the low cost of HIV testing when done routinely in the context of prenatal care (as recommended in this report) affects cost-effectiveness calculations in this setting.

In support of the recommendations in Chapter 7, this appendix estimates the predictive value of prenatal HIV testing, reviews existing economic evaluations of prenatal screening programs, and develops a simple model to evaluate prenatal HIV testing in clinical and economic terms. The primary difference between this and existing models is that the costs of initial ELISA (enzyme-linked immunosorbent assay) tests are limited to the marginal costs of including HIV in the standard panel of prenatal blood tests with no additional blood samples, and there is no cost for office visits or counseling (since the testing is done in the context of prenatal care).

Predictive Value of Prenatal HIV Testing

The positive predictive value (PPV) of a test is the probability that an individual with a positive test result is truly infected with HIV. The key assumptions for this calculation are the following. First, a two-stage testing procedure is used, as described by Pins and colleagues (1997). One specimen is subjected to an initial ELISA test, and, if positive, to a second. If repeatedly positive, the same specimen is subjected to a confirmatory Western blot test. Second, the sensitivity of the repeated ELISA test is 100%, and the specificity is 0.999 (Pins et al., 1997). Third, the prevalence of HIV in pregnant women ranges from 1 per 10,000 to 100 per 10,000 (or 1%). This range parallels the range of values found in the 1994 Survey of Childbearing Women.

Table K.1 displays the number of true positives (women truly HIV-positive) and the number of positive ELISA tests that would result for every 10,000 pregnant women tested for a given HIV prevalence rate. The table also shows the PPV for a range of prevalence values. As is generally the case, the positive predictive value of the test is lower where the prevalence of HIV is also low. If the prevalence of HIV in the population tested is above 20 per 10,000 (as is the case in about seven states, the District of Columbia, and Puerto Rico), the PPV exceeds 67%. If the prevalence is as low as 2 per 10,000 (as is the case in Utah or Oklahoma), the PPV is only about 17%. This means that there is less than a one

TABLE K.1 Cost-Effectiveness of HIV Screening Incorporated into Prenatal Care

Per 10,000 Women Tested				Cost of ELISA (dollars)			
				At $5/Test		At $3/Test	
Prevalence	TRUE Positives	Positive ELISA	PPV	Total	$/True +	Total	$/True +
0.0001	1	11	0.091	51,100	51,100	31,100	31,100
0.0002	2	12	0.167	51,200	25,600	31,200	15,600
0.0005	5	15	0.333	51,500	10,300	31,500	6,300
0.001	10	20	0.500	51,999	5,200	31,999	3,200
0.002	20	30	0.667	52,998	2,650	32,998	1,650
0.005	50	60	0.834	55,995	1,120	35,995	720
0.01	100	110	0.910	60,990	610	40,990	410
0.02	200	210	0.953	70,980	355	50,980	255
0.05	500	510	0.981	100,950	202	80,950	162

in five chance that a women with a repeatedly positive ELISA test is truly infected with HIV. Note that these rates apply to repeated ELISA testing only. When the original blood samples are subjected to Western blot confirmatory testing, most of the false positive results would test negative. Some fraction of Western blot results are indeterminate (depending on the testing procedure used and the laboratory), but some of these indicate an early-stage infection (Pins et al., 1997).

Economic Evaluations of HIV Testing and Treatment in Pregnancy

There have been numerous economic evaluations of HIV testing and treatment in pregnancy, each with different assumptions and different specific questions. Taken as a group, however, they generally establish the cost-effectiveness of prenatal HIV screening and treatment programs.

Mauskopf and colleagues (1996) have estimated the economic impact of treating pregnant women who are HIV-positive with ZDV (zidovudine), and have found that such treatment is cost saving over a wide range of assumptions. They further find that voluntary prenatal HIV screening programs are cost saving if the prevalence exceeds 4.6 per 1,000 (under certain assumptions). Under the assumption that the prevalence rate is 1.7 per 1,000 (the national average), the cost per case avoided of a voluntary screening program with comprehensive counseling and 100% acceptance is $155,000. The same program with limited pre-test counseling is actually cost saving.

In their base case analysis, assuming a prevalence rate of 1.7 per 1,000 in pregnant women, Gorsky and colleagues (1996) find that implementation of the Public Health Service (PHS) counseling and testing guidelines nationally would prevent 656 pediatric HIV infections annually and would result in a medical care cost saving of $105.6 million. Varying the maternal seroprevalence rate, they find that screening is cost saving as long as the prevalence rate is above 1.1 per 1,000.

Myers and colleagues (1998) have determined the cost-effectiveness of mandatory versus voluntary prenatal HIV screening. They conclude that mandatory screening will prevent more cases of pediatric AIDS, but at a somewhat higher cost than voluntary screening. Under their base assumptions, including a maternal seroprevalence rate of 1.7 per 1,000, the cost per case averted was $255,000 for mandatory screening and $367,000 for voluntary screening. The incremental cost-effectiveness of mandatory compared with voluntary screening was $29,500.

Cost-Effectiveness of Universal, Routine HIV Testing in Prenatal Care

Two additional assumptions are needed for this calculation. First, the marginal cost of including an HIV test in the standard prenatal panel is $3 to $5. Costs of testing vary markedly according to the circumstances in which the testing is done. ELISA tests done by private laboratories range from $15 to $65, but the cost to state laboratories is about $5. It costs the U.S. Army only $2.50 per serum specimen in its routine screening of all recruits because of the number tested and the established infrastructure for transporting specimens to the laboratory (all of these figures are from Mauskopf). In New York, the marginal cost of testing infant heel-stick samples for HIV is only about one dollar (Birkhead, 1998). Second, the follow-up cost for a repeatedly positive ELISA test (including the cost of the Western blot test and counseling those who are positive, but not treatment costs) is $100.

Table K.1 also shows the marginal cost of prenatal testing (per 10,000 women in prenatal care) and the cost per true positive case found. The results show that in high-prevalence areas the cost per case found is extremely low—hundreds of dollars. Even in low-prevalence areas the cost exceeds $50,000 per case found only if the marginal cost per ELISA test is $5 and the prevalence is 1 per 10,000. In a more reasonable low-prevalence scenario ($3 dollars per test and a prevalence of 2 per 10,000), the cost per case found is only $15,600.

While these numbers are not precise, they clearly indicate that universal routine HIV testing integrated into prenatal care can be very cost-effective, even in low-prevalence areas.

STRATEGIES TO REDUCE PERINATAL HIV TRANSMISSION

Inadequate prenatal care among women at high risk for HIV, health care providers' lack of adherence to PHS guidelines, and women's rejection of HIV testing and ZDV use all limit the ability to further reduce perinatal transmission. This section provides estimates of each potential barrier to HIV transmission reduction and presents a simplified model with which to assess the implications of different intervention strategies.

If a hypothetical population of 7,000 HIV-infected pregnant women all obtained early prenatal care; if their providers were in complete compliance with PHS recommendations regarding counseling, testing, and ZDV treatment; and if women all accepted HIV tests and ZDV treatment, and all pregnancies resulted in a live birth—the committee estimates that 350 HIV-infected babies would be born (i.e., the risk of transmission under optimal care is 5%). If, however, the onset of prenatal care, provider behavior, or other factors affecting perinatal HIV transmission are not optimal, the number of HIV-infected babies increases. Table K.2 shows the effects of varying some of the factors affecting perinatal HIV transmission. Column 2 shows the committee's estimates of the current environment: an estimated 85% of HIV-positive women seek prenatal care, 75% of women are counseled regarding HIV testing, 80% of women accept the test, 90% of HIV-positive women are offered ZDV, and 90% of women accept and comply with ZDV treatment when it is offered. Given this scenario, 1,172 babies would be born to the hypothetical cohort of 7,000 HIV-infected women, a 235% in-

TABLE K.2 Alternative Prenatal Transmission Scenarios for 7,000 HIV-infected Pregnant Women—Change Current Environment

Factors Affecting HIV Transmission Rates	Currently Achievable (1)	Estimate of Current Environment (2)	Increase Prenatal Care Attendance (3)	Increase Providers' Offering of Test (4)
Women with prenatal care (%)	100.00	85.00	**100.00**	85.00
Women counseled (%)	100.00	75.00	75.00	**100.00**
Women accepting HIV test (%)	100.00	80.00	80.00	80.00
Women offered ZDV treatment (%)	100.00	90.00	90.00	90.00
Women accepting/ complying with ZDV treatment (%)	100.00	90.00	90.00	90.00
Babies exposed to low transmission rate (.05) (%)	100.00	41.31	48.60	55.08
Babies exposed to high transmission rate (.25) (%)	0.00	58.69	51.40	44.92
Expected number HIV-infected babies	350.00	1,071.66	1,069.60	978.88
Reduction in number HIV-infected babies from current scenario (%)	70.13	NA	8.71	16.45
Increase in number of HIV-infected babies from achievable scenario (%)	NA	234.76	205.60	179.68

NOTE: Model assumes no fetal loss and two perinatal HIV transmission rates (.25 and .05); NA = not applicable.

crease over the currently achievable state (i.e., from 350 to 1,172 HIV-infected babies).[1] If we hold all but one condition constant, and change one parameter at a time, the impact of changes in the current environment can be assessed.

---

[1]The model assumes only two HIV transmission rates, .25 if women are not treated and .05 if they are treated. These transmission rates actually vary according to the HIV-infected woman's clinical state, and the onset and completeness of treatment. The model also assumes that testing rates for HIV-positive women are similar to those observed in the general population of pregnant women.

Increase Women's Test Acceptance (5)	Increase Providers' Offering of ZDV (6)	Increase Women's Acceptance of/Compliance with ZDV (7)	Increase Provider's Offering of Test and ZDV (8)	Increase Women's Acceptance of Test/ZDV (9)
85.00	85.00	85.00	85.00	85.00
75.00	75.00	75.00	**100.00**	75.00
100.00	80.00	80.00	80.00	**100.00**
90.00	**100.00**	90.00	**100.00**	90.00
90.00	90.00	**100.00**	90.00	**100.00**
51.64	45.90	45.90	61.20	57.38
48.36	54.10	54.10	38.80	42.63
1,027.08	1,107.40	1,107.40	893.20	946.75
12.34	5.48	5.48	23.77	19.20
193.45	216.40	216.40	155.20	170.50

- Increasing the receipt of prenatal care from 85% to 100% reduces the number of HIV-infected babies by 9% (i.e., from 1,172 to 1,070) (column 3).
- Increasing the rate at which providers offer HIV tests from 75% to 100% reduces the number of HIV-infected babies by 16% (i.e., from 1,172 to 979) (column 4).
- Increasing women's acceptance of HIV tests from 80% to 100% reduces the number of HIV-infected babies by 12% (i.e., from 1,172 to 1,027) (column 5).
- Increasing the providers offering ZDV treatment from 90% to 100% reduces the number of HIV-infected babies by 5% (from 1,172 to 1,107) (column 6).

TABLE K.3 Alternative Prenatal Transmission Scenarios for 7,000
HIV-Positive Pregnant Women—Change Current Environment

Factors Affecting HIV Transmission Rates	Currently Achievable (1)	Estimate of Current Environment (2)	Increase All but Prenatal Care Attendance (3)	Close Gap Between Current and Achievable by 10% (4)
Women with prenatal care (%)	100.00	85.00	85.00	86.50
Women counseled (%)	100.00	75.00	100.00	77.50
Women accepting HIV test (%)	100.00	80.00	100.00	82.00
Women offered ZDV treatment (%)	100.00	90.00	100.00	91.00
Women accepting/complying with ZDV treatment (%)	100.00	90.00	100.00	91.00
Babies exposed to low transmission rate (.05) (%)	100.00	41.31	85.00	45.52
Babies exposed to high transmission rate (.25) (%)	0.00	58.69	15.00	54.48
Expected number HIV-infected babies	350.00	1,171.66	560.00	1,112.70
Reduction in number HIV-infected babies from current scenario (%)	70.13	NA	52.20	5.03
Increase in number of HIV-infected babies from achievable scenario (%)	NA	234.76	60.00	217.91

NOTE: Model assumes no fetal loss and two perinatal HIV transmission rates (.25 and .05);
NA = not applicable.

• Increasing women's acceptance of ZDV treatment from 90% to 100%
reduces the number of HIV-infected babies by 5% (i.e., from 1,172 to 1,107)
(column 7).

Given the current environment, the most effective single intervention to
reduce perinatal transmission is to increase the number of providers offering HIV
tests (reduces perinatal HIV transmission by 16%). If providers were in complete
compliance with the PHS guidelines (i.e., they offered HIV tests and ZDV treatment to all women), there would be a 24% decrease in the number of HIV-
infected babies (from 1,172 to 893) (column 8). Alternatively, if the current
environment remained the same, but all HIV-infected women accepted HIV test-

Close Gap Between Current and Achievable by 20% (5)	Close Gap Between Current and Achievable by 30% (6)	Close Gap Between Current and Achievable by 40% (7)	Close Gap Between Current and Achievable by 50% (8)	Close Gap Between Current and Achievable by by 78% (9)
88.00	89.50	91.00	92.50	96.70
80.00	82.50	85.00	87.50	94.50
84.00	86.00	88.00	90.00	95.60
92.00	93.00	94.00	95.00	97.80
92.00	93.00	94.00	95.00	97.80
50.05	54.92	60.14	65.74	83.56
49.95	45.08	39.86	34.26	16.44
1,049.26	981.10	907.97	829.62	580.17
10.45	16.26	22.51	29.19	50.48
199.79	180.31	159.42	137.03	65.76

ing when offered, and accepted and complied with ZDV treatment, there would be a 19% reduction in the number of HIV-infected babies (i.e., from 1,172 to 947) (column 9). If both providers and HIV-infected women had optimal rates (i.e., if all but prenatal care is set to 100%), there would be a 52% decline in the number of HIV-infected babies (i.e., from 1,172 to 560) (Table K.3, column 3).

This simplified model illustrates the need for multifaceted approaches to significantly reduce perinatal HIV transmission. But even with a multifaceted approach, significant further reductions in the number of HIV-infected babies will be difficult to achieve. Table K.3 shows the effects of closing the gap between current and optimal rates by 10% to 50% (columns 4 through 8). Even if the gap was reduced by 50% (e.g., prenatal care increases from 85% to 92.5%), there would be only a 29% decline in the number of HIV-infected babies (i.e., from 1,172 to 830). Here it is assumed that 92.5% of HIV-infected pregnant women obtained early prenatal care, 87.5% of women were offered HIV testing, 90% of women accepted testing, 95% of HIV-positive women were offered ZDV, and 95% of women accepted and complied with ZDV therapy. To achieve a further 50% decline in the number of HIV-infected babies (i.e., from 1,172 to 580 infected babies) and be within reach of the currently achievable state (i.e., 350 infected babies), the gap between observed and achievable rates would have to close by 78%, and rates for factors related to transmission would have to be very high (e.g., 96.7% of women with prenatal care) (column 9).

REFERENCES

Birkhead GS. New York State AIDS Institute. Personal communication. 1998.

Gorsky RD, Farnham PG, Straus WL, Caldwell B, Holtgrave DR, Simonds RJ, Rogers MF, Guinan ME. Preventing perinatal transmission of HIV: Costs and effectiveness of a recommended intervention. *Public Health Rep* 111(4):335–341, 1996.

Mauskopf JA, Paul JE, Wichman DS, White AD, Tilson HH. Economic impact of treatment of HIV-positive pregnant women and their newborns with zidovudine. Implications for HIV screening. *JAMA* 276(2):132–138, 1996.

Myers ER, Thompson JW, Simpson K. Cost–effectiveness of mandatory compared with voluntary screening for human immunodeficiency virus in pregnancy. *Obstet Gynecol* 91(2):164–181,1998.

Pins MR, Teruya J, Stowell CP. Human immunodeficiency virus testing and case detection: pragmatic and techincal issues. In: Cotton D and Watts DH, eds. *The Medical Management of AIDS in Women.* Wiley-Liss: New York City, 1996.

APPENDIX

L

Passing the Test: New York's Newborn HIV Testing Policy, 1987–1997

David Abramson

INTRODUCTION

This appendix traces the evolution of policy in New York State regarding the screening of newborns for HIV antibodies, from the introduction of the blinded newborn seroprevalence survey in November 1987 through the implementation of the mandatory newborn testing and notification begun in February 1997. It is intended to provide the reader with the context in which key policies were debated or enacted and a sense of who the key players were. A caveat for the reader: since this material spans over a decade's worth of activity and discourse around a highly charged emotional issue, as a chronological accounting it can only touch upon key events and personalities. Moreover, an effort has been made to present the issues and decisions objectively by outlining the arguments advanced for certain decisions or policies, rather than arguing the merits of one point of view over another.

Data for this appendix were collected through confidential key informant interviews, literature reviews, and archival material review (such as program documentation and newspaper reports). Because many of the informants are currently involved in policy making and public health activities and might otherwise feel constrained from being completely candid if their comments would be publicly attributed, individuals' insights and comments have been intertwined within the narrative without identifiable attribution.

This particular case of newborn screening policy in New York offers insights into the state's broader politics and policy making surrounding HIV/AIDS. Several of the key lessons include the following:

• Policies and advocacy efforts from the 1960s through the 1990s produced a confluence of the patients' right movement, community engagement models, and categorical funding streams that resulted in a public health environment far more sensitive to individual privacy rights, patient autonomy, special interests and particularized communities than the more traditional mandate of public health operating solely for a majoritarian "public good."

• Advocates for people affected by HIV/AIDS have consistently challenged the traditional public health roles of surveillance, resource distribution, and case finding—and particularly the consequences of these traditional policies and programs for disenfranchised populations—and in so doing have compelled "exceptionalist" policies regarding HIV/AIDS that differ in many important aspects from other communicable or sexually transmitted diseases (STDs). New York's newborn screening debate embodied the struggle between the traditional and the exceptionalist approaches.

• As the issue of newborn surveillance evolved from an insular public health issue to one of political moment, who framed the issue and how the issue was framed became the two most important predictors of public opinion.

• The locus of decision making shifted over the course of a decade, as did the arena in which debate was engaged. Once public health policy was being debated in a political arena (and particularly once it reached a certain crescendo), the ultimate decisions and considerations were more often related to their political consequences than to their health consequences. When the testing policy changed in 1996 and 1997 (first with "consented" testing and then with mandatory testing), this occurred primarily because of shifting political winds and not because of scientific sea changes.

• As originally conceived, the state's newborn screening program addressed "public health uncertainty" about the epidemiology of HIV, but could not resolve the "medical uncertainty" of a clinician unaware of a patient's status, and therefore reinforced the divide between the population orientation of the state and the patient orientation of the clinician.

• Although New York's initial newborn testing policy revolved around surveillance and its epidemiological utility for charting the epidemic and for program planning, the legislative battle focused on newborn testing for the purposes of case finding. ***When the political debate was first engaged in 1993, there was scant evidence that mandatory testing would result in any decrease in perinatal transmission.*** Although there was a consensus regarding secondary prevention of *Pneumocystis carinii* pneumonia (PCP) among infants using pentamidine prophylactically, and the Centers for Disease Control and Prevention (CDC) had issued guidelines regarding HIV-positive mothers abstaining from breast-feeding (which might be delayed up to six weeks awaiting test results and follow-up), the medical and public health communities were divided on the absolute benefit of newborn testing as a means of reducing perinatal transmission. Even as the scientific landscape changed (particularly concerning the clear evidence for intervening in the prenatal period) the terms of the newborn testing debate remained fixed. Given the advent of rapid testing and the potential value of zidovudine (ZDV) therapy antenatally, medical science is only now beginning to demonstrate any evidence for proactively identifying HIV-antibody-carrying infants at birth. The cornerstones of the political discourse on the testing policy, though, were predicated on emotional and political issues, not scientific ones. Furthermore, as a case finding tool, newborn testing was principally effective only in identifying the mother. When the issue was first raised legislatively in 1993, there was no system of follow-up care or any reliable way to assure that all HIV-positive babies were accurately identified when they seroconverted.

• Given the players, the program, and the shifting political environment, it is likely that mandatory testing was inevitable in New York State. The mandatory newborn testing policy has also facilitated the successful passage of other HIV legislation in New York, such as mandatory partner notification and named HIV reporting.

The chronology of newborn testing policy unfolded in a shifting context of decision making and debate: from insular public health (the pragmatic era), to the population/clinical split (the era of mounting clinical frustration), to the political arena (marked by polarization, issue framing, and political "processes" of negotiation and pressure), to clinical optimism (retroviral therapy and protease inhibitors), and a return to public health pragmatism (the implementation of a political decision).

There were two points of strong federal state interaction regarding newborn screening, and the nature of each reveals a great deal about the shifting eras. In 1987, the CDC strongly supported New York's surveillance efforts as a complement to its "Family of Surveys" and provided half the ongoing funding for New York's newborn screening program. This was clearly the era of public health pragmatism, particularly in the face of uncertainty about the epidemic's future path. In 1995–1996, there was increasing political momentum at the federal level (evidenced by amendments to the Ryan White Reauthorization Act proposed by Congressmen Tom Coburn and Gary Ackerman) for mandatory newborn testing. With the sweep of Republicans into U.S. Congress, and similar Republican inroads in the New York State legislature (and the change at the executive level from a Democratic to a Republican governor), the Democratic-controlled Assembly faced increasing political pressure to conform to the governor's wishes for a mandatory newborn testing program. In 1996, after quiet negotiations between several key legislative players, the New York State Assembly speaker reversed his three-year opposition to mandatory testing and helped pass the "Baby AIDS" bill.

The framing and marketing of the issue of newborn screening and testing played a significant part in the decisions and actions taken. The early blinded screening program publicized its findings of high seroprevalence rates among

women in inner-city communities, and the news was presented as that of epidemiologic discovery. The emerging pattern of HIV transmission—with its growing impact on communities of heterosexual women and their offspring, in some
neighborhoods as high as 4%—served as the impetus for a number of prevention
and education efforts. In contrast, once the issue entered the political arena, the
debate was waged in the realm of public opinion. Those who favored mandatory
newborn testing presented the issue as one of villains and victims. The villain in
this case was "Big Brother" government, armed with specific knowledge about a
baby that could save his/her life, thwarting the victims—dedicated doctors and
caring mothers—from saving HIV-infected babies. The counterarguments were
far subtler, often relying upon biostatistical arguments, legal or ethical frameworks, or advocacy on behalf of minority women. Although those opposed to
mandatory testing advocated a model of voluntary HIV testing, which presumably worked to foster trust between a health care provider and a mother and
capitalized on maternal instincts to protect a baby's welfare, the images could not
compete with those of HIV-infected babies being denied treatment by an uncar-
ing government.

Finally, what state public health officials had recognized early on—that
using the sentinel event of birth as a primary epidemiological marker because it
was universal, occurred in an institutional setting over which the state had considerable regulatory power, and was built upon a successful newborn genetic
screening program—carried equal appeal for policy makers. Whether the state
was interested in HIV surveillance or case finding, the birth of a baby appeared to
provide a perfect opportunity.

THE PUBLIC HEALTH ENVIRONMENT, 1980–1986

New York's city and state health departments confronted a number of sensitive issues in the first few years of the AIDS epidemic: the regulation of sexual
behavior in commercial bathhouses, clean needle exchanges for injection drug
users, and the development of voluntary HIV testing programs, among others.
Each issue posed its own policy challenge. In considering bathhouse closures,
public health officials weighed the benefit of using their police powers against
the consequence of threatening a particular group's civil liberties. With proposed
needle exchange programs, they tried to balance the moralism of antidrug policies and politics with the pragmatism of stemming an avenue of transmission. As
HIV tests became available in 1985, officials had the task of inspiring trust
among groups that were wary of a government's ability to preserve an individual's
privacy and confidentiality. From the debates that arose among public health
officials, interest groups and affected individuals, health care providers, and political leaders, a general strategy of voluntary risk reduction and HIV prevention
programs emerged. Rather than use their prerogative to close gay bathhouses,
bars, and other public venues, public health officials first sought voluntary com-

pliance from the gay community. Only after the voluntary effort had failed did the state compel the closure of commercial bathhouses. The health commissioners had less success with needle exchange programs. Although sequential New York City Health Commissioners David Sencer and Stephen Joseph both endorsed needle exchange programs, and New York State Health Commissioner David Axelrod was also willing—albeit reluctantly—to experiment with such approaches, the proposed programs generated too much political opposition. It was not until 1989 that a limited needle exchange demonstration was approved for New York City. The lessons reinforced by these two issues were clear: individual rights matter and politics matter. To craft strategic programs, public health officials had to appease civil libertarians and advocacy groups at one end of the political spectrum and political conservatives at the other end.

The HIV antibody test developed in 1985 as a means of safeguarding the blood supply raised the greatest specter of government intrusion into an individual's private domain. Although public health officials did not universally endorse a voluntary HIV testing program initially (it was, in fact, opposed initially by the city health commissioner), by the end of 1985 most health officials acknowledged the test's utility for preventing transmission of the virus. The HIV test, however, was regarded by its opponents as the linchpin for a number of potentially intrusive measures—registries of HIV-infected individuals (which could both stigmatize and lead to discrimination if the names were ever revealed), mandatory partner notification programs, impingement of women's reproductive choices, and potential deportation of infected immigrants. In response to these concerns, public health officials and policy makers reinforced the exceptionalist nature of AIDS policy—rather than using the traditional reporting requirements and contact tracing associated with sexually transmitted and other communicable diseases, New York health officials carved out explicit informed consent requirements and voluntary HIV testing and notification policies. Behind such policies was an implicit quid pro quo. In return for relying upon various risk groups' voluntary compliance with these prevention strategies, public health officials would withhold a compulsory approach. Given the absence of any reliable treatment in the mid-1980s, public health officials' reliance upon voluntary prevention efforts seemed the most prudent course of action.

New York's innovative administration of its AIDS programs further reflected its awareness that this disease required a different approach than others. The AIDS Institute was established as an independent center within the state health department in 1982, at first reporting to the director of the Center for Community Health (an umbrella unit for all community-based public health activities) and later reporting directly to the commissioner of health. The broad mandate of the AIDS Institute included strategic planning, the oversight of community and clinical programs, the synthesis of epidemiological and evaluation data for planning purposes, and policy development. The Bureau of HIV/AIDS Surveillance operated separately from the AIDS Institute and worked as a component of the state's epidemiology unit. The surveillance group was responsible for analyzing data provided by the state's Wadsworth Laboratory, which represented the third leg of the administrative tripod. Finally, the state legislature created the AIDS Advisory Council (staffed by the AIDS Institute) as a forum to provide the health commissioner with input from both health care providers and communities affected by AIDS. The AIDS Advisory Council served as a buffer between vocal community advocacy groups, program planners within the health department, and the state legislature. Among the council's roles were developing proposed statewide AIDS budgets, identifying special needs populations, and lobbying politicians on designated "Legislators Days." According to one knowledgeable observer, "The AIDS budget is unique. It is laid out in lines that are more specific than the overall department's budget, because of visibility and political action. Each group of constituencies is represented in a separate line, such as a budget line for 'High risk women and children.' " Prior to the current administration, which began in 1995, the AIDS Institute also had its own policy office, distinct from the health department's, which oversaw an interagency policy committee that coordinated the AIDS policy work of a number of state agencies and units. AIDS policy in New York was clearly exceptional and political, and the locus of decision making was in the hands of Dr. David Axelrod, the state's health commissioner.

PUBLIC HEALTH PRAGMATISM, 1987–1990

At the Third International AIDS Conference in Washington, D.C. in the summer of 1987, the State of Massachusetts reported on its anonymous newborn screening program for HIV antibodies, which had been operational for a year. The first state in the nation to conduct such surveillance, Massachusetts had capitalized on its newborn screening program for genetic and metabolic disorders in order to test for the presence or absence of maternal HIV antibodies in a baby's blood. Two high-ranking New York public health officials, Lloyd Novick, the director of the Center for Community Health (which oversaw both the epidemiology unit and the AIDS Institute at the time), and Donald Berns, the assistant director of the state-run Wadsworth Center for Laboratories and Research, were very impressed by Massachusetts's presentation. Berns assured Novick that they had the laboratory capacity to conduct such a surveillance effort in New York. They returned to New York intent on developing an even more sophisticated screening program. The two met with Health Commissioner David Axelrod and Herbert Dickerman, the head of the Wadsworth Labs, and began planning the newborn surveillance program. From the onset, the four determined to improve on the Massachusetts surveillance program by also collecting demographic data, including the zip code of the mother (or the hospital if the mother's zip code was unavailable), maternal age, and the race/ethnicity of the infant.

Although the planners' principal concerns at first were those of logistics and capacity—securing a sufficient blood sample from a newborn heel-stick; design-ing the data form for accurate coding; removing identifiers; developing the epide-miological framework to use the data collected by the labs, conduct small- and large-area analyses, and report findings—the health department officials acknowl-edged in their meetings that the issue of dealing with HIV-positive results was of some concern. The universal newborn screening program had to be built on research conducted on anonymous blood samples. If mothers were approached for consent to test their newborn's blood it would raise issues of potential bias, since not all mothers would consent and the resultant sample might not be repre-sentative of the population of childbearing women. Since the surveillance there-fore had to be conducted in anonymous fashion, "blinded" to those drawing the blood and those analyzing the blood, the health department had no legal authority or capacity to then identify those babies testing HIV-positive and notify the mother. In addition to the planned newborn serosurvey, New York public health officials were also designing serosurveys that provided epidemological data among population "windows" for whom blood was routinely collected—drug users, state prisoners, runaways and homeless teens referred to medical examina-tions, and family planning and STD clients, in addition to newborns.

The decision to launch the blinded newborn seroprevalence survey and re-lated serosurveys rested with these four public health officials, and principally with Health Commissioner Axelrod. As one of Governor Cuomo's most trusted cabinet members, Axelrod was afforded a great deal of latitude in formulating public health policy and was well respected by members of the state legislature. Axelrod's management style was such that he relied upon a close circle of high-ranking deputies for their counsel, and all major decisions funneled up to him. To assure himself that his strategies were sound both scientifically and ethically, Axelrod often convened committees of outside experts to consider the effective-ness, consequence, or significance of particular policies or programs. In mid-Sep-tember 1987, Axelrod brought together clinicians and ethicists to review the gamut of proposed seroprevalence surveys—the "windows" into various populations—and particularly the newborn screening study. The Advisory Committee (composed of Elaine Abrams of Harlem Hospital, Daniel Callahan of the Hastings Center, Victor DeGruttola of Harvard School of Public Health, Richard Kaslow from the National Institute for Allergy and Infectious Diseases, the CDC's Magarite Pappaioanou, and Warren Winkelstein from the University of California at Berke-ley) unanimously supported the universal newborn screening program.

The blinded newborn seroprevalence study built upon the state's established Newborn Screening Program (NSP), which tested infants at hospital discharge for seven inherited disorders (phenylketonuria [PKU], congenital hyperthyroid-ism, and maple sugar urine disease, among others) by drawing blood through a heel-stick. The NSP had been developed in New York State in the early 1960s by a Buffalo microbiologist Dr. Robert Guthrie. He had watched in horror as his niece had gone undiagnosed with PKU until she was 16 months old; she grew up retarded and schizophrenic, which he attributed to the initially undiagnosed PKU. His impetus to develop the newborn screening was that if PKU was detected early enough after birth, babies could be put on a special low-protein diet and go on to lead perfectly normal lives. On average, New York screens over 300,000 infants each year and identifies approximately 12 children with PKU. (In contrast, in a nine-month period from February 1, 1997, through October 31, 1997, of 185,540 births there were 779 infants born with maternal HIV antibodies.)

The state health department began collecting newborn HIV seroprevalence data on November 30, 1987. "What I recall quite vividly," said one of the study planners, "is that after the first two weeks we were taken aback by the results. They had quite an impact on us." Several earlier newborn studies conducted in municipal hospitals in New York City had revealed seroprevalence rates of 2.4% to 2.5%. The study planners expected to find similar data in high-risk neighborhoods and were stunned to find rates of 4% seroprevalence in Harlem, the South Bronx, and the Bedford Stuyvesant section of Brooklyn. "This meant that 1 of every 25 women [delivering a baby] was infected," noted a public health official, "and when we reported that we expected a big outcry, and a large media push, for us to immediately unblind the survey." To their surprise, newspaper coverage focused on the epidemiological significance of the findings—on the spread of HIV infection across the state and the depth of HIV seroprevalence in particular communities.

Within four weeks of starting the newborn seroprevalence study, the state health department had amended the contracts of state-regulated family planning programs and prenatal care clinics, which served over 300,000 women annually, requiring them to provide on-site HIV counseling and testing services. The state also stepped up its efforts to reach pregnant women in high-risk neighborhoods through its Community Health Worker program and through targeted education campaigns, and advised obstetricians and other physicians throughout the state of the compelling need to provide HIV counseling and testing services to women of reproductive age. In his State of the State message on January 6, 1988, Governor Mario Cuomo told the assembled legislators, "There is no greater tragedy than the birth of a child condemned to death, yet estimates indicate 1,000 infants will be born with the AIDS virus in 1988. . . . The initial results of the prevalence studies have only served to heighten our sense of urgency and to focus dramatically upon our most vulnerable populations. Results on the first 11,000 newborn blood specimens demonstrate an alarming statewide HIV seroprevalence rate of almost 1% among women of childbearing age."

At the same time that New York was beginning its seroprevalence studies, the CDC was initiating its Family of Surveys seroprevalence sample studies in 45 states. The CDC funded states to conduct anonymous seroprevalence studies on representative samples of injection drug users, STD and tuberculosis clinic patients, hospital admissions, patients at clinics serving women of reproductive age, and newborns. New York public health officials decided to conduct universal, anonymous screening rather than sampled screening, since it was piggybacking the study on the universal Newborn Screening Program and the additional cost was warranted by the greater predictive power of conducting a universal test. The CDC contributed funding that covered half of New York's seroprevalence studies, and the state made up the difference (by 1996, the state was paying three-quarters of the cost of the seroprevalence surveys, and CDC one-quarter of the $2 million program).

As Novick was to write later (Novick, 1991), the newborn seroprevalence survey provided the state health department with three critical elements: currency, relevance, and focus. The "currency" allowed the state to monitor the real-time spread of the infection without having to account for the lag time between HIV infection and a reported AIDS case (and it enabled the state to conduct analyses of HIV trends over time without adjusting for the CDC's expanded definition of AIDS in 1993); the "relevance" of the universal screening test enabled the state to report actual, rather than projected, infection rates among childbearing women and to closely estimate the rate among all women ages 15–44; and the "focus" derived from the small-area planning that could be conducted given the sociodemographic variables of maternal age, race/ethnicity, and zip code. The last was perhaps the most important to state public health officials, since it served as an early-warning system that alerted them to what communities the virus was moving into, and thereby provided an opportunity for targeted prevention and education efforts.

In March 1988, Commissioner Axelrod reconvened a special advisory committee to review the preliminary results of the newborn serosurvey. The committee (composed of Elaine Abrams and Margaret Heagarty of Harlem Hospital, NIAID's Richard Kaslow, the CDC's Timothy Dondero and Margaret Oxtoby, Myron Essex and Harvey Fineberg of Harvard School of Public Health, Keith Krasinski of Bellevue Hospital, Peter Selwyn of Montefiore Hospita;, and Isaac Weisfuse of the New York City Department of Health) strongly recommended continuing the serosurvey, particularly for purposes of monitoring the epidemic.

Only days before the advisory committee met, an article in *Newsday* (a major New York daily) featured an interview with Dr. Rodney Hoff, the architect of the Massachusetts health department's blinded newborn survey. Even as he presented the rationale for the blinded serosurvey, ". . . so that we can monitor HIV infection trends in women," he did sound a cautionary note, saying that, "there is a trade-off here between the legal issue of consent and ethical issue of duty to inform." Since there was no accepted treatment at the time, Hoff said he considered it ethically acceptable to not identify individual patients (a position adopted by Bayer and others (1986), and by the journal *Nature's* editorialists in a 1987 article). "Once there is an effective treatment for infected infants," he concluded, "we will very quickly convert to a case-detection system."

Between 1988 and 1990, the New York State health department pursued a number of measures predicated on voluntary adherence to primary and secondary prevention practices. In the absence of a treatment or vaccine, public health strategies focused first on preventing initial infection (primary prevention) by modifying risk behaviors and, for those infected, on preventing further spread of the virus (secondary prevention). Tertiary prevention efforts, focused on limiting the progression of the disease within an infected individual, were for the most part limited to PCP prophylaxis and experimental antiretroviral therapies. As has been extensively documented, since HIV/AIDS raised so many issues of the authority of the public health officials to intervene in the private affairs of selected communities (e.g., gay bathhouse closures, mandatory partner notification) and since there had been sufficient numbers of cases of HIV/AIDS discrimination in housing, public schools, and employment to warrant a genuine concern, public health officials generally believed that the most expeditious prevention strategy had to be voluntarily elicited, rather than coerced or mandated. Furthermore, such an approach followed the principle of the "least restrictive alternative" in gauging appropriate public health action.[1] Particularly given some of the early successes in persuading the homosexual male population to voluntarily reduce risky behaviors, it seemed sensible to public health officials and legislators to pursue measures that educated and engaged the communities most at risk, rather than potentially alienating these communities and driving them away from the health care system.

In keeping with this approach, the state legislature passed New York State's confidentiality statute in 1988, which imposed strict penalties for disclosure of confidential HIV information and required written informed consent prior to any HIV testing. According to one of the key legislators involved in drafting the law, "We recognized that there was an urgent public health need to have people come forward and be tested, to be counseled, and to cooperate, and since there was no lure of treatment we had to offer a guarantee of confidentiality." One key provision of the statute gave physicians treating HIV-infected individuals the "power" to warn others who might be at risk of HIV infection, but not the "duty" to warn. This was in keeping with the balance between prevention and case finding, as was the language of the informed consent. Rather than adopting a "directed" approach that recommended HIV testing, the language of the informed consent was "non-directed," spelling out all the potential negative consequences of testing and leaving the formulation of a decision entirely up to the individual. This approach to informed consent was based on 20 years of success in the field of

---

[1]In one of the most cogent articles examining the legal capacity of public health authorities to constrain individual behavior through the regulation of public meeting places or contact tracing, Gostin and Curran (1987, p. 217) concluded in 1987 that, "even stricter scrutiny will be applied to public health measures which affect liberty, autonomy, or privacy of human beings. These measures should not be promulgated without searching examinations as to public health need, specificity of the targeted population, and adherence to the principle of the least restrictive alternative."

genetic counseling and was driven by various consumer movements promoting both patients' rights and autonomy, and a shared medical decision making model that regarded the patient as an active partner along with his or her health care provider.

The state health department codified its strategy in two key planning documents: (1) the January 1989 five-year interagency plan, "AIDS: New York's Response," which introduced a number of new initiatives aimed at education (such as HIV/AIDS education incorporated into the core curricula of all public schools and colleges), voluntary counseling and testing, expansion of health services, and preservation of human rights through antidiscrimination legislation and adherence to the principles of informed consent; and (2) the "New York State Principles for the Care of Women and Children with HIV Infection," (New York State AIDS Institute, 1990) drafted after a three day symposium in 1990 at the Mohonk Mountain House in New Paltz, and thereafter known as the "Mohonk Principles." The Mohonk symposium, led by the AIDS Institute's Nick Rango, brought together key staff from a number of state agencies, as well as health professionals involved in AIDS-related services and women affected by the epidemic. The document clearly stipulated the state's voluntarist approach. The consensus document urged "routine counseling and voluntary testing of all women of reproductive age," which should be provided in all health care settings; it asserted each woman's right to make her own reproductive choices; and it recommended a program of routine counseling and voluntary testing of postpartum women who may not have received adequate counseling or testing opportunities prior to giving birth. The document further clarified a consensus position opposing mandatory newborn screening, arguing that involuntary testing of the mother (the practical consequence of newborn testing) must be weighed against the state's interest in safeguarding the health and welfare of the infant. It presented the criteria that had to be met before unblinding the newborn screening: "(1) substantial clinical benefit of treatment in HIV-infected newborns has been demonstrated; (2) appropriate clinical services are available to all HIV-infected family members regardless of family resources; (3) a definitive laboratory test becomes available allowing for the detection of HIV infection in newborns (as opposed to the presence of maternal antibodies), or the indicated clinical intervention for infants with HIV infection has been proven to be sufficiently nontoxic to uninfected infants who would receive it because of the presence of maternal HIV antibodies; and (4) a system of voluntary counseling and testing of all women of reproductive age has failed to be effective."

The voluntary counseling and testing program at family planning clinics and prenatal care programs was emblematic of this approach. The state intended that every woman of reproductive age seen in a state-regulated facility would be provided with sufficient information to protect herself from being infected and that every woman would also voluntarily take the HIV test in an effort to inform reproductive choices (such as whether to have an abortion or to pursue future pregnancies) and to encourage other secondary prevention efforts. In 1990, state health officials also rejected the CDC's 1989 recommendation for risk-based assessments—which attempted to concentrate efforts on encouraging testing among individuals in specific self-reported high-risk categories—in favor of a broader, universal approach that sought to gain the consent to test among all women at state-regulated clinics. In September 1990, the health department sent out a "Dear Colleague" letter to all physicians in the state, urging them to counsel any patient who had sex with more than one person in the last ten years, or who had ever used illicit drugs, to be tested for HIV. Furthermore, the state launched the OB Initiative in 1990, a postpartum program at 24 hospitals in high-seroprevalence areas to counsel and test women who indicated they had not been tested during their pregnancies.

The results of these voluntary programs, though, proved disappointing. Testing rates in 1991 and 1992 ranged from 14% to 66% (Healton et al., 1996) at the women's clinics, and except for Harlem Hospital's program, which persuaded over 90% of postpartum women to test, the OB Initiative was equally ineffective. Although the merits of case finding versus prevention were debated, it was increasingly evident to public health officials in the early 1990s that such voluntary case finding strategies needed strengthening.

At the same time that these programs directed at individual behavior change were being initiated, a number of efforts were undertaken by the state health department to more accurately focus community-wide prevention and treatment efforts. One innovation developed by the AIDS Institute and the state's epidemiology unit was a Community Needs Index, which took into account newborn seroprevalence rates and hospital discharge data in constructing a profile of high-, medium-, and low-risk neighborhoods. The index was then used in program development, the expansion of specially designated AIDS centers at hospitals and community health centers, and the distribution of state funds to community-based organizations in high-risk neighborhoods.

From an epidemiological perspective, universal newborn screening was still regarded as effective and relevant. Beginning in 1990, though, as treatment options for HIV-infected infants became more widely accepted, the tension between the epidemiological and the clinical utility of newborn screening (in very broad terms, the polarization of surveillance and prevention versus case finding and treatment) grew within the state health department. These issues had percolated within the larger health care community since 1988 (Krasinski et al., 1988), but now they were gaining a wider audience. What began as an internal debate within the health care community in the late 1980s evolved into a very public debate by 1993.

THE SEEDS OF DISCONTENT, 1990–1993

By 1990, Commissioner Axelrod was having second thoughts about the state's blinded seroprevalence study. The Fifth International AIDS Conference in

Montreal the previous summer had featured a number of promising studies suggesting the value of specific prophylactic therapies directed at infants, and the CDC was in the process of formulating new guidelines for PCP prophylaxis for infants and children that would be released in 1991. The efficacy of such treatment, as with antiretroviral therapy in adults, was dependent upon early detection of the viral infection. Axelrod convened his chief deputies and discussed the possibility of replacing the blinded newborn screening program with one in which newborns carrying the HIV antibody would be mandatorily identified and a parent notified. Nick Rango, director of the AIDS Institute, was vehemently opposed and urged Axelrod instead to redouble his efforts on the voluntary testing program. As the data continued to show, though, women were not voluntarily stepping forward to be tested. In late 1990, Axelrod asked one of his key deputies to assemble a small team and draw up a plan for unblinding the newborn study. The plan was to include how notification would be made, how to bring women back for comprehensive care and treatment, and how to assure sufficient capacity at existing designated AIDS centers to care for the women and children. At first, the team considered an approach that involved giving each woman the "right of refusal," but rejected that as having too many problems. It settled instead on a plan of mandatory newborn testing and notification, along with assured treatment for all who tested positive. The AIDS Institute's Rango continued to object to the approach.

In February 1991, Axelrod suffered an incapacitating stroke. Despite its advocates within the health department, the plan to unblind the newborn testing was shelved. "We had no commissioner," said one veteran public health official who favored the plan, "and no one with the political resources to pull it off."

Outside the health department, indeed outside the medical community, there was an increasing interest in revisiting the newborn testing issue. In mid-1991, Gretchen Buchenholz, executive director of the Association to Benefit Children (ABC), a New York City-based foster care agency, approached her legal counsel to lead a lobbying campaign to unblind the newborn screening study. After several cases in which foster children had gone undiagnosed with HIV infection despite their caregivers' interest in obtaining an HIV test for the infant, and which was attributed to the restrictiveness of the state's confidentiality statute in not allowing foster parents to order an HIV test without the natural parents' consent,[2] the agency decided that the most effective strategy would be mandatory HIV screening of all newborns, with a guaranteed provision of care for all who tested

---

[2]This was actually an artifact of rule making by the local governmental child welfare agency and not the state statute, which in fact gave each local governmental child welfare agency the authority to test foster children without the natural parents' consent. The New York City Child Welfare Administration's policy was to require that every effort be made to acquire the natural parents' consent prior to testing the foster child.

positive. The special counsel and the executive director of ABC approached a number of agencies to enlist them in the campaign. According to their published accounting of these lobbying efforts, they were rebuffed by the state AIDS Institute, the Lambda Legal Defense and Education Fund, and the Gay and Lesbian Rights Project of the American Civil Liberties Union. But they did receive positive support from certain children's rights groups. For three years, ABC continued to seek common cause with other HIV/AIDS providers, and it was not until 1994 that ABC decided to use a litigation strategy to advance its position.

Some of the strongest dissenting voices opposed to blinded newborn screening study in 1992 came from Nassau County on Long Island, a predominantly conservative area just east of New York City, and in the reportage of the area's leading daily newspaper, *Newsday*. In the summer of 1992, the Nassau HIV Commission recommended to the local board of health that it petition the state to allow mothers to consent to be notified if their infants tested positive for HIV. The commission also lobbied the Nassau County Board of Health to recommend to the state that all physicians throughout the state be required to offer an HIV test to their pregnant patients. One Nassau County Board of Health member, Dr. Larry Ravich, said during the board meeting at which the commission's recommendations were presented, "I think we are approaching this with little slippers on." He pressed for mandatory HIV testing of all pregnant women, a position adopted by the board. Several days later, *Newsday* columnist Bob Wiemer endorsed the board's push for mandatory HIV testing. He referred to the 1988 confidentiality statute that stood in the way of such mandatory testing as "criminally foolish," and argued that under the existing laws, "the rights of the carrier are held superior to the rights of the uninfected." Although the Nassau County Board of Health's recommendations did not alter state policy, they did demonstrate a breach within the public health community. And the columnist's sentiments, however inflammatory they appeared at first glance, would soon gain currency in the legislative efforts to unblind newborn screening.

In January 1993, *Newsday* ran a series of articles by reporter Nina Bernstein that documented the failure of voluntary partner notification to protect unsuspecting women from HIV-infected husbands. The articles were powerful and dramatic, and the stories the reporter recounted of women learning their husbands' diagnoses as they lay on their deathbeds—sometimes as a result of an inadvertent slip by a social worker or physician caring for the husband—made a strong case for stronger partner notification policies. The state health department and the state legislature were implicated in the failure to protect these women, and it so infuriated state Assemblywoman Nettie Mayersohn as she read the newspaper series that she grew determined to change state law. Within weeks of reading the newspaper articles, at the start of the legislative session, Mayersohn, a Democratic majority member of the Assembly's Health Committee, proposed amending the public health code. Her proposed legislation would require named reporting of HIV-infected individuals to the local health department and mandatory partner notification if the infected individual voluntarily released the names of sexual contacts. As a politician and community activist with a long history of supporting women's rights, Mayersohn perceived herself to be operating from a similar position, that of protecting women from unfair policies and inequitable relationships. She sought support for her position from a variety of women's groups and gay activists, and was surprised at their rebuff. Next, she went to the medical community. After a presentation at the Medical Society of the State of New York, a physician approached her and told her about the state's policy of blinded newborn screening. He presented it as the greatest travesty of the state's confidentiality statute—that the state knew the HIV status of infected babies, but would not let either the mothers or the physicians know. Notwithstanding the inaccuracies of such a portrayal—the state did not maintain the identities of the HIV-infected babies, nor was it preventing or denying the ability of mothers to test or physicians to strongly counsel their patients to test—this captured Mayersohn's attention completely. After verifying the facts of the blinded newborn screening policy, she decided to shelve her partner notification legislation and devote all her legislative energy towards the passage of the "Baby AIDS" bill she introduced in May 1993, which would unblind newborn screening and mandatorily notify the parents of the baby's status. "The secret is out," Mayersohn wrote in one of her first newsletters on the subject in 1993, "the State of New York has been using babies for statistical purposes—but has been denying them treatment and the protection they need to save their lives." Her legislation was mirrored in the state senate in a bill sponsored by Guy Velella, a Republican from the Bronx.

Given the response to her partner notification legislation, Mayersohn was hardly surprised by the vehement opposition she encountered from gay activists, civil libertarians, and feminist groups. Still, she was confident that her constituency of middle-class, mostly Jewish homeowners in Queens would support her position as one consonant with her "pro-family" stance. She set aside virtually all other legislative business to focus on the newborn testing issue. According to Mayersohn, "This was an issue that people would respond to. I was horrified. I couldn't focus on any other political agenda." Her doggedness was not overlooked by her fellow Assembly members, especially those who opposed her legislation. According to one legislative leader, "It is rare to see a legislator focus her career down to one question. She was irrelevant to the legislative process [once she began pursuing the Baby AIDS legislation], but that fixation contributed to her success. It was clear to me from the start that it would be extremely difficult to overcome her position."

Mayersohn's proposed legislation to mandate newborn testing proved to be a turning point in the evolution of policy. Whereas the locus of decision making control over newborn testing had resided within the state health department from 1987 through 1992, the debate and decision making over newborn testing now entered the public and political realms. Public health officials had become secondary actors in the policy making process. Whatever their personal inclinations to advocate or oppose mandatory newborn testing, their role became that of functionaries rather than trusted advisers. Public health officials would provide the legislators and advisory committees with data, and would work on the implementation of the interim and final policies regarding newborn testing, but they would no longer steer the process.

POLITICAL MANEUVERINGS, 1993–1994

Mayersohn introduced her 1993 legislation in the political environment of a Democratic Assembly (100 of 150 seats); a Republican Senate; and a three-term liberal governor, Mario Cuomo, as the state executive. Both state houses operate under protocols of centralized leadership: the Assembly speaker and the Senate majority leader each have the power to move legislation out of committee for a floor vote or to block votes from coming up the floor. Until procedural reforms were enacted in the 1998 legislative session, the legislative leaders also controlled budgetary decisions; the state budget was determined by negotiation among the Assembly speaker, the Senate majority leader, and the governor. In 1993, Mayersohn had little influence either with Speaker Sheldon Silver, a Manhattan Democrat, or with Governor Cuomo.

A former community activist who first ran for political office when she was in her mid-fifties, Mayersohn's greatest political assets were her persistence and the image she presented of herself as a plain-speaking Jewish grandmother. In her home district in Queens, Mayersohn had been a tenant organizer, president of the PTA, and a Democratic district leader. She had returned to college after raising a family and graduated from Queens College alongside her youngest son. Although she had run against a Democratic incumbent to gain her Assembly seat, Mayersohn fostered some key political ties amongst fellow Queens Democrats. When she was a district leader, Mayersohn helped Gary Ackerman campaign successfully for a state Senate seat, and the two kept in contact after he became a U.S. Congressman. In 1995, Ackerman would play a pivotal role in the shifting national debate about newborn testing when he introduced a bill modeled on Mayersohn's New York bill.

The populist image Mayersohn cultivated was that of an independent thinker, not beholden to the party line, who was devoted to protecting those without power (such as women and babies). Also, based on the relative homogeneity of her home district and her strong record of constituent service, Mayersohn enjoyed very strong electoral support. In order to bolster her position and gain the endorsement of her fellow legislators, Mayersohn would photocopy relevant medical journal articles and newspaper reports that supported her arguments and circulate them to all of her colleagues.

Mayersohn was well aware that her bill faced an uphill battle, particularly given what she called the "Manhattan constituency," by which she meant legislators whose most vocal leftist constituents constrained the legislators from voting

their consciences and who instead favored special protections and undue entitle-
ments. Chief among her opponents was Richard Gottfried, a Manhattan Democrat who chaired the Assembly's Health Committee. As one of the original draft-
ers of the 1988 confidentiality statute, he was a staunch supporter of voluntary
programs. After several newspaper editorials came out in favor of Mayersohn's
proposed legislation (including the *New York Times* and *Newsday*), and there was
mounting legislative support for her bill, Gottfried moved to table her bill pending a report by a panel of clinicians and ethicists constituted as a subcommittee of
the AIDS Advisory Council and known as the "Blue Ribbon panel." The motion
to table the bill barely passed by a 10–9 vote in August 1993. The Blue Ribbon
panel was expected to deliver its report in early 1994.

"At the beginning," said one legislative leader who favored voluntary testing, "we were trying to buy time, to build an opposition. When [Mayersohn]
raised the issue in Spring 1993, Jim Tallon [the Assembly majority leader] came
up with the idea to reach out to [Dr. David] Rogers [the chair of the AIDS
Advisory Council] to create a subcommittee to study the issue. It had support
from the Speaker. If the Blue Ribbon panel had not been there the bill might have
passed into law that year."

Between September and December 1993 the Blue Ribbon panel held five
public meetings and a public hearing in a packed Manhattan conference room. In
late January 1994, the chair of the Assembly's Health Committee, Richard
Gottfried, wrote an op-ed piece reaffirming the importance of voluntary testing
programs. "Treating a patient with consideration and respect—which includes
relying on informed consent—is the best way to win that patient's cooperation."
He reiterated his position that counseling every pregnant woman would find and
treat more HIV-positive babies than a mandatory approach because it would
involve the women in their care, and he concluded with a call for mandatory
counseling of all women.

On February 10, 1994, the Blue Ribbon panel issued its recommendations.
During its deliberations, the panel had considered the range of mandatory and
voluntary testing options, the potential timing of such HIV testing (prenatally or
antenatally), and the available treatment opportunities for women and infants
identified as HIV-positive. Furthermore, the panel had considered the effects of
various treatment options on two outcomes: (1) increasing the percentage of
HIV-positive women and infants who were tested and (2) increasing the rate at
which infected and exposed women and infants could be expected to enter treatment. Given that HIV testing during the prenatal period provided greater opportunities for counseling and informing mothers, avoided the possibility of losing
as many cases to follow-up if HIV test results were delayed postpartum, and
offered the greater opportunity for preventing perinatal transmission if the ZDV
clinical trial proved successful, a majority of the panel rejected the mandatory
newborn testing policy and instead recommended mandatory HIV counseling for
all pregnant and postpartum women. The panel further urged the development of

intensive counseling programs similar to that of Harlem Hospital, which routinely persuaded over 90% of its obstetrical patients to accept HIV testing. Four physicians on the panel—the public health commissioner from Westchester County and three pediatricians—dissented. One of them, Dr. Lou Cooper, the head of the New York chapter of the American Academy of Pediatrics, told the *New York Times*, "Reliance on counseling that encourages voluntary testing ignores the unacceptably high failure rate of such an approach. In addition, it siphons off resources which could be focused more effectively for needed care."

Within days after the Blue Ribbon panel released its report, the Data Safety Monitoring Board of the NIAID interrupted AIDS Clinical Trials Group protocol number 076 (ACTG 076) when it became clear that ZDV administered to pregnant women and newborns could reduce vertical transmission of HIV by 69%. Citing the dramatic, incontrovertible value to intervening prenatally, Cooper reversed his position and sided with the majority view of the panel to focus prevention and case finding efforts on pregnant women rather than newborns.

On February 24, 1994, the AIDS Advisory Council adopted the Blue Ribbon panel's recommendation and advised the state to pursue universal voluntary testing. On the same day, a joint Senate–Assembly bill was proposed by Michael Tully, the chair of the Senate Health Committee and Assembly Speaker Sheldon Silver, calling for mandatory counseling and voluntary testing of pregnant women. The sponsors pointed to the recent reports of ZDV's efficacy as a clear mandate to focus efforts on enlisting pregnant women in the detection and care of their HIV-infected babies. The battle over Mayersohn's bill had clearly been joined.

Newsday columnist Jim Dwyer, who would later win a Pulitzer Prize for his series of columns on the Baby AIDS legislation, published a column in April, 1994, "A Silence that Kills Children," prompted by a conversation he had with Mayersohn that transpired after he had attended the funeral of a baby who died from AIDS complications (Mayersohn, 1994a). In the column, he quoted pediatrician Stephen Nicholas of Columbia Presbyterian Medical Center as favoring "routine newborn testing, the same we do for syphilis testing." Nicholas, who had been involved in the design and implementation of Harlem Hospital's much-touted High Risk Pregnancy Clinic, told the columnist that he felt that even 90% voluntary agreement to test was not sufficient, "because you're still missing 10%."

Throughout the early spring, there was considerable political discussion and negotiation over possible terms of compromise between the Silver–Tully sponsors and the Mayersohn–Velella sponsors. One compromise being considered was directed counseling that urged HIV testing and the written acceptance or refusal of testing at delivery. At the same time, the foster-care agency ABC had renewed its advocacy for allowing HIV testing of foster children without explicit consent of the birth parents, a policy that many saw as linked with the mandatory newborn testing proposals because both would amend the state's confidentiality statute and both would be undertaken on behalf of HIV-infected children. ABC and its pro bono counsel had made it clear to the state commissioners of social services and health that they would pursue a lawsuit against Governor Cuomo and the state. On June 6, 1994, only days before the lawsuit was to be filed, the commissioner of social services announced new regulations that would allow foster children to be tested after a good-faith effort to locate the natural parents had been made. The regulations would be adopted on an emergency basis, which meant that within a year the agency would have to hold hearings and adopt the regulations permanently. ABC, satisfied with the compromise, dropped its plans for a lawsuit.

Throughout June, the battle over the Baby AIDS bill intensified, particularly since the end of the legislative session was scheduled for the first week of July and there was a major election looming in November. *Newsday* columnist Dwyer wrote one column referring to the "corrosive influence of a Religious Left" backed by well-paid Albany lobbyists, which was marked by dogma that held that any threat to a woman's right to privacy was a threat to abortion, that any abrogation of the state's confidentiality statute was the first step on a slippery slope to the persecution of people with AIDS, and that mandatory testing would drive mothers away from medical care.

New York Times columnist Anna Quindlen (1994) took the opposing view: "The word on the mandatory reporting measure is that it is opposed only by special interest groups, gay organizations obsessed with privacy, and feminists concerned only with women. Why then is it opposed by Lorraine Hale, whose Hale House has been caring for sick and abandoned babies for years?" Quindlen concluded that "the Baby Bill sounds so right; the mothers, with all their many problems, are not so sympathetic. But winning their trust and cooperation, not coercing and blindsiding them, is how real change will occur."

The results of ACTG 076 had changed the terms of the debate for a number of individuals and organizations. Both the New York chapter of the American Academy of Pediatrics and the Medical Society of the State of New York reversed their positions on mandatory testing, favoring instead a policy of mandatory counseling for pregnant women and voluntary testing. Given the existence of an effective treatment, a number of clinicians were loathe to institute a policy that might drive any women from care, and a number had seen the clinical opportunity shift from the delivery setting—which many regarded as too late for effective intervention—to the prenatal setting.

The Republican candidate for governor, State Senator George Pataki, announced in early June that he favored mandatory HIV testing of newborns, a position that was echoed by the candidate for state attorney general, Dennis Vacco, running on Pataki's ticket. Governor Cuomo had still not taken a public stand. In early spring, months after the AIDS Advisory Council had released its recommendations, Governor Cuomo charged the Task Force on Life and the Law with reviewing the issue of mandatory HIV newborn testing. According to one member of that advisory panel, which often addressed ethical issues of concern to the governor, Cuomo wanted to delay his decision until after the gubernatorial reelection campaign.

Right up to the end of the legislative session in early July, supporters of the Silver–Tully bill calling for mandatory counseling and voluntary testing believed their bill would pass in the final hours. Even Mayersohn had accepted the likelihood of her opponents' bill passing. "I left at midnight [on the last night of the legislative session] thinking this would pass. [*Newsday* columnist] Dwyer called me the next morning to say the bill wasn't introduced. It was never put up for a vote. That left an opening for our bill to be reintroduced in the 1995 session." Mayersohn harbored no illusions as to the impact of the upcoming gubernatorial elections. "With Pataki, I had no doubt that if he won we would see a different force at work. The activists would not have the same influence they had under Cuomo."

In November 1994, George Pataki narrowly defeated Mario Cuomo for governor.

POLITICAL MANEUVERINGS, 1995–1996

Shortly after Pataki assumed office, he held to one of his campaign promises to limit government by placing a moratorium on the promulgation of any new regulations. Ironically, this included the Department of Social Services' effort to create permanent rules for the HIV testing of foster children after its emergency rule making of 1994. The Association to Benefit Children felt that its negotiated victory was in jeopardy and began preparing another lawsuit. In mid-March, ABC sued the governor on behalf of "Baby Girl" seeking routine HIV testing for all newborns, and treatment and counseling for all HIV-positive infants, mothers, and other family members. Mayersohn had encouraged the lawsuit, since she felt it would help advance the cause of mandatory testing. The HIV Law Project, a legal advocacy group representing HIV-infected women, petitioned the court to be added as a "defendant–intervenor" since it felt that the state would not adequately represent its own interest in maintaining the voluntary testing program, given the campaign statements of both Pataki and Attorney General Dennis Vacco.

There was little doubt as to the new administration's agenda concerning newborn testing. When Pataki's nominee for health commissioner, Dr. Barbara DeBuono, commented in an appointment hearing that she supported voluntary testing over mandatory testing approaches, Mayersohn placed a call to the governor. Within a couple of days, DeBuono had reversed her position and proffered her support for pursuing mandatory newborn testing.

Actions at the federal level in the spring of 1995 were felt at the state level as well. In March, Congressmen Ackerman and Coburn introduced H.R.-1289, an amendment to the Ryan White Comprehensive AIDS Resources Emergency (CARE) Act which would require states to disclose the HIV status of newborns.

The amendment gained broad bipartisan support, including from the congressional Black Caucus and such progressive representatives as Ronald Dellums and Patricia Schroeder. In response, in May 1995 the CDC suspended its anonymous HIV Survey of Childbearing Women. According to one senior New York public health official, the state health department decided to continue its program of newborn surveillance without the $500,000 provided by the CDC. "After Mayersohn began agitating," the official noted, sharply contrasting the state response to that of the federal public health agency, "it would not have been politically astute to pull it."

After Mayersohn and Velella reintroduced their mandatory testing bills, there was again a great deal of movement to strike a compromise before the end of the legislative session in early July. Late in the evening on one of the last nights of the session, a member of Assembly Speaker Silver's staff approached Mayersohn. The speaker was willing to amend the law to allow the health commissioner to order the HIV test, rather than mandate it by law. Mayersohn readily accepted the compromise. This time, as the legislative session drew to a close, Mayersohn was convinced that her position would prevail. As happened the previous year, though, the legislation that everyone expected to pass was not brought to the floor. According to various accounts, the speaker had been approached by Assembly Democrats opposed to mandatory testing, so he had decided instead to await the resolution of the Ackerman–Coburn amendment in the House of Representatives.

In September 1995, the state attorney general approached ABC to settle its lawsuit. Since the governor could not change the confidentiality statute by executive order, the state was limited to working within the bounds of an arrangement that included written informed consent. The two sides (absent the HIV Law Project) settled upon a compromise. The state would propose rules by which postpartum women would be approached for consent to have their infant's HIV status disclosed, and there would be a provision allowing a physician to conduct HIV testing if he or she determined that an emergency existed. According to ABC counsel Colin Crawford, in retrospect ABC "could have considered the possibility of voluntary testing following a compelled choice either to learn the results or not, far earlier than we did. We could have come to this realization, moreover, from working even harder than we did to try and accommodate the confidentiality and civil liberties of our opponents."

Richard Gottfried, chair of the Assembly Health Committee, was not unhappy with the settlement. "For some people, the ABC lawsuit gave legitimacy to Nettie's position. But, in fact, it was almost exactly what I would have wanted to have as state law." The only critical difference, according to Gottfried, was that the proposed rules would mandate directed HIV counseling only in state-regulated facilities (such as hospitals, clinics, and certain HMO practices), whereas the Silver–Tully bill he had cosponsored would require all physicians—whether regulated or not, public or private—to provide mandatory counseling.

In settling the lawsuit, Governor Pataki was quoted in the *New York Times* as saying, "This is as far as we can go in the absence of legislative action." Mayersohn announced she would reintroduce her bill in January 1996. Pataki, supporting Mayersohn, said he would sign the bill if it crossed his desk.

Over a period of five months, the state health department worked with the governor's office to develop rules and an implementation plan for what was being called the "Consented Newborn HIV Testing Program." As implemented on May 1, 1996, the regulations required that women in labor must sign a written consent form, and if neither consent nor refusal is present a physician may order the HIV test. If the woman provided written consent, she would receive the results of her newborn's HIV test, would consent to follow-up testing of the baby after discharge to determine if the baby was truly infected, and would authorize the disclosure of the baby's test result to appropriate programs and the state health department to ensure that the baby received follow-up and specialty medical care. The facility providing maternity services would be responsible for identifying a physician to receive the HIV test results, preferably the baby's pediatrician. Post-test counseling would be provided at the time the woman was notified of the test results, and the pediatrician was required to order a polymerase chain reaction (PCR) test on the newborn to determine if the infant was HIV infected or was only manifesting the mother's antibodies. If the state newborn screening program did not receive the PCR specimen within five to six weeks after birth, it would contact the hospital designee or pediatrician for further follow-up.

Women could refuse notification of results, in which case the screening would remain anonymous and be used for epidemiologic purposes only. If a woman in the newborn setting did not provide written consent or refusal, her physician could act in the absence of parental consent "when a medical emergency exists for the infant." According to state health department officials, over the nine-month period of the Consented Newborn HIV Testing Program, this emergency provision was exercised only four times—in two cases the babies had been separated from their mothers, and in one case the mother was comatose.

Notwithstanding the compromise reached over the lawsuit, in the months surrounding the implementation of the Consented Testing Program the mandatory testing legislation reintroduced by Mayersohn and Velella gained considerable momentum. In late April, House and Senate negotiators came to an agreement over mandatory testing as part of the Ryan White CARE Act reauthorization. House Republicans agreed to support the position of the Senate conference committee, the American Medical Association, and the National Governor's Association calling for a five-year trial period of voluntary testing before instituting mandatory newborn testing. As signed in June, the Ryan White CARE Reauthorization Act required states to demonstrate that they had satisfied one of the following criteria, or face the loss of their Title II funding: either (1) a 50% reduction in AIDS cases from perinatal transmission compared with 1993 data; (2) HIV testing of at least 95% of pregnant women who had received at least two prenatal visits prior to 34 weeks gestation; or (3) a program of mandatory testing of all newborns whose mothers had not undergone prenatal HIV testing.

Also in June 1996, Assembly Speaker Sheldon Silver reversed his position on mandatory testing legislation and allowed the bill to pass the legislature. According to one legislative insider, "The Assembly leadership did not want to go into 1996 elections with this as an open issue. In 1994, the U.S. House and Senate went Republican, as did the New York governor. In 1996, the Speaker was very concerned this [opposition to mandatory testing] would lead to a loss of a significant number of Assembly seats, and that would then invigorate the Republicans. We could potentially lose majority control. That got played out on a long list of issues, whether criminal justice, or welfare reform, or mandatory testing." On June 26, 1996, Pataki signed the Baby AIDS bill into law. The new law gave the health commissioner the authority to impose newborn HIV tests. According to Speaker Silver, "We're leaving it to the health professionals to make the determination."

As expected, Health Commissioner Barbara DeBuono issued a call for developing regulations to put the mandatory newborn HIV screening program into place, and on February 1, 1997, the Comprehensive Newborn Testing Program was implemented.

EPILOGUE

In the wake of the mandatory newborn testing policy which began in 1997, Mayersohn returned to her original proposed partner notification legislation from 1993. According to one observer, "The success of the Baby AIDS program [mandatory newborn testing] was a major arguing point in the efforts to pass partner notification, and the lines of support were parallel." A number of county health officials, the state medical society, and a number of physicians supported the effort; similarly, a number of community groups, civil libertarians, and physicians opposed to mandatory newborn testing also opposed the partner notification legislation. The case of Nushawn Williams, an HIV-positive Brooklyn man who infected a number of underage teenage girls through sexual contacts in rural Chautauqua County in 1997, further fueled public debate and interest in the partner notification legislation. According to public reports about the case, although Williams was aware of his HIV-positive status he did not disclose it to the girls with whom he had intercourse. A number have since tested positive for HIV.

Mayersohn's reintroduced bill requires providers to solicit the names of sexual contacts and injection drug-using contacts from individuals who test positive for HIV. Physicians, laboratories, coroners, and medical examiners are required to report the names of individuals testing positive and their contacts (if known) to the state health commissioner. In turn, the state will then forward the information to the local health commissioner or district health officer. Local health officers are required to trace the sexual and/or drug-sharing contacts of

HIV-positive individuals, inform them of their risk, provide counseling, and direct them to testing and treatment centers. Rigorous confidentiality standards are required, and the identity of the index case may not be revealed to the partners who are traced. Furthermore, a special protocol would be developed for individuals at risk of domestic violence. In addition to the "duty to warn," the legislation also allows the commissioner to establish a named HIV registry similar to that in effect in 27 other states. Mayersohn's bill was tabled for further discussion in 1997 and passed both houses of the legislature in the closing days of the 1998 session. The bill was signed into law by Governor Pataki on the last day of the legislative session in June 1998. After regulations are drafted and comments received, the law will go into effect on January 1, 1999.

The combined partner notification–named HIV registry legislation signified a further breach of New York's exceptionalist HIV policy. With some notable exceptions—such as the development of Special Needs Plans for HIV-positive Medicaid recipients, rather than pooling them with the rest of the Medicaid managed care population—public health policy regarding HIV-positive individuals has tended toward the more traditional approaches of case finding, containment, and chronic disease management.

Under the Pataki administration, the composition of the AIDS Advisory Council has changed as well, since the governor can appoint 9 of the 17 council members. There is less representation from advocacy groups and community interests, and a greater voice of traditionalist public health as represented by several suburban health commissioners. The governor also appointed Mayersohn's legislative counsel, William Viskovitch, to serve on the council.

Mayersohn herself has continued to support her agenda on a national scale, through a growing electronic network that includes contacts in Delaware, a medical society in California, congressional staff, an Indiana-based children's publisher, and a number of physicians who treat HIV-positive patients.

The state health department's AIDS Institute is no longer entrenched in the HIV policy arena, as it was under Axelrod and, particularly, Rango's direction. As one observer pointed out about the AIDS Institute, "There is no policy agenda now." All policy matters department-wide have been consolidated under a single office reporting directly to the commissioner, such that there is no AIDS policy distinct from that of the entire department.

Although the legislative battle over mandatory newborn testing in New York State is over, the legal battle continues. The HIV Law Project, a legal advocacy service for low-income HIV-positive individuals in the Bronx and Manhattan, has pursued a dual strategy: (1) malpractice suits against providers and institutions whose failure to carry out timely and appropriate testing and notification represent an abrogation of the standard of care; and (2) a lawsuit against the state health department for failure to carry out the law fairly, equitably, and with adequate protections. Despite the fact that the former strategy targets individual providers, the objective—as in the latter—is to implicate the law. Since a ruling on the HIV Law Project's request for a preliminary injunction against the state has not yet been issued, as of July 1998 New York remained the only state to mandatorily test newborns for HIV and notify the mother of the results. According to data released by the state health department, in the first 11 months of the newborn testing program (February through December 1997), 957 HIV-positive infants were identified out of 236,663 tested. These 957 infants were born to 923 HIV-positive mothers, of whom 96 (10.4%) had not known their HIV status prior to delivery.[3] Seventy-seven cases were referred back to the state health department for follow-up when the hospitals or physicians were unable to locate the mothers or persuade them to return for follow-up care. Using AIDS Institute staff in New York City and communicable disease specialists in upstate New York, the state was able to directly locate and notify 68 of the 77 mothers; 5 mothers had moved out of state, and 4 were lost to follow-up.

REFERENCES

American Healthline. Stateline—New York: Mothers Will Know Babies' HIV Test Results. October 10, 1995. [www document] URL http://cloakroom.com/pubs/healthline.

American Healthline. Politics & policy—Ryan White Act: Includes Mandatory Newborn HIV Testing, May 1, 1996. [www document] URL http://cloakroom.com/pubs/healthline.

American Healthline. Politics & Policy—Ryan White Act: House Passes Reauthorization Bill. May 2,1996. [www document] URL http://cloakroom.com/pubs/healthline.

American Healthline. Stateline—New York: Pataki Signs Newborn HIV Testing Law, June 27, 1996. [www document] URL http://cloakroom.com/pubs/healthline.

American Healthline. Stateline—New York: Pataki and Legislators Agree on HIV Testing Law. June 6, 1996. [www document] URL http://cloakroom.com/pubs/healthline.

Avery GB. Editorial: Out of the vortex—neonatologists' treatment decisions for newborns at risk for HIV. *AJPH* 85(11):1484–1485,1995.

Baby Girl Doe v. Pataki, Index No. 95-106661 (SupCt NY County, filed July 18, 1997).

Bayer R. Perinatal transmission of HIV infection: The ethics of prevention. In: Gostin LO, ed. *AIDS and the Health Care System*. New Haven: Yale University Press, 1990.

Bayer R. AIDS and the future of reproductive freedom. In: Nelkin D, Willis D, Parris S, eds. *A Disease of Society*. Cambridge, England: Cambridge University Press, 1991.

Bayer R. *Private Acts, Social Consequences*. New Brunswick, NJ: Rutgers University Press, 1991.

Bayer R. Public health policy and the AIDS epidemic: An end to exceptionalism? *NEJM* 324:1500–1504, 1991.

Bayer R. Women's rights, babies' interests: Ethics, politics, and science in the debate of newborn HIV screening. In: Minkoff HL, DeHovitz JA, Duerr A, eds. *HIV Infection in Women*. New York: Raven Press, 1995.

Bayer R. Rethinking the testing of babies and pregnant women for HIV infection. *Journal of Clinical Ethics* 7(1):85–87, 1996.

---

[3]Since the conversion of the infant's HIV status is unknown, one can only estimate the actual numbers of babies who will seroconvert to HIV positivity. Given a range of 10%–25% who might seroconvert, the number of HIV-positive babies ranges from 96 to 239; similarly, the number of HIV-positive infants whose mothers learned their status as a result of the mandatory testing program could range from 10 to 24 in the 11-month reporting period.

Bayer R, Levine C, Wolf SM. HIV antibody screening: An ethical framework for evaluating proposed programs. *JAMA* 256(13):1768–1774,1986.

Berger J, Rosner F, Farnsworth P. The ethics of mandatory HIV testing in newborns. *Journal of Clinical Ethics* 7(1):77–84, 1996.

Bernstein N. The secret life of AIDS. *Newsday*, Jan. 15, 1993.

Bernstein N. 'No one would tell me': Wife of AIDS victim was kept in dark. *Newsday*, Jan. 15, 1993.

Bernstein N. Death by silence: A failure to notify costs lives. *Newsday*, Jan. 15, 1993.

Bernstein N. Doctors' orders: No obligation to warn. *Newsday*, Jan. 17, 1993.

Bernstein N. 'Who wants to know they're going to die?' *Newsday*, Jan. 17, 1993.

Bernstein N. In grave danger: NY's partner-notification policy puts women at risk. *Newsday*, Jan. 17, 1993.

Bernstein A. The *Newsday* interview with Barbara DeBuono. *Newsday*, p. A23, Mar. 27, 1995.

Bunis D, Slackman M. NY plan: AIDS test for all newborns. *Newsday* p. A4, June 6, 1996.

Centers for Disease Control and Prevention. Update: HIV counseling and testing using rapid tests—United States, 1995. *MMWR* 47(11):211–215, 1998.

Chavkin W, Breitbart V, Wise P. Finding common ground: The necessity of an integrated agenda for women's and children's health. *Journal of Law, Medicine & Ethics* 22(3):262–269, 1994.

Chavkin W, Breitbart V, Wise P. Efforts to reduce perinatal mortality, HIV, and drug addiction: Survey of the states. *Journal of the American Medical Womens Association* 50(5):164–166, 1995.

Connor EM, Sperling RS, Gelber R, Kiselev P, Scott G, O'Sullivan MJ, VanDyke R, Bey M, Shearer W, Jacobson RL, Jimenez E, O'Neill E, Bazin B, Delfraissy JF, Culnane M, Coombs R, Elkins M, Moye J, Stratton P, Balsley J. Reduction of maternal–infant transmission of human immunodeficiency virus type 1 with zidovudine treatment. Pediatric AIDS Clinical Trials Group Protocol 076 Study Group. *N Engl J Med* 331(18):1173–1180, 1994.

Crossley M. Of diagnoses and discrimination: Discriminatory nontreatment of infants with HIV infection. *Columbia Law Review* 93(7):1581–1667, 1993.

Curnin K. Newborn HIV screening and NY Assembly bill 6747-B: Privacy and equal protection of pregnant women. *Fordham Urban Law Journal* 21(3):857–926, 1994.

Dwyer J. A silence that kills children. *Newsday* p. A2, Apr. 15, 1994.

Dwyer J. That dirty HIV secret. *Newsday*, June 1, 1994.

Dwyer J. State stands by as babies die. *Newsday* p. A2, June 8, 1994.

Dwyer J. Baby fodder for HIV data. *Newsday* p. A2, June 27, 1994.

Dwyer J. A devastation we didn't stop. *Newsday* p. A2, May 19, 1995.

Dwyer J. No silver lining for AIDS kids. *Newsday* p. A2, July 5, 1995.

Dwyer J. HIV results not positive. *Newsday*, July 14, 1996.

Fleischman A, Dumois A. HIV Testing is not health care. *Newsday*, Jan. 18, 1994.

Fleischman AR, Farber Post L, Neveloff Dubler N. Mandatory newborn screening for HIV. *Bull of the NY Academy of Medicine* 71(1):5–17, 1994.

Goodman E. Need change of attitude on HIV testing. *Albany Times Union* p. A11, July 18, 1995.

Gostin LO, Curran WJ. Legal control measures for AIDS: Reporting requirements, surveillance, quarantine, and regulation of public meeting places. *AJPH* 77(2):214–218, 1987.

Gostin LO, Webber DW. HIV infection and AIDS in the public health and health care systems: The role of law and litigation. *JAMA* 279(14):1108–1113, 1998.

Gottfried RN. The great importance of testing newborns for HIV. *Albany Times Union* p. A10, Jan. 21, 1994.

Gottfried R. Wiser moms, healthier kids. *Newsday* p. A38, Apr. 26, 1994.

Gottfried R. Make counseling mandatory. *Newsday* p. A40, June 9, 1994.

Grondahl P. Screening eases baby disorders. *Albany Times-Union* p. G1, Dec. 16, 1990.

Healton C, Messeri P, Abramson D, Howard J, Sorin MD, Bayer R. A balancing act: The tension between case finding and primary prevention strategies in New York State's voluntary HIV counseling and testing program in women's health care settings. *American Journal of Preventive Medicine* 12 (4 Suppl):53–60, 1996.

Hentoff N. Silence = Death. *Village Voice,* May 11, 1994.

Hentoff N. Gary Ackerman's multicultural liberators. *Village Voice,* May 17, 1995.

Hentoff N. The shame of Sheldon Silver. *Village Voice,* Aug. 1, 1995.

Hentoff N. Breakthrough for HIV-positive babies. *Washington Post,* July 1996.

Institute of Medicine. *HIV Screening of Pregnant Women and Newborns.* Washington, DC: National Academy Press, 1991.

Krasinski K, Borkowsky W, Bebenroth T. Failure of voluntary testing for human immunodeficiency virus to identify infected parturient women in a high-risk population (letter to the editor). *New Engl J Med* 318(3):185, 1988.

Landesman S, Minkoff H, Holman S, McCalla S, Sijin O. Serosurvey of HIV infection in parturients. *JAMA* 258(19):2701–2703, 1987.

Lester P, Partridge J, Chesney M, Cooke M. The consequences of a positive prenatal HIV antibody test for women. *Journal of Acquired Immune Deficiency Syndromes and Human Retrovirology* 10(3):341–349, 1995.

Levin BW, Krantz DH, Driscoll JM, Fleischman AR. The treatment of non-HIV-related condition in newborns at risk for HIV: A survey of neonatalogists. *AJPH* 85(11):1507–1513, 1995.

Mason-Draffen C. A vote for AIDS tests: Nassau recommends screening pregnant women. *Newsday,* July 22, 1992.

Mayersohn N. It's a baby, not a statistic, stupid. News from Assemblywoman Nettie Mayersohn, 27th Assembly District, 1993.

Mayersohn N. The "Baby AIDS" bill. *Fordham Urban Law Journal* 24(4):721–727, 1997.

McFadden RD. David Axelrod, health chief under Cuomo, is dead at 59. *NY Times* p. D14, July 5, 1994.

Minkoff H, Willoughby A. Pediatric HIV disease, zidovudine in pregnancy, and unblinding heelstick surveys. *JAMA* 274(14):1165–1168, 1995.

Nature. Editorial. AIDS and illiberal measures. *Nature* 325:647, 1987.

New York State AIDS Advisory Council. Report of the Subcommittee on Newborn HIV Screening. February 10, 1994.

New York State AIDS Institute. Principles for the Care of Women and Children with HIV Infection (the "Mohonk Principles"). 1990.

New York State Assembly—Nettie Mayersohn, 1998. [www document] URL http://assembly.state.ny.us/ members/bios/mayersn.html.

New York State Assembly Bill 6629-A, Senate Bill 4422-A, "HIV Partner Notification Bill," June 18, 1998.

New York State Department of Health. HIV counseling and testing of pregnant women and newborns. Memorandum 96-7, Apr. 8, 1996.

New York State Department of Health. Maternal–pediatric HIV prevention and care program: HIV counseling and voluntary testing of pregnant women; routine HIV testing of newborns as part of the Comprehensive Newborn Testing Program. Memorandum 97-2, Jan. 24, 1997.

New York State Public Health Law. AIDS Institute Advisory Council. Article 27-E, Sec. 2778, amended 1990.

Newsday. Editorial. State should tell moms their infants have HIV. *Newsday,* Aug. 14, 1995.

New York Times. Editorial. AIDS babies deserve testing. *NY Times* p. A16, June 27, 1994.

Novick LF, Berns D, Stricof R, Stevens R, Pass K, Wethers J. HIV seroprevalence in newborns in New York State. *JAMA* 261(12):1745–1750, 1989.

Novick LF. HIV seroprevalence surveys: Impetus for preventive activities. *AJPH* 81(Suppl):15–21, 1991.

Novick LF. New York State HIV seroprevalence project: Goals, windows, and policy consideration. *AJPH* 81(Suppl):11–14, 1991.

Novick LF, Glebatis DM, Stricof RL, MacCubbin PA, Lessner L, Berns DS. Newborn seroprevalence study: Methods and results. *AJPH* 81(Suppl):15–21, 1991.

Perez-Rivas M. The Baby AIDS bill: On a crusade—lawmaker's profile grows. *Newsday,* Mar. 31, 1994.

Quindlen A. Take a good, hard look at infant AIDS legislation. *Albany Times Union* p. A11, June 8, 1994.

R.Z. v. Pataki, Index No. 97-112960 (SupCt NY County, filed July 18, 1997).

Richardson L. HIV testing project draws complaints. *NY Times,* June 16, 1997.

Riley J. AIDS baby bill favored by GOP guv hopeful. *Newsday* p. A12, June 11, 1994.

Sack K. Battle lines drawn over newborn HIV disclosure. *NY Times* p. A23, June 26, 1994.

Sontag D. HIV testing for newborns debated anew. *NY Times* p. A1, Feb. 10, 1997.

Taylor CL. Baby AIDS test bill fizzling: But deal may be in works. *Newsday,* May 24, 1994.

Teare C, English A. Women, girls, and the HIV epidemic. In: Moss KL, ed. *Man-Made Medicine: Women's Health, Public Policy, and Reform.* Durham, NC: Duke University Press, 1996.

Truog R. Is 'Informed right of refusal' the same as informed consent? *Journal of Clinical Ethics* 7(1):87–89, 1996.

Vacco D. Turning a 'blind' eye to dying babies. *Albany Times Union* p. A9, Sept. 12, 1995.

Wiemer B. Conspiracy of Silence Aids AIDS' spread. *Newsday,* July 27, 1992.

Excerpts from the Ryan White CARE Act Amendments of 1996

110 STAT. 1368   PUBLIC LAW 104-146—MAY 20, 1996

SEC. 7. PERINATAL TRANSMISSION OF HIV DISEASE.

42 USC 300ff-33
note.

(a) FINDINGS.—The Congress finds as follows:

(1) Research studies and statewide clinical experiences have demonstrated that administration of anti-retroviral medication during pregnancy can significantly reduce the transmission of the human immunodeficiency virus (commonly known as HIV) from an infected mother to her baby.

(2) The Centers for Disease Control and Prevention have recommended that all pregnant women receive HIV counseling; voluntary, confidential HIV testing; and appropriate medical treatment (including anti-retroviral therapy) and support services.

(3) The provision of such testing without access to such counseling, treatment, and services will not improve the health of the woman or the child.

(4) The provision of such counseling, testing, treatment, and services can reduce the number of pediatric cases of acquired immune deficiency syndrome, can improve access to and provision of medical care for the woman, and can provide opportunities for counseling to reduce transmission among adults, and from mother to child.

(5) The provision of such counseling, testing, treatment, and services can reduce the overall cost of pediatric cases of acquired immune deficiency syndrome.

(6) The cancellation or limitation of health insurance or other health coverage on the basis of HIV status should be impermissible under applicable law. Such cancellation or limitation could result in disincentives for appropriate counseling, testing, treatment, and services.

(7) For the reasons specified in paragraphs (1) through (6)—

(A) routine HIV counseling and voluntary testing of pregnant women should become the standard of care; and

(B) the relevant medical organizations as well as public health officials should issue guidelines making such counseling and testing the standard of care.

(b) ADDITIONAL REQUIREMENTS FOR GRANTS.—Part B of title XXVI (42 U.S.C. 300ff-21 et seq.) is amended—

(1) by inserting after the part heading the following:

"Subpart I—General Grant Provisions";

42 USC 300ff-21.

(2) in section 2611(a), by adding at the end the following sentence: "The authority of the Secretary to provide grants under part B is subject to section 2626(e)(2) (relating to the decrease in perinatal transmission of HIV disease)."; and

PUBLIC LAW 104–146—MAY 20, 1996   110 STAT. 1369

(3) by adding at the end thereof the following new subpart:

"Subpart II—Provisions Concerning Pregnancy and Perinatal Transmission of HIV

"**SEC. 2625. CDC GUIDELINES FOR PREGNANT WOMEN.**   42 USC 300ff–33.

"(a) REQUIREMENT.—Notwithstanding any other provision of   Certification.
law, a State shall, not later than 120 days after the date of enactment of this subpart, certify to the Secretary that such State has
in effect regulations or measures to adopt the guidelines issued
by the Centers for Disease Control and Prevention concerning recommendations for human immunodeficiency virus counseling and
voluntary testing for pregnant women.

"(b) NONCOMPLIANCE.—If a State does not provide the certification required under subsection (a) within the 120-day period
described in such subsection, such State shall not be eligible to
receive assistance for HIV counseling and testing under this section
until such certification is provided.

"(c) ADDITIONAL FUNDS REGARDING WOMEN AND INFANTS.—

"(1) IN GENERAL.—If a State provides the certification
required in subsection (a) and is receiving funds under part
B for a fiscal year, the Secretary may (from the amounts
available pursuant to paragraph (2)) make a grant to the State
for the fiscal year for the following purposes:

"(A) Making available to pregnant women appropriate
counseling on HIV disease.

"(B) Making available outreach efforts to pregnant
women at high risk of HIV who are not currently receiving
prenatal care.

"(C) Making available to such women voluntary HIV
testing for such disease.

"(D) Offsetting other State costs associated with the
implementation of this section and subsections (a) and
(b) of section 2626.

"(E) Offsetting State costs associated with the
implementation of mandatory newborn testing in accordance with this title or at an earlier date than is required
by this title.

"(2) FUNDING.—For purposes of carrying out this subsection, there are authorized to be appropriated $10,000,000
for each of the fiscal years 1996 through 2000. Amounts made
available under section 2677 for carrying out this part are
not available for carrying out this section unless otherwise
authorized.

"(3) PRIORITY.—In awarding grants under this subsection
the Secretary shall give priority to States that have the greatest
proportion of HIV seroprevalance among child bearing women
using the most recent data available as determined by the
Centers for Disease Control and Prevention.

"**SEC. 2626. PERINATAL TRANSMISSION OF HIV DISEASE; CONTINGENT**   42 USC 300ff–34.
**REQUIREMENT REGARDING STATE GRANTS UNDER THIS
PART.**

"(a) ANNUAL DETERMINATION OF REPORTED CASES.—A State
shall annually determine the rate of reported cases of AIDS as
a result of perinatal transmission among residents of the State.

"(b) CAUSES OF PERINATAL TRANSMISSION.—In determining the rate under subsection (a), a State shall also determine the possible causes of perinatal transmission. Such causes may include—

"(1) the inadequate provision within the State of prenatal counseling and testing in accordance with the guidelines issued by the Centers for Disease Control and Prevention;

"(2) the inadequate provision or utilization within the State of appropriate therapy or failure of such therapy to reduce perinatal transmission of HIV, including—

"(A) that therapy is not available, accessible or offered to mothers; or

"(B) that available therapy is offered but not accepted by mothers; or

"(3) other factors (which may include the lack of prenatal care) determined relevant by the State.

"(c) CDC REPORTING SYSTEM.—Not later than 4 months after the date of enactment of this subpart, the Director of the Centers for Disease Control and Prevention shall develop and implement a system to be used by States to comply with the requirements of subsections (a) and (b). The Director shall issue guidelines to ensure that the data collected is statistically valid.

Guidelines.

Federal Register, publication.

"(d) DETERMINATION BY SECRETARY.—Not later than 180 days after the expiration of the 18-month period beginning on the date on which the system is implemented under subsection (c), the Secretary shall publish in the Federal Register a determination of whether it has become a routine practice in the provision of health care in the United States to carry out each of the activities described in paragraphs (1) through (5) of section 2627. In making the determination, the Secretary shall consult with the States and with other public or private entities that have knowledge or expertise relevant to the determination.

"(e) CONTINGENT APPLICABILITY.—

"(1) IN GENERAL.—If the determination published in the Federal Register under subsection (d) is that (for purposes of such subsection) the activities involved have become routine practices, paragraph (2) shall apply on and after the expiration of the 18-month period beginning on the date on which the determination is so published.

"(2) REQUIREMENT.—Subject to subsection (f), the Secretary shall not make a grant under part B to a State unless the State meets not less than one of the following requirements:

"(A) A 50 percent reduction (or a comparable measure for States with less than 10 cases) in the rate of new cases of AIDS (recognizing that AIDS is a suboptimal proxy for tracking HIV in infants and was selected because such data is universally available) as a result of perinatal transmission as compared to the rate of such cases reported in 1993 (a State may use HIV data if such data is available).

"(B) At least 95 percent of women in the State who have received at least two prenatal visits (consultations) prior to 34 weeks gestation with a health care provider or provider group have been tested for the human immunodeficiency virus.

"(C) The State has in effect, in statute or through regulations, the requirements specified in paragraphs (1) through (5) of section 2627.

PUBLIC LAW 104-146—MAY 20, 1996   110 STAT. 1371

"(f) LIMITATION REGARDING AVAILABILITY OF FUNDS.—With respect to an activity described in any of paragraphs (1) through (5) of section 2627, the requirements established by a State under this section apply for purposes of this section only to the extent that the following sources of funds are available for carrying out the activity:

"(1) Federal funds provided to the State in grants under part B or under section 2625, or through other Federal sources under which payments for routine HIV testing, counseling or treatment are an eligible use.

"(2) Funds that the State or private entities have elected to provide, including through entering into contracts under which health benefits are provided. This section does not require any entity to expend non-Federal funds.

"SEC. 2627. TESTING OF PREGNANT WOMEN AND NEWBORN INFANTS.   42 USC 300ff-35.

"An activity or requirement described in this section is any of the following:

"(1) In the case of newborn infants who are born in the State and whose biological mothers have not undergone prenatal testing for HIV disease, that each such infant undergo testing for such disease.

"(2) That the results of such testing of a newborn infant be promptly disclosed in accordance with the following, as applicable to the infant involved:

"(A) To the biological mother of the infant (without regard to whether she is the legal guardian of the infant).

"(B) If the State is the legal guardian of the infant:

"(i) To the appropriate official of the State agency with responsibility for the care of the infant.

"(ii) To the appropriate official of each authorized agency providing assistance in the placement of the infant.

"(iii) If the authorized agency is giving significant consideration to approving an individual as a foster parent of the infant, to the prospective foster parent.

"(iv) If the authorized agency is giving significant consideration to approving an individual as an adoptive parent of the infant, to the prospective adoptive parent.

"(C) If neither the biological mother nor the State is the legal guardian of the infant, to another legal guardian of the infant.

"(D) To the child's health care provider.

"(3) That, in the case of prenatal testing for HIV disease that is conducted in the State, the results of such testing be promptly disclosed to the pregnant woman involved.

"(4) That, in disclosing the test results to an individual under paragraph (2) or (3), appropriate counseling on the human immunodeficiency virus be made available to the individual (except in the case of a disclosure to an official of a State or an authorized agency).

"(5) With respect to State insurance laws, that such laws require—

"(A) that, if health insurance is in effect for an individual, the insurer involved may not (without the consent of the individual) discontinue the insurance, or alter the terms of the insurance (except as provided in subparagraph

(C)), solely on the basis that the individual is infected with HIV disease or solely on the basis that the individual has been tested for the disease or its manifestation;

"(B) that subparagraph (A) does not apply to an individual who, in applying for the health insurance involved, knowingly misrepresented the HIV status of the individual; and

"(C) that subparagraph (A) does not apply to any reasonable alteration in the terms of health insurance for an individual with HIV disease that would have been made if the individual had a serious disease other than HIV disease.

For purposes of this subparagraph, a statute or regulation shall be deemed to regulate insurance for purposes of this paragraph only to the extent that such statute or regulation is treated as regulating insurance for purposes of section 514(b)(2) of the Employee Retirement Income Security Act of 1974.

42 USC 300ff–36. **"SEC. 2628. REPORT BY THE INSTITUTE OF MEDICINE.**

"(a) IN GENERAL.—The Secretary shall request that the Institute of Medicine of the National Academy of Sciences conduct an evaluation of the extent to which State efforts have been effective in reducing the perinatal transmission of the human immuno deficiency virus, and an analysis of the existing barriers to the further reduction in such transmission.

"(b) REPORT TO CONGRESS.—The Secretary shall ensure that, not later than 2 years after the date of enactment of this section, the evaluation and analysis described in subsection (a) is completed and a report summarizing the results of such evaluation and analysis is prepared by the Institute of Medicine and submitted to the appropriate committees of Congress together with the recommendations of the Institute.

42 USC 300ff–37. **"SEC. 2629. STATE HIV TESTING PROGRAMS ESTABLISHED PRIOR TO OR AFTER ENACTMENT.**

"Nothing in this subpart shall be construed to disqualify a State from receiving grants under this title if such State has established at any time prior to or after the date of enactment of this subpart a program of mandatory HIV testing.".

1995 U.S. Public Health Service Recommendations for Human Immunodeficiency Virus Counseling and Testing for Pregnant Women

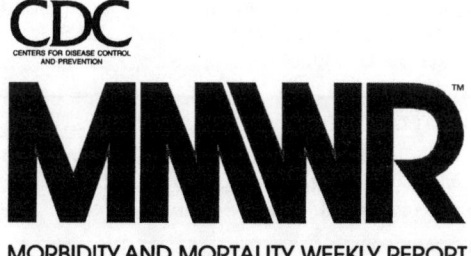

July 7, 1995 / Vol. 44 / No. RR-7

*Recommendations
and
Reports*

MORBIDITY AND MORTALITY WEEKLY REPORT

U.S. Public Health Service Recommendations for Human Immunodeficiency Virus Counseling and Voluntary Testing for Pregnant Women

U.S. DEPARTMENT OF HEALTH AND HUMAN SERVICES
Public Health Service
Centers for Disease Control
and Prevention (CDC)
Atlanta, Georgia 30333

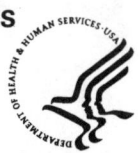

The *MMWR* series of publications is published by the Epidemiology Program Office, Centers for Disease Control and Prevention (CDC), Public Health Service, U.S. Department of Health and Human Services, Atlanta, GA 30333.

SUGGESTED CITATION

Centers for Disease Control and Prevention. U.S. Public Health Service recommendations for human immunodeficiency virus counseling and voluntary testing for pregnant women. MMWR 1995;44(No. RR-7):[inclusive page numbers].

Centers for Disease Control and Prevention .... David Satcher, M.D., Ph.D.
Director

The material in this report was prepared for publication by:

National Center for HIV/STD/TB Prevention .... Helene D. Gayle, M.D., M.P.H.
Acting Director

Division of HIV/AIDS Prevention ....James W. Curran, M.D., M.P.H.
Acting Director

The production of this report as an *MMWR* serial publication was coordinated in:

Epidemiology Program Office.................................... Stephen B. Thacker, M.D., M.Sc.
Director

Richard A. Goodman, M.D., M.P.H.
Editor, MMWR *Series*

Scientific Information and Communications Program

Recommendations and Reports.................................. Suzanne M. Hewitt, M.P.A.
Managing Editor

Rachel J. Wilson
Project Editor

Morie M. Higgins
Peter M. Jenkins
Visual Information Specialists

Copies can be purchased from Superintendent of Documents, U.S. Government Printing Office, Washington, DC 20402-9325. Telephone: (202) 783-3238.

351

Contents

Use of AZT to Prevent Perinatal Transmission (ACTG 076): Workshop on Implications for Treatment, Counseling, and HIV Testing

In February 1994, the National Institutes of Health announced interim results from a multicenter, placebo-controlled clinical trial (AIDS Clinical Trials Group [ACTG] protocol 076), indicating that administration of zidovudine (ZDV) to a selected group of pregnant women infected with human immunodeficiency virus (HIV) and to their newborns reduced the risk for perinatal HIV transmission by approximately two thirds. On June 6–7, 1994, the U.S. Public Health Service (PHS) convened a workshop in Bethesda, Maryland, to a) develop recommendations for the use of ZDV to reduce the risk for perinatal HIV transmission and b) discuss the implications of these recommendations for treatment, counseling, and HIV testing of women and infants. PHS published recommendations regarding ZDV therapy for pregnant women and their newborns in August 1994.* The following persons either served as consultants at the workshop for developing the recommendations for HIV counseling and voluntary testing for pregnant women or were members of the U.S. Public Health Service Task Force on the Use of Zidovudine to Reduce Perinatal Transmission of Human Immunodeficiency Virus.

Consultants

James R. Allen, M.D., M.P.H.
American Medical Association
Chicago, IL

Arthur J. Ammann, M.D.
Pediatric AIDS Foundation
Novato, CA

Kela Ammons-Blenman
Multicultural AIDS Coalition, Inc.
Boston, MA

Barbara Aranda-Naranjo, R.N., M.S.N.
The University of Texas Health Science
   Center at San Antonio
San Antonio, TX

Marian D. Banzhaf
New Jersey Women and AIDS Network
New Brunswick, NJ

Mary Beth Caschetta, M.A.
HIV Law Project
New York, NY

Louis Z. Cooper, M.D.
St. Luke's-Roosevelt Hospital Center
New York, NY

Rosemary Davis
National Medical Association
Washington, DC

Clemente Diaz, M.D.
University of Puerto Rico Children's
   Hospital
San Juan, PR

Ana O. Dumois, Ph.D., D.S.W.
Community Family Planning Council
New York, NY

*CDC. Recommendations of the U.S. Public Health Service Task Force on the Use of Zidovudine to Reduce Perinatal Transmission of Human Immunodeficiency Virus. MMWR 1994;43 (No. RR-11).

Vol. 44 / No. RR-7   MMWR   iii

Consultants — Continued

Kathleen Edwards, M.D.
Department of Health and Mental
    Hygiene
Baltimore, MD

I. Celine Hanson, M.D.
Baylor College of Medicine
Houston, TX

Cheryl Healton, Dr.P.H.
Columbia School of Public Health
New York, NY

Lisa Hernandez
For AIDS Children Everywhere
Cincinnati, OH

Richard Hoffman, M.D., M.P.H.
Council of State and Territorial
    Epidemiologists
Denver, CO

Linda Horton
Baltimore, MD

Jeannette Ickovics, Ph.D.
Yale University
New Haven, CT

Paul Kawata
National Minority AIDS Council
Washington, DC

Joep M.A. Lange, M.D.
World Health Organization
Geneva, Switzerland

Michael K. Lindsay, M.D., M.P.H.
Emory University
Atlanta, GA

Patricia Loftman, C.N.M., M.S.
Harlem Hospital Center
New York, NY

Laurene Mascola, M.D.
Los Angeles County Department of
    Health Services
Los Angeles, CA

Herman Mendez, M.D.
State University of New York at
    Brooklyn
Brooklyn, NY

Howard Minkoff, M.D.
State University of New York at
    Brooklyn
Brooklyn, NY

Janet L. Mitchell, M.D., M.P.H.
Harlem Hospital Center
New York, NY

Cynthia Newbille
National Black Women's Health Project
Atlanta, GA

Robert H. Pantell, M.D.
University of California
San Francisco, CA

Sallie Perryman
New York State Department of Health
New York, NY

Merlene Robb
National Coalition of Hispanic Health
    and Human Services
Washington, DC

Merlin Robb, M.D.
Walter Reed Army Institute of Research
Rockville, MD

Gary Rose
National Association of Persons with
    AIDS
Washington, DC

George Rutherford, M.D.
California Department of Health
    Services
Sacramento, CA

Consultants — Continued

Gwendolyn B. Scott, M.D.
University of Miami School of Medicine
Miami, FL

Maureen Shannon, C.N.M., F.N.P.
San Francisco General Hospital
San Francisco, CA

Gloria Spears
Powder Springs, GA

Pauline Thomas, M.D.
New York City Department of Health
New York, NY

Mary Kay Whitaker
Cooper Hospital
Pleasantville, NJ

Stanley Zinberg, M.D.
The American College of Obstetricians
   and Gynecologists
Washington, DC

Carmen Zorrilla, M.D.
University of Puerto Rico School of
   Medicine
San Juan, PR

U.S. Public Health Service Task Force on the Use of Zidovudine to Reduce Perinatal Transmission of Human Immunodeficiency Virus

Lynne M. Mofenson, M.D. (chair)
National Institutes of Health
Bethesda, MD

James Balsley, M.D., Ph.D.
National Institutes of Health
Bethesda, MD

Patricia S. Fleming
Office of the Secretary
U.S. Department of Health and Human
   Services
Washington, D.C.

Helene D. Gayle, M.D., M.P.H.
Centers for Disease Control and
   Prevention
Atlanta, GA

Steve Gitterman, M.D., Ph.D.
Food and Drug Administration
Rockville, MD

David Lanier, M.D.
Agency for Health Care Policy and
   Research
Rockville, MD

Frances E. Page, M.P.H.
Office of National AIDS Policy
Washington, DC

Martha F. Rogers, M.D.
Centers for Disease Control and
   Prevention
Atlanta, GA

Patricia Salomon, M.D.
Health Resources and Services
   Administration
Rockville, MD

The following CDC staff members prepared this report:

Martha F. Rogers, M.D.
Robin R. Moseley, M.A.T.
Robert J. Simonds, M.D.
Janet S. Moore, Ph.D.
Marta Gwinn, M.D., M.P.H.
Linda G. Elsner
James W. Curran, M.D., M.P.H.
Division of HIV/AIDS Prevention
National Center for HIV/STD/TB Prevention

Amy S. Bloom, M.D.
Herbert B. Peterson, M.D.
Division of Reproductive Health
National Center for Chronic Disease Prevention
and Health Promotion

in collaboration with

Lynne M. Mofenson, M.D.
Center for Research for Mothers and Children
National Insititute of Child Health and Human Development
National Institutes of Health

U.S. Public Health Service Recommendations for Human Immunodeficiency Virus Counseling and Voluntary Testing for Pregnant Women

Summary

These recommendations were developed by the U.S. Public Health Service to address the increasing epidemic of human immunodeficiency virus (HIV) infection among women and their infants. The recommendations stress the importance of early diagnosis of HIV infection for the health of both women and their infants and are based on advances made in HIV-related treatment and prevention. The most significant advance for this population has been the results from a placebo-controlled, clinical trial that indicated that administration of zidovudine to HIV-infected pregnant women and their newborns reduced the risk for perinatal transmission of HIV by approximately two thirds (1). This document recommends routine HIV counseling and voluntary testing for all pregnant women and is intended to serve as guidance for health-care providers in educating women about the importance of knowing their HIV infection status. For uninfected women, such HIV counseling and testing programs can provide information that can reduce their risk for acquiring HIV; for women who have HIV infection, these programs can enable them to receive appropriate and timely medical interventions for their own health and for reducing the risk for perinatal (i.e., mother to infant) and other modes of HIV transmission. These programs also can facilitate appropriate follow-up care and services for HIV-infected women, their infants, and other family members.

INTRODUCTION

During the past decade, human immunodeficiency virus (HIV) infection has become a leading cause of morbidity and mortality among women, the population accounting for the most rapid increase in cases of acquired immunodeficiency syndrome (AIDS) in recent years. As the incidence of HIV infection has increased among women of childbearing age, increasing numbers of children have become infected through perinatal (i.e., mother to infant) transmission; thus, HIV infection has also become a leading cause of death for young children. To reverse these trends, HIV education and services for prevention and health care must be made available to all women. Women who have HIV infection or who are at risk for infection need access to current information regarding a) early interventions to improve survival rates and quality of life for HIV-infected persons, b) strategies to reduce the risk for perinatal HIV transmission, and c) management of HIV-infection in pregnant women and perinatally exposed or infected children. Results from a randomized, placebo-controlled clinical trial have indicated that the risk for perinatal HIV transmission can be substantially reduced by administration of zidovudine (ZDV [also referred to as AZT]) to HIV-infected pregnant women and their newborns (1). To optimally benefit from this therapy, HIV-infection must be diagnosed in these women before or during early pregnancy.

The U.S. Public Health Service (PHS) encourages all women to adopt behaviors that can prevent HIV infection and to learn their HIV status through counseling and voluntary testing. Ideally, women should know their HIV infection status before becoming pregnant. Thus, sites serving women of childbearing age (e.g., physicians' offices, family planning clinics, sexually transmitted disease clinics, and adolescent clinics) should counsel and offer voluntary HIV testing to women, including adolescents—regardless of whether they are pregnant. Because specific services must be offered to HIV-infected pregnant women to prevent perinatal transmission, PHS is recommending routine HIV counseling and voluntary testing of all pregnant women so that interventions to improve the woman's health and the health of her infant can be offered in a timely and effective manner.

The recommendations in this report were developed by PHS as guidance for health-care providers in their efforts to a) encourage HIV-infected pregnant women to learn their infection status; b) advise infected pregnant women of methods for preventing perinatal, sexual, and other modes of HIV transmission; c) facilitate appropriate follow-up for HIV-infected women, their infants, and their families; and d) help uninfected pregnant women reduce their risk for acquiring HIV infection. Increased availability of HIV counseling, voluntary testing, and follow-up medical and support services is essential to ensure successful implementation of these recommendations. These services can be optimally delivered through a readily available medical system with support services designed to facilitate ongoing care for patients.

BACKGROUND

HIV Infection and AIDS in Women and Children

HIV infection is a major cause of illness and death among women and children. Nationally, HIV infection was the fourth leading cause of death in 1993 among women 25–44 years of age (*2*) and the seventh leading cause of death in 1992 among children 1–4 years of age (*3*). Blacks and Hispanics have been disproportionately affected by the HIV epidemic. In 1993, HIV infection was the leading cause of death among black women 25–44 years of age and the third leading cause of death among Hispanic women in this age group (*2*). In 1991, HIV infection was the second leading cause of death among black children 1–4 years of age in New Jersey, Massachusetts, New York, and Florida and among Hispanic children in this age group in New York (CDC, unpublished data).

By 1995, CDC had received reports of >58,000 AIDS cases among adult and adolescent women and >5,500 cases among children who acquired HIV infection perinatally. Approximately one half of all AIDS cases among women have been attributed to injecting-drug use and one third to heterosexual contact. Nearly 90% of cumulative AIDS cases reported among children and virtually all new HIV infections among children in the United States can be attributed to perinatal transmission of HIV. An increasing proportion of perinatally acquired AIDS cases has been reported among children whose mothers acquired HIV infection through heterosexual contact with an infected partner whose infection status and risk factors were not known by the mother.

Data from the National Survey of Childbearing Women indicate that in 1992, the estimated national prevalence of HIV infection among childbearing women was

1.7 HIV-infected women per 1,000 childbearing women (*4*). Approximately 7,000 HIV-infected women gave birth annually for the years 1989–1992 (*5*). Given a perinatal transmission rate of 15%–30%, an estimated 1,000–2,000 HIV-infected infants were born annually during these years in the United States. Although urban areas, especially in the northeast, generally have the highest seroprevalence rates, data from this survey have indicated a high prevalence of HIV infection among childbearing women who live in some rural and small urban areas—particularly in the southern states (*6*).

Perinatal Transmission of HIV

HIV can be transmitted from an infected woman to her fetus or newborn during pregnancy, during labor and delivery, and during the postpartum period (through breastfeeding), although the percentage of infections transmitted during each of these intervals is not precisely known (*7–9*). Although transmission of HIV to a fetus can occur as early as the 8th week of gestation (*7*), data suggest that at least one half of perinatally transmitted infections from non-breastfeeding women occur shortly before or during the birth process (*10–12*). Breastfeeding may increase the rate of transmission by 10%–20% (*9, 13, 14*).

Several prospective studies have reported perinatal transmission rates ranging from 13% to 40% (*15–19*). Transmission rates may differ among studies depending on the prevalence of various factors that can influence the likelihood of transmission. Several maternal factors have been associated with an increased risk for transmission, including low CD4+ T-lymphocyte counts, high viral titer, advanced HIV disease, the presence of p24 antigen in serum, placental membrane inflammation, intrapartum events resulting in increased exposure of the fetus to maternal blood, breastfeeding, low vitamin A levels, premature rupture of membranes, and premature delivery (*8, 11, 15, 20–23*). Factors associated with a decreased rate of HIV transmission have included cesarean section delivery, the presence of maternal neutralizing antibodies, and maternal zidovudine therapy (*11, 24–26*).

HIV Prevention and Treatment Opportunities for Women and Infants

HIV counseling and testing for women of childbearing age offer important prevention opportunities for both uninfected and infected women and their infants. Such counseling is intended to a) assist women in assessing their current or future risk for HIV infection; b) initiate or reinforce HIV risk reduction behavior; and c) allow for referral to other HIV prevention services (e.g., treatment for substance abuse and sexually transmitted diseases) when appropriate. For infected women, knowledge of their HIV infection status provides opportunities to a) obtain early diagnosis and treatment for themselves and their infants, b) make informed reproductive decisions, c) use methods to reduce the risk for perinatal transmission, d) receive information to prevent HIV transmission to others, and e) obtain referral for psychological and social services, if needed.

Interventions designed to reduce morbidity in HIV-infected persons require early diagnosis of HIV infection so that treatment can be initiated before the onset of opportunistic infections and disease progression. However, studies indicate that many HIV-infected persons do not know they are infected until late in the course of illness. A survey of persons diagnosed with AIDS between January 1990 and December 1992 indicated that 57% of the 2,081 men and 62% of the 360 women who participated in the survey gave illness as the primary reason for being tested for HIV infection; 36% of survey participants first tested positive within 2 months of their AIDS diagnosis (*27*).

Providing HIV counseling and testing services in gynecologic and prenatal and other obstetric settings presents an opportunity for early diagnosis of HIV infection because many young women frequently access the health-care system for obstetric- or gynecologic-related care. Clinics that provide prenatal and postnatal care, family planning clinics, sexually transmitted disease clinics, adolescent-health clinics, and other health-care facilities already provide a range of preventive services into which HIV education, counseling, and voluntary testing can be integrated. When provided appropriate access to ongoing care, HIV-infected women can be monitored for clinical and immunologic status and can be given preventive treatment and other recommended medical care and services (*28*).

Diagnosis of HIV infection before or during pregnancy allows women to make informed decisions regarding prevention of perinatal transmission. Early in the HIV epidemic, strategies to prevent perinatal HIV transmission were limited to either avoiding pregnancy or avoiding breastfeeding (for women in the United States and other countries that have safe alternatives to breast milk). More recent strategies to prevent perinatal HIV transmission have focused on interrupting in utero and intrapartum transmission. Foremost among these strategies has been administration of ZDV to HIV-infected pregnant women and their newborns (*1*). Results from a multicenter, placebo-controlled clinical trial (the AIDS Clinical Trials Group [ACTG] protocol number 076) indicated that administration of ZDV to a selected group of HIV-infected women during pregnancy, labor, and delivery and to their newborns reduced the risk for perinatal HIV transmission by approximately two thirds: 25.5% of infants born to mothers in the placebo group were infected, compared with 8.3% of those born to mothers in the ZDV group (*1*). The ZDV regimen caused minimal adverse effects among both mothers and infants; the only adverse effect after 18 months of follow-up was mild anemia in the infants that resolved without therapy. As a result of these findings, PHS issued recommendations regarding ZDV therapy to reduce the risk for perinatal HIV transmission (*29*). In addition, the Food and Drug Administration (FDA) has approved the use of ZDV for this therapy.

Despite the substantial benefits and short-term safety of the ZDV regimen, however, the results of the trial present several unresolved issues, including a) the long-term safety of the regimen for both mothers and infants, b) ZDV's effectiveness in women who have different clinical characteristics (e.g., CD4+ T-lymphocyte count and previous ZDV use) than those who participated in the trial, and c) the likelihood of the mother's adherence to the lengthy treatment regimen. The PHS recommendations for ZDV therapy emphasize that HIV-infected pregnant women should be informed of both benefits and potential risks when making decisions to receive such therapy. Discussions of treatment options should be noncoercive—the final decision to accept or reject ZDV treatment is the responsibility of the woman. Decisions concerning treatment can be complex and adherence to therapy, if accepted, can be difficult; therefore, good rapport and a trusting relationship should be established between the health-care provider and the HIV-infected woman.

Several other possible strategies to reduce the risk for perinatal HIV transmission are under study or are being planned (*30*); however, their efficacies have not yet been determined. These strategies include a) administration of HIV hyperimmune globulin to infected pregnant women and their infants, b) efforts to boost maternal and infant immune responses through vaccination, c) virucidal cleansing of the birth canal before and during labor and delivery, d) modified and shortened antiretroviral regimens, e) cesarean section delivery, and f) vitamin A supplementation.

Knowledge of HIV infection status during pregnancy also allows for early identification of HIV-exposed infants, all of whom should be appropriately tested, monitored, and treated (*28*). Prompt identification and close monitoring of such children (particularly infants) is essential for optimal medical management (*28,31,32*). Approximately 10%–20% of perinatally infected children develop rapidly progressive disease and die by 24 months of age (*33,34*). *Pneumocystis carinii* pneumonia (PCP) is the most common opportunistic infection in children who have AIDS and is often fatal. Because PCP occurs most commonly among perinatally infected children 3–6 months of age (*35*), effective prevention requires that children born to HIV-infected mothers be identified promptly, preferably through prenatal testing of their mothers, so that prophylactic therapy can be initiated as soon as possible. CDC and the National Pediatric & Family HIV Resource Center have published revised guidelines for prophylaxis against PCP in children that recommend that all children born to HIV-infected mothers be placed on prophylactic therapy at 4–6 weeks of age (*32*). Careful follow-up of these children to promptly diagnose other potentially treatable HIV-related conditions (e.g., severe bacterial infections or tuberculosis) can prevent morbidity and reduce the need for hospitalization (*28*). Infants born to HIV-infected women also require changes in their routine immunization regimens as early as 2 months of age (*36*).

Despite the potential benefits of HIV counseling and testing to both women and their infants, some persons have expressed concerns about the potential for negative effects resulting from widespread counseling and testing programs in prenatal and other settings. These concerns include the fear that a) such programs could deter pregnant women from using prenatal-care services if testing is not perceived as voluntary and b) women who have been tested but who choose not to learn their test results may be reluctant to return for further prenatal care. Other potential negative consequences following a diagnosis of HIV infection can include loss of confidentiality, job- or health-care–related discrimination and stigmatization, loss of relationships, domestic violence, and adverse psychological reactions. Although cases of discrimination against HIV-infected persons and loss of confidentiality have been documented (*37*), data concerning the frequency of these events for women are limited. Reported rates of abandonment, loss of relationships, severe psychological reactions, and domestic violence have ranged from 4% to 13% (*38–41*). Providing infected women with or referring them to psychological, social, or legal services may help minimize such potential risks and enable women to benefit from the many health advantages of early HIV diagnosis.

Counseling and Testing Strategies

Guidelines published in 1985 (*42*) regarding HIV counseling and testing of pregnant women recommended a targeted approach directed to women known to be at increased risk for HIV infection (e.g., injecting-drug users and women whose sex partners were HIV-infected or at risk for infection). However, several studies have indicated that counseling and testing strategies that offer testing only to those women who report risk factors fail to identify and offer services to many HIV-infected women (i.e.,

50%–70% of infected women in some studies) (*43–45*). Women may be unaware of their risk for infection if they have unknowingly had sexual contact with an HIV-infected person (*46*). Other women may refuse testing to avoid the stigma often associated with high-risk sexual and injecting-drug–use behaviors.

Because of the advances in prevention and treatment of opportunistic infections for HIV-infected adults and children during the past 10 years, several professional organizations (*47,48*) and others (*49*) have recommended a more widespread approach of offering HIV counseling and testing for pregnant women. This approach can be applied nationally to all pregnant women or to women in limited geographic areas based on the prevalence of HIV infection among childbearing women in those areas. However, a counseling and testing recommendation based on a prevalence threshold (e.g., one HIV-infected woman per 1,000 childbearing women) could delay or discourage implementation of counseling and testing services in areas (e.g., states) where prevalence data are inadequate, outdated, or unavailable, and would miss substantial numbers of HIV-infected pregnant women in areas with lower seroprevalence rates but high numbers of births (e.g., California). A prevalence-based approach also could lead to potentially discriminating testing practices, such as singling out a geographic area or racial/ethnic group. A universal approach of offering HIV counseling and testing to all pregnant women—regardless of the prevalence of HIV infection in their community or their risk for infection—provides a uniform policy that will reach HIV-infected pregnant women in all populations and geographic areas of the United States. Although this universal approach will necessitate increased resources (e.g., funding), effective implementation of HIV counseling and testing services for pregnant women and the ensuing medical interventions will reduce HIV-related morbidity in women and their infants and could ultimately reduce medical costs.

Counseling and testing policies also must address issues associated with provision of consent for testing. Data from universal, routine HIV counseling and voluntary testing programs in several areas indicate that high test-acceptance levels can be achieved without mandating testing (*50–52*). Mandatory testing may increase the potential for negative consequences of HIV testing and result in some women avoiding prenatal care altogether. In addition, mandatory testing may adversely affect the patient-provider relationship by placing the provider in an enforcing rather than facilitating role. Providers must act as facilitators to adequately assist women in making decisions regarding HIV testing and ZDV preventive therapy. Although few studies have addressed the issue of acceptance of HIV testing, higher levels of acceptance have been found in clinics where testing is voluntary but recommended by the health-care provider than in clinics that use a nondirective approach to HIV testing (i.e, patients are told the test is available, but testing is neither encouraged nor discouraged) (*52*).

Laboratory Testing Considerations

The HIV-1 testing algorithm recommended by PHS comprises initial screening with an FDA-licensed enzyme immunoassay (EIA) followed by confirmatory testing of repeatedly reactive EIAs with an FDA-licensed supplemental test (e.g., Western blot or immunofluorescence assay [IFA]) (*53*). Although each of these tests is highly sensitive and specific, the use of both EIA and supplementary tests further increases the accuracy of results.

Indeterminate Western blot results can be caused by either incomplete antibody response to HIV in sera from infected persons or non-specific reactions in sera from uninfected persons (*54–56*). Incomplete antibody responses that produce negative or indeterminate results on Western blot may occur in persons recently infected with HIV who are seroconverting, persons who have end-stage HIV disease, and perinatally exposed infants who are seroreverting (i.e., losing maternal antibody). In addition, non-specific reactions producing indeterminate results in uninfected persons have occurred more frequently among pregnant or parous women than among persons in other groups characterized by low HIV seroprevalence (*55,56*). No large-scale studies to estimate the prevalence of indeterminate test results in pregnant women have been conducted. However, a survey testing more than 1 million neonatal dried-blood specimens for maternally acquired HIV-1 antibody indicated a relatively low rate of indeterminate Western blot results (i.e., <1 in every 4,000 specimens tested by EIA); overall, 1,044,944 EIAs and 2,845 Western blots were performed (*56*).

IFA can be used to resolve an EIA-positive, Western blot-indeterminate sample. The FDA-licensed IFA kit is highly sensitive and specific and is less likely than Western blot to yield indeterminate results. Data from one study indicated that 211 of 234 Western blot-indeterminate samples were negative for HIV-1 antibody by IFA (*57*).

False-positive Western blot results (especially those with a majority of bands) are extremely uncommon. For example, in a study of >290,000 blood donors that used a sensitive culture technique, no false-positive Western blot results were detected (*58*). In a study of the frequency of false-positive diagnoses among military applicants from a low prevalence population (i.e., <1.5 infections per 1,000 population), one false-positive result among 135,187 persons tested was detected (*59*).

Incorrect HIV test results occur primarily because of specimen-handling errors, laboratory errors, or failure to follow the recommended testing algorithm. However, patients may report incorrect test results because they misunderstood previous test results or misperceive that they are infected (*60*). Although these occurrences are uncommon, increased testing of pregnant women will result in additional indeterminate, false-positive, and incorrect results. Because of a) the significance of an HIV-positive test result for the mother and its impact on her reproductive decisions and b) the potential toxicity of HIV therapeutic drugs for both the pregnant woman and her infant, HIV test results must be obtained and interpreted correctly. In some circumstances, correct interpretation may require consideration of not only additional or repeat testing, but also the woman's clinical condition and history of possible exposure to HIV.

In addition to the standard antibody assays used for older children and adults, definitive diagnosis of HIV infection in infants requires the use of other assays (e.g., polymerase chain reaction [PCR] or virus culture). Virtually all infants born to HIV-infected mothers acquire maternal antibody and will test antibody positive for up to 18 months of age (*61*). Uninfected infants will gradually lose maternally derived antibody during this time, whereas infected infants generally remain antibody positive. Diagnosis of HIV infection in early infancy can be made on the basis of two or more positive assays (e.g., viral culture, PCR, or p24 antigen test) (*62*).

RECOMMENDATIONS

The following recommendations have been developed to provide guidance to health-care workers when educating women about HIV infection and the importance of early diagnosis of HIV. The recommendations are based on the advances made in treatment and prevention of HIV infection and stress the need for a universal counseling and voluntary testing program for pregnant women. These recommendations address a) HIV-related information needed by infected and uninfected pregnant women for their own health and that of their infants, b) laboratory considerations involved in HIV testing of this population, and c) the importance of follow-up services for HIV- infected women, their infants, and other family members.

HIV Counseling and Voluntary Testing of Pregnant Women and Their Infants

- Health-care providers should ensure that all pregnant women are counseled and encouraged to be tested for HIV infection to allow women to know their infection status both for their own health and to reduce the risk for perinatal HIV transmission. Pretest HIV counseling of pregnant women should be done in accordance with previous guidelines for HIV counseling (*63,64*). Such counseling should include information regarding the risk for HIV infection associated with sexual activity and injecting-drug use, the risk for transmission to the woman's infant if she is infected, and the availability of therapy to reduce this risk. HIV counseling, including any written materials, should be linguistically, culturally, educationally, and age appropriate for individual patients.

- HIV testing of pregnant women and their infants should be voluntary. Consent for testing should be obtained in accordance with prevailing legal requirements. Women who test positive for HIV or who refuse testing should not be a) denied prenatal or other health-care services, b) reported to child protective service agencies because of refusal to be tested or because of their HIV status, or c) discriminated against in any other way (*65*).

- Health-care providers should counsel and offer HIV testing to women as early in pregnancy as possible so that informed and timely therapeutic and reproductive decisions can be made. Specific strategies and resources will be needed to communicate with women who may not obtain prenatal care because of homelessness, incarceration, undocumented citizenship status, drug or alcohol abuse, or other reasons.

- Uninfected pregnant women who continue to practice high-risk behaviors (e.g., injecting-drug use and unprotected sexual contact with an HIV-infected or high-risk partner) should be encouraged to avoid further exposure to HIV and to be retested for HIV in the third trimester of pregnancy (*64*).

- The prevalence of HIV infection may be higher in women who have not received prenatal care (*66*). These women should be assessed promptly for HIV infection. Such an assessment should include information regarding prior HIV testing, test results, and risk history. For women who are first identified as being HIV infected during labor and delivery, health-care providers should consider offering intrapartum and neonatal ZDV according to published recommendations (*29*). For women whose HIV infection status has not been determined, HIV counseling should be provided and HIV testing offered as soon as the mother's medical condition permits. However, involuntary HIV testing should never be substituted for counseling and voluntary testing.

- Some HIV-infected women do not receive prenatal care, choose not to be tested for HIV, or do not retain custody of their children. If a woman has not been tested for HIV, she should be informed of the benefits to her child's health of knowing her child's infection status and should be encouraged to allow the child to be tested. Counselors should ensure that the mother provides consent with the understanding that a positive HIV test for her child is indicative of infection in herself. For infants whose HIV infection status is unknown and who are in foster care, the person legally authorized to provide consent should be encouraged to allow the infant to be tested (with the consent of the biologic mother, when possible) in accordance with the policies of the organization legally responsible for the child and with prevailing legal requirements for HIV testing.

- Pregnant women should be provided access to other HIV prevention and treatment services (e.g., drug-treatment and partner-notification services) as needed.

Interpretation of HIV Test Results

- HIV antibody testing should be performed according to the recommended algorithm, which includes the use of an EIA to test for antibody to HIV and confirmatory testing with an additional, more specific assay (e.g., Western blot or IFA) (53). All assays should be performed and conducted according to manufacturers' instructions and applicable state and federal laboratory guidelines.

- HIV infection (as indicated by the presence of antibody to HIV) is defined as a repeatedly reactive EIA and a positive confirmatory supplemental test. Confirmation or exclusion of HIV infection in a person with indeterminate test results should be made not only on the basis of HIV antibody test results, but with consideration of a) the person's medical and behavioral history, b) results from additional virologic and immunologic tests when performed, and c) clinical follow-up. Uncertainties regarding HIV infection status, including laboratory test results, should be resolved before final decisions are made concerning pregnancy termination, ZDV therapy, or other interventions.

- Pregnant women who have repeatedly reactive EIA and indeterminate supplemental tests should be retested immediately for HIV antibody to distinguish between recent seroconversion and a negative test result. Additional tests (e.g., viral culture, PCR, or p24 antigen test) to diagnose or exclude HIV infection may be required for women whose test results remain indeterminate—especially women who have behavioral risk factors for HIV, have had recent exposure to HIV, or have clinical symptoms compatible with acute retroviral illness. In such situations, confirmation by an FDA-licensed IFA kit may be helpful because IFA is less likely to yield indeterminate results than Western blot.

- Women who have negative EIAs and those who have repeatedly reactive EIAs but negative supplemental tests should be considered uninfected.

Recommendations for HIV-Infected Pregnant Women

- HIV-infected pregnant women should receive counseling as previously recommended (*64*). Posttest HIV counseling should include an explanation of the clinical implications of a positive HIV antibody test result and the need for, benefit of, and means of access to HIV-related medical and other early intervention services. Such counseling should also include a discussion of the interaction between pregnancy and HIV infection (*67*), the risk for perinatal HIV transmission and ways to reduce this risk (*29*), and the prognosis for infants who become infected.

- HIV-infected pregnant women should be evaluated according to published recommendations to assess their need for antiretroviral therapy, antimicrobial prophylaxis, and treatment of other conditions (*28,68,69*). Although medical management of HIV infection is essentially the same for pregnant and nonpregnant women, recommendations for treating a patient who has tuberculosis have been modified for pregnant women because of potential teratogenic effects of specific medications (e.g., streptomycin and pyrazinamide) (*70*). HIV-infected pregnant women should be evaluated to determine their need for psychological and social services.

- HIV-infected pregnant women should be provided information concerning ZDV therapy to reduce the risk for perinatal HIV transmission. This information should address the potential benefit and short-term safety of ZDV and the uncertainties regarding a) long-term risks of such therapy and b) effectiveness in women who have different clinical characteristics (e.g., CD4+ T-lymphocyte count and previous ZDV use) than women who participated in the trial. HIV-infected pregnant women should not be coerced into making decisions about ZDV therapy. These decisions should be made after consideration of both the benefits and potential risks of the regimen to the woman and her child. Therapy should be offered according to the appropriate regimen in published recommendations (*29*). A woman's decision not to accept treatment should not result in punitive action or denial of care.

- HIV-infected pregnant women should receive information about all reproductive options. Reproductive counseling should be nondirective. Health-care providers should be aware of the complex issues that HIV-infected women must consider when making decisions about their reproductive options and should be supportive of any decision.

- To reduce the risk for HIV transmission to their infants, HIV-infected women should be advised against breastfeeding. Support services should be provided when necessary for use of appropriate breast-milk substitutes.

- To optimize medical management, positive and negative HIV test results should be available to a woman's health-care provider and included on both her and her infant's confidential medical records. After obtaining consent, maternal health-care providers should notify the pediatric-care providers of the impending birth of an HIV-exposed child, any anticipated complications, and whether ZDV should be administered after birth. If HIV is first diagnosed in the child, the child's health-care providers should discuss the implication of the child's diagnosis for the woman's health and assist the mother in obtaining care for herself. Providers are encouraged to build supportive health-care relationships that can facilitate the discussion of pertinent health information. Confidential HIV-related information should be disclosed or shared only in accordance with prevailing legal requirements.

- Counseling for HIV-infected pregnant women should include an assessment of the potential for negative effects resulting from HIV infection (e.g., discrimination, domestic violence, and psychological difficulties). For women who anticipate or experience such effects, counseling also should include a) information on how to minimize these potential consequences, b) assistance in identifying supportive persons within their own social network, and c) referral to appropriate psychological, social, and legal services. In addition, HIV-infected women should be informed that discrimination based on HIV status or AIDS regarding matters such as housing, employment, state programs, and public accommodations (including physicians' offices and hospitals) is illegal (*65*).

- HIV-infected women should be encouraged to obtain HIV testing for any of their children born after they became infected or, if they do not know when they became infected, for children born after 1977. Older children (i.e., children >12 years of age) should be tested with informed consent of the parent and assent of the child. Women should be informed that the lack of signs and symptoms suggestive of HIV infection in older children may not indicate lack of HIV infection; some perinatally infected children can remain asymptomatic for several years.

Recommendations for Follow-Up of Infected Women and Perinatally Exposed Children

- Following pregnancy, HIV-infected women should be provided ongoing HIV-related medical care, including immune-function monitoring, antiretroviral therapy, and prophylaxis for and treatment of opportunistic infections and other HIV-related conditions (*28,68,69*). HIV-infected women should receive gynecologic care, including regular Pap smears, reproductive counseling, information on how to prevent sexual transmission of HIV, and treatment of gynecologic conditions according to published recommendations (*28,47,71,72*).

- HIV-infected women (or the guardians of their children) should be informed of the importance of follow-up for their children. These children should receive follow-up care to determine their infection status, to initiate prophylactic therapy to prevent PCP, and, if infected, to determine the need for antiretroviral and other prophylactic therapy and to monitor disorders in growth and development, which often occur before 24 months of age (*28,31,32,73*). HIV-infected children and other children living in households with HIV-infected persons should be vaccinated according to published recommendations for altered schedules (*36*).

- Because the identification of an HIV-infected mother also identifies a family that needs or will need medical and social services as her disease progresses, health-care providers should ensure that referrals to these services focus on the needs of the entire family.

References
1. Connor EM, Sperling RS, Gelber R, et al. Reduction of maternal-infant transmission of human immunodeficiency virus type 1 with zidovudine treatment. N Engl J Med 1994;331:1173–80.
2. National Center for Health Statistics. Annual summary of births, marriages, divorces, and deaths: United States, 1993. Hyattsville, MD: US Department of Health and Human Services, Public Health Service, CDC, 1994. (Monthly vital statistics report, vol. 42, no. 13).
3. National Center for Health Statistics. Advanced report of final mortality statistics, 1992. Hyattsville, MD: US Department of Health and Human Services, Public Health Service, CDC, 1994. (Monthly vital statistics report; vol. 43, no. 6S).
4. CDC. National HIV seroprevalence summary: results through 1992. Atlanta, GA: US Department of Health and Human Services, Public Health Service, CDC, 1994.
5. Davis S, Gwinn M, Wasser S, Fleming P, Karon J. HIV prevalence among U.S. childbearing women, 1989-1992 [Abstract]. First National Conference on Human Retroviruses and Related Infections, Washington, DC, 1993.
6. Wasser SC, Gwinn M, Fleming P. Urban-nonurban distribution of HIV infection in childbearing women in the United States. J Acquir Immune Defic Syndr 1993;6:1035–42.
7. Lewis SH, Reynolds-Kohler C, Fox HE, Nelson JA. HIV-1 in trophoblastic and villous Hofbauer cells, and haematological precursors in eight-week fetuses. Lancet 1990;335:565–8.
8. Mofenson LM, Wolinsky SM. Current insights regarding vertical transmission. In: Pizzo PA, Wilfert CM, eds. Pediatric AIDS: the challenge of HIV infection in infants, children, and adolescents. 2nd ed. Baltimore, MD: Williams & Wilkins, 1994:179–203.
9. Dunn DT, Newell ML, Ades AE, Peckham CS. Risk of human immunodeficiency virus type 1 transmission through breastfeeding. Lancet 1992;340:585–8.
10. Rogers MF, Ou C-Y, Rayfield M, et al. Use of the polymerase chain reaction for early detection of the proviral sequences of human immunodeficiency virus in infants born to seropositive mothers. N Engl J Med 1989;320:1649–54.
11. Boyer PJ, Dillon M, Navaie M, et al. Factors predictive of maternal-fetal transmission of HIV-1: preliminary analysis of zidovudine given during pregnancy and/or delivery. JAMA 1994; 271:1925–30.
12. Rouzioux C, Costagliola D, Burgard M, et al. Timing of mother-to-child HIV-1 transmission depends on maternal status. AIDS 1993;7(suppl 2):S49–S52.
13. St. Louis ME, Kalish M, Kamenga M, et al. The timing of perinatal HIV-1 transmission in an African setting [Abstract]. First National Conference on Human Retroviruses and Related Infections, Washington, DC, 1993.
14. Ekpini E, Wiktor SZ, Sibailly T, et al. Late postnatal mother-to-child HIV transmission in Abidjan, Côte d'Ivoire [Abstract]. Xth International Conference on AIDS, Yokohama, Japan, August 1994.
15. Ryder RW, Nsa W, Hassig SE, et al. Perinatal transmission of the human immunodeficiency virus type I to infants of seropositive women in Zaire. N Engl J Med 1989;320:1637–42.
16. Blanche S, Rouzioux C, Moscato MG, et al. A prospective study of infants born to women seropositive for human immunodeficiency virus type 1. N Engl J Med 1989;320:1643-8.
17. European Collaborative Study. Risk factors for mother-to-child transmission of HIV-1. Lancet 1992;339:1007–12.
18. Gabiano C, Tovo P-A, de Martino M, et al. Mother-to-child transmission of human immunodeficiency virus type 1: risk of infection and correlates of transmission. Pediatrics 1992;90:369–74.
19. Dabis F, Msellati P, Dunn D, et al. Estimating the rate of mother-to-child transmission of HIV: report of a workshop on methodological issues—Ghent, Belgium, February 17–20, 1992. AIDS 1993;7:1139–48.
20. St. Louis ME, Kamenga M, Brown C, et al. Risk for perinatal HIV-1 transmission according to maternal immunologic, virologic, and placental factors. JAMA 1993;269:2853–9.
21. Burns DN, Landesman S, Muenz LR, et al. Cigarette smoking, premature rupture of membranes, and vertical transmission of HIV-1 among women with low CD4+ levels. J Acquir Immune Defic Syndr 1994;7:718–26.
22. Weisner B, Nachman S, Tropper P, et al. Quantitation of human immunodeficiency virus type 1 during pregnancy: relationship of viral titer to mother-to-child transmission and stability of viral load. Proc Natl Acad Sci USA 1994;91:8037–41.
23. Semba RD, Miotti PG, Chiphangwi JD, et al. Maternal vitamin A deficiency and mother-to-child transmission of HIV-1. Lancet 1994;343:1593–7.

24. Dunn DT, Newell ML, Mayaux MJ, et al. Mode of delivery and vertical transmission of HIV-1: a review of prospective studies. J Acquir Immune Defic Syndr 1994;7:1064–6.
25. Scarlatti G, Albert J, Rossi P, et al. Mother-to-child transmission of human immunodeficiency virus type 1: correlation with neutralizing antibodies against primary isolates. J Infect Dis 1993;168:207–10.
26. Thomas PA, Weedon J, Krasinski K, et al. Maternal predictors of perinatal HIV transmission. Pediatr Infect Dis J 1994;13:489–95.
27. Wortley PM, Chu SY, Diaz T, et al. HIV testing patterns: where, why and when were persons with AIDS tested for HIV? AIDS 1995;9:487–92.
28. El-Sadr W, Oleske JM, Agins BD, et al. Evaluation and management of early HIV infection. Rockville, MD: US Department of Health and Human Services, Public Health Service, Agency for Health Care Policy and Research, January 1994. DHHS publication no. (AHCPR)94-0572. (Clinical Practice Guideline no. 7).
29. CDC. Recommendations of the U.S. Public Health Service Task Force on the Use of Zidovudine to Reduce Perinatal Transmission of Human Immunodeficiency Virus. MMWR 1994;43(No. RR-11).
30. Peckham CS, Newell M-L, eds. Measures to decrease the risk of mother-to-child transmission of HIV infection: highlights of a seminar meeting, January 11–13, 1993, London, UK. London: Colwood House Medical Publications, 1993.
31. Working Group on Antiretroviral Therapy: National Pediatric HIV Resource Center. Antiretroviral therapy and medical management of the human immunodeficiency virus-infected child. Pediatr Infect Dis J 1993;12:513–22.
32. CDC. 1995 Revised guidelines for prophylaxis against *Pneumocystis carinii* pneumonia for children infected with or perinatally exposed to human immunodeficiency virus. MMWR 1995;44(No. RR-4).
33. Blanche S, Mayaux M-J, Rouzioux C, et al. Relation of the course of HIV infection in children to the severity of the disease in their mothers at delivery. N Engl J Med 1994;330:308–12.
34. Byers B, Caldwell B, Oxtoby M, Pediatric Spectrum of Disease Project. Survival of children with perinatal HIV infection: evidence for two distinct populations [Abstract]. IXth International Conference on AIDS, Berlin, June 1993.
35. Simonds RJ, Oxtoby MJ, Caldwell MB, Gwinn ML, Rogers MF. *Pneumocystis carinii* pneumonia among U.S. children with perinatally acquired HIV infection. JAMA 1993;270:470–3.
36. ACIP. Recommendations of the Advisory Committee on Immunization Practices (ACIP): use of vaccines and immune globulins in persons with altered immunocompetence. MMWR 1993;42(No. RR-4).
37. New York City Commission on Human Rights (The AIDS Discrimination Division). Report on discrimination against people with AIDS and people perceived to have AIDS, January 1986–June 1987.
38. Moore J, Solomon L, Schoenbaum E, et al. Factors associated with stress and distress among HIV-infected and uninfected women [Abstract]. HIV Infection in Women Conference, Washington DC, February 1995.
39. Gielen A, O'Campo P, Faden R, Eke A. Women with HIV: disclosure, concerns, and experiences [Abstract]. HIV Infection in Women Conference, Washington DC, February 1995.
40. Perry SW, Jacobsberg LB, Fishman B, et al. Psychological responses to serological testing for HIV. AIDS 1990;4:145–52.
41. Brown GR, Rundell JR. A prospective study of psychiatric aspects of early HIV disease in women. Gen Hosp Psychiatry 1993;15:139–47.
42. CDC. Recommendations for assisting in the prevention of the perinatal transmission of human T-lymphotropic virus type III/lymphadenopathy-associated virus and acquired immunodeficiency syndrome. MMWR 1985;34:721–6, 731–2.
43. Barbacci MB, Dalabetta GA, Repke JT, et al. Human immunodeficiency virus infection in women attending an inner-city prenatal clinic: ineffectiveness of targeted screening. Sex Transm Dis 1990;Jul–Sept:122–6.
44. Fehrs LJ, Hill D, Kerndt PR, Rose TP, Henneman C. Targeted HIV screening at a Los Angeles prenatal/family planning health center. Am J Public Health 1991;81:619–22.

45. Lindsay MK, Adefris W, Peterson HB, et al. Determinants of acceptance of routine voluntary human immunodeficiency virus testing in an inner-city prenatal population. Obstet Gynecol 1989;78:678–80.
46. Ellerbrock TV, Lieb S, Harrington PE, et al. Heterosexually transmitted human immunodeficiency virus infection among pregnant women in a rural Florida community. N Engl J Med 1992;327:1704–9.
47. ACOG Technical Bulletin. Human Immunodeficiency Virus Infections. June 1992;169.
48. Task Force on Pediatric AIDS. Perinatal human immunodeficiency virus (HIV) testing. Pediatrics 1992;89:791–4.
49. Hardy LM, ed. HIV screening of pregnant women and newborns. Washington, DC: National Academy Press, 1991.
50. Barbacci M, Repke JT, Chaisson RE. Routine prenatal screening for HIV infection. Lancet 1991; 337:709–11.
51. Lindsay MK, Peterson HB, Feng TI, Slade BA, Willis S, Klein L. Routine antepartum human immunodeficiency virus infection screening in an inner-city population. Obstet Gynecol 1989; 74:289–94.
52. Cozen W, Mascola L, Enguidanos R, et al. Screening for HIV and hepatitis B virus in Los Angeles County prenatal clinics: a demonstration project. J Acquir Immune Defic Syndr 1993;6:95–8.
53. CDC. Public Health Service guidelines for counseling and antibody testing to prevent HIV infection and AIDS. MMWR 1987;36:509–15.
54. Celum CL, Coombs RW, Lafferty W, et al. Indeterminate human immunodeficiency virus type 1 Western blots: seroconversion risk, specificity of supplemental tests, and an algorithm for evaluation. J Infect Dis 1991;164:656–64.
55. Celum CL, Coombs RW, Jones JM, et al. Risk factors for repeatedly reactive HIV-1 EIA and indeterminate Western blots: a population-based case-control study. Arch Intern Med 1994; 154:1129–37.
56. Gwinn M, Redus MA, Granade TC. HIV-1 serologic test results for one million newborn dried-blood specimens: assay performance and implications for screening. J Acquir Immune Defic Syndr 1992;5:505–12.
57. Mucke H, Schinkinger M, Haushofer A, Fischer M, et al. Evaluation of a novel anti-HIV immunoflourescence assay in comparison with ELISA and Western blot. AIDS-Forschung 1990; 191–9.
58. MacDonald KL, Jackson JB, Bowman RJ, et al. Performance characteristics of serologic tests for human immunodeficiency virus type 1 (HIV-1) antibody among Minnesota blood donors: public health and clinical implications. Ann Intern Med 1989;110:617–21.
59. Burke DS, Brundage JF, Redfield RR, et al. Measurement of the false positive rate in a screening program for human immunodeficiency virus infections. N Engl J Med 1988;319:961–4.
60. Sheon AR, Fox HE, Alexander G, et al. Misdiagnosed HIV infection in pregnant women: implications for clinical care. Public Health Rep 1994;109:694–9.
61. Rogers MF, Schochetman G, Hoff R. Advances in diagnosis of HIV infection in infants. In: Pizzo PA, Wilfert CM, eds. Pediatric AIDS: the challenge of HIV infection in infants, children, and adolescents. 2nd ed. Baltimore, MD: Williams & Wilkins, 1994:219–38.
62. CDC. 1994 Revised classification system for human immunodeficiency virus infection in children less than 13 years of age; Official authorized addenda—human immunodeficiency virus infection codes and official guidelines for coding and reporting ICD-9-CM. MMWR 1994;43(No. RR-12).
63. CDC. Recommendations for HIV testing services for inpatients and outpatients in acute-care hospital settings; and Technical guidance on HIV counseling. MMWR 1993;42(No. RR-2).
64. CDC. HIV counseling, testing, and referral: standards & guidelines. Atlanta, GA: US Department of Health & Human Services, Public Health Service, CDC, 1994.
65. Americans With Disabilities Act, 29 U.S.C. § 706 and 42 U.S.C. 12101 et seq.
66. Lindsay MK, Feng TI, Peterson HB, Slade BA, Willis S, Klein L. Routine human immunodeficiency virus infection screening in unregistered and registered inner-city parturients. Obstet Gynecol 1991;77:599–603.
67. Minkoff HL, Duerr A. Obstetric issues—relevance to women and children. In: Pizzo PA, Wilfert CM, eds. Pediatric AIDS: the challenge of HIV infection in infants, children, and adolescents. 2nd ed. Baltimore, MD: Williams & Wilkins, 1994:773–84.

68. Sande MA, Carpenter CCJ, Cobbs CG, et al. Antiretroviral therapy for adult HIV-infected patients: recommendations from a state-of-the-art conference. JAMA 1993;270:2583–9.
69. CDC. Recommendations for prophylaxis against *Pneumocystis carinii* pneumonia for adults and adolescents infected with human immunodeficiency virus. MMWR 1992;41(No. RR-4).
70. CDC. Initial therapy for tuberculosis in the era of multidrug resistance: recommendations of the Advisory Council for the Elimination of Tuberculosis. MMWR 1993;42(No. RR-7).
71. CDC. 1993 Sexually transmitted diseases treatment guidelines. MMWR 1993;42(No. RR-14).
72. CDC. Update: barrier protection against HIV infection and other sexually transmitted diseases. MMWR 1993;42:589–91,597.
73. Report of a Consensus Workshop, Siena, Italy, January 17–18, 1992. Early Diagnosis of HIV Infection in Infants. J Acquir Immune Defic Syndr 1992;5:1169–78.

MMWR

The *Morbidity and Mortality Weekly Report (MMWR)* Series is prepared by the Centers for Disease Control and Prevention (CDC) and is available free of charge in electronic format and on a paid subscription basis for paper copy. To receive an electronic copy on Friday of each week, send an e-mail message to *lists@list.cdc.gov.* The body content should read *subscribe mmwr-toc.* Electronic copy also is available from CDC's World-Wide Web server at *http://www.cdc.gov/* or from CDC's file transfer protocol server at *ftp.cdc.gov.* To subscribe for paper copy, contact Superintendent of Documents, U.S. Government Printing Office, Washington, DC 20402; telephone (202) 783-3238.

Data in the weekly *MMWR* are provisional, based on weekly reports to CDC by state health departments. The reporting week concludes at close of business on Friday; compiled data on a national basis are officially released to the public on the following Friday. Address inquiries about the *MMWR* Series, including material to be considered for publication, to: Editor, *MMWR* Series, Mailstop C-08, CDC, 1600 Clifton Rd., N.E., Atlanta, GA 30333; telephone (404) 332-4555.

All material in the *MMWR* Series is in the public domain and may be used and reprinted without permission; citation as to source, however, is appreciated.

☆U.S. Government Printing Office: 1995-633-175/05081 Region IV

APPENDIX
O

Acronyms and Glossary

ACRONYMS

AAFP	American Academy of Family Physicians
AAP	American Academy of Pediatrics
ACNM	American College of Nurse Midwives
ACOG	American College of Obstetricians and Gynecologists
ACTG 076	AIDS Clinical Trials Group protocol number 076
ADA	American with Disabilities Act
ADAP	AIDS Drug Assistance Program
AETC	AIDS Education and Training Center
AFDC	Aid to Families with Dependent Children
AFP	alpha-fetoprotein
AHEC	AIDS Health Education Center
AIDS	acquired immune deficiency syndrome
AMA	American Medical Association
AMCHP	Association of Maternal and Child Health Programs
APIDS	AIDS Public Information Data Set
APPCYF	AIDS Policy Center for Children, Youth and Families
AWHONN	Association of Women's Health, Obstetric and Neonatal Nurses
BPHC	Bureau of Primary Care
BRFSS	Behavioral Risk Factor Surveillance System
CARE	(Ryan White) Comprehensive AIDS Resources Emergency (Act)

CDC	Centers for Disease Control and Prevention
CHIP	Child Health Insurance Program
CIP	consumer information program
CPCRA	Terry Beirn Community Programs for Clinical Research on AIDS
DHHS	Department of Health and Human Services
DSH	disproportionate share hospital
ELISA	enzyme-linked immunosorbent assay
FDA	Food and Drug Administration
HCFA	Health Care Financing Administration
HEDIS	Health Plan Employer Data and Information Set
HIPAA	Health Insurance Portability and Accountability Act
HIV	human immunodeficiency virus
HRSA	Health Resources and Services Administration
IOM	Institute of Medicine
IDU	injection drug users
JCAHO	Joint Commission on Accreditation of Health Care Organizations
MCHB	Maternal and Child Health Bureau
MCO	managed care organization
MSA	metropolitan statistical area
MSAFP	maternal serum alpha-fetoprotein
NAS	National Academy of Sciences
NCQA	National Committee for Quality Assurance
NIH	National Institutes of Health
NMA	National Medical Association
NRC	National Research Council
NTD	neural tube defect
OPA	Office of Population Affairs
PACTG	Pediatric AIDS Clinical Trials Group
PCP	*Pneumocystis carinii* pneumonia
PCR	polymerase chain reaction
PGEP	Perinatal Guidelines Evaluation Project

PHS	Public Health Service
PKU	phenylketonuria
PRAMS	Pregnancy Risk Assessment Monitoring System
PRWORA	Personnel Responsibility and Work Opportunity Reconciliation Act of 1996
PSD	Pediatric Spectrum of Disease
SAMHSA	Substance Abuse and Mental Health Services Administration
SCBW	Survey of Childbearing Women
SCD	sickle cell disease
SPNS	Special Projects of National Significance
SSDI	Social Security Disability Insurance
SSI	Supplemental Security Income
SSIDCP	SSI Disabled Children's Program
STD	sexually transmitted disease
STEP	Surveillance to Evaluate Prevention
TANF	Temporary Assistance for Needy Families
WIC	Special Supplemental Nutrition Program for Women, Infants, and Children
WIN	Women's Initiative for HIV Care and Reduction of Perinatal Transmission
WORLD	Women Organized to Respond to Life-threatening Diseases
ZDV	zidovudine, previously known as AZT

GLOSSARY

acquired immune deficiency syndrome (AIDS): an acquired, as opposed to inherited (congenital), disease characterized by the progressive deterioration of host immune defenses that renders the affected individual susceptible to an array of infectious and malignant disorders that do not normally afflict persons with intact immune systems. AIDS results from infection with human immunodeficiency virus, and is formally defined by a case definition issued by the Centers for Disease Control and Prevention (CDC).

AIDS exceptionalism: phenomenon where HIV/AIDS is treated differently from other diseases, especially with regard to clinical testing and public health screening programs.

alpha-fetoprotein (AFP): normal fetal protein that is usually present in maternal serum, used to diagnose neural tube defects and other conditions during pregnancy.

case finding: identifying a previously unknown or unrecognized condition in apparently healthy or asymptomatic persons and offering presymptomatic treatment to those so identified.

completely mandatory: situation in which a government agency requires citizens to undergo a screening test, and sanctions those who do not comply.

conditionally mandatory: situation in which either government or a private institution makes access to a designated service or opportunity contingent on participation in a screening program.

counseling: communication process by which individuals and their family members are given information about the nature, risks, burden and benefits of testing, and the meaning of test results.

HIV: the retrovirus, human immunodeficiency virus, that is responsible for most cases of AIDS worldwide.

Neural tube defect (NTD): major birth defect affecting the brain and spinal column.

Non-directive patient choice: situation in which individuals are provided information about a test and the choice is explicitly left to them.

phenylketonuria (PKU): hereditary metabolic disorder, in which a deficiency of an enzyme leads to the accumulation of the amino acid phenylalanine, resulting in severe mental retardation if not appropriately treated.

routine with notification: situation in which individuals are informed that a certain test is a standard part of prenatal care, and of their right to refuse before the testing is done.

routine without notification: situation in which individuals are routinely and automatically tested unless they expressly ask that a test not be done.

screening: application of a test to all individuals in a defined population.

sickle cell disease (SCD): an autosomal recessive hemolytic anemia occurring most frequently in African Americans, but also in persons of Mediterranean origin and others.

surveillance: monitoring the incidence or prevalence of a disease in a defined population over time, or comparing the incidence or prevalence among different populations.

testing: application of a test or measurement to selected individuals for the purpose of identifying a disease or medical condition.

zidovudine (ZDV) (also knows as AZT): antiretroviral drug found to significantly reduce perinatal transmission of HIV.

Index

A

Abortion, 17, 26, 45, 102-103, 269, 278, 324
Accountability
    clinical policy performance measures, 18,
        117-118, 125, 133, 196
    health care plans/providers, general, 8, 62-
        63, 65, 89, 187
    state programs, federally funding criteria, 1,
        4-5, 10, 16-17, 57, 59, 61, 122-123,
        125-126, 173, 175, 177, 181, 343-
        346
    see also Cost and cost-benefit factors
ACTG (AIDS Clinical Trials Group)
    ACTG 076 (AIDS Clinical Trials Group
        protocol number 076) 34, 39, 48,
        120, 127, 359
    awareness of, 75, 114
    compliance with, 96, 107, 121-122, 208,
        209, 243, 264
    general, 49, 62
    impact of, general, *vii*, 1, 4, 5, 14, 15-16,
        68, 106, 128, 213, 331
    Medicaid managed care, 66
    rapid testing, 13, 52
    steps involved in implementation, 206
    unintended pregnancies, 12
    see also *"counseling guidelines" and
        "testing guidelines" under Public
        Health Service*

Adolescents, 103, 176, 180, 212, 242, 243-244
    attitudes, 243-244
    community-level services, 56, 62, 131-132,
        156, 161, 243-244
    injection drug users, 131, 244
    Medicaid, 131, 244
    rapid tests, 13, 130
    testing of, 13, 117, 130, 131-132, 243-244
    see also School-based programs
Advocacy, *vii*, 34, 314, 336
AFP, *see* Alpha-fetoprotein
African Americans
    patient vignettes, 246-247
    prenatal care trends, 74
    prevalence, 3, 38, 40-41, 204, 228, 357
    sickle cell disease, 19, 25, 27-28
    testing of newborns, 333
    testing of women, 34-35, 74, 87, 89, 93, 95,
        207, 226, 288, 290, 293, 296, 298,
        300, 302
Age factors
    AIDS development in infants/children, 37,
        205
    epidemiology, 39, 41, 53, 321
    incarcerated women, 129
    polymerase chain reaction tests, 52
    service provision, 214
    testing of women, 87, 207, 289, 290, 293,
        297, 299, 300
    ZDV use, 238